Overview Volume 1 and 2

Sobotta

Atlas of Human Anatomy

Volume 2
Trunk, Viscera, Lower Limb

Sobotta

Atlas of Human Anatomy

Edited by R. Putz and R. Pabst

In collaboration with Renate Putz

Translation by S. Bedoui

Volume 2
Trunk, Viscera, Lower Limb

14th edition, newly edited
704 colour plates with 914 figures

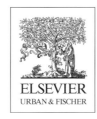

ELSEVIER
URBAN & FISCHER

URBAN & FISCHER
München · Jena

Correspondence and feedback should be addressed to:

Elsevier GmbH, Urban & Fischer Verlag, Department for Medical Student Information, Alexander Gattnarzik, Karlstraße 45, 80333 Munich, Germany
e-mail: medizinstudium@elsevier.de

Addresses of the editors:

Professor Dr. med. Reinhard Putz
Vorstand des Anatomischen Instituts
der Ludwig-Maximilians-Universität
Pettenkoferstraße 11
80336 München
Germany
e-mail: reinhard.putz@med.uni-muenchen.de

Professor Dr. med. Reinhard Pabst
Leiter der Abteilung
Funktionelle und Angewandte Anatomie
Medizinische Hochschule Hannover
Carl-Neuberg-Straße 1
30625 Hannover
Germany
e-mail: pabst.reinhard@mh-hannover.de

Bibliographic information published by Die Deutsche Bibliothek

Die Deutsche Bibliothek lists this publication in the Deutsche National-bibliografie; detailed bibliographic data is available in the Internet at http://dnb.ddb.de.

The 14th edition of the Sobotta Atlas consists of two volumes and a booklet containing tables (enclosed in Volume 1):

Volume 1: Head, Neck, Upper Limb

Volume 2: Trunk, Viscera, Lower Limb

Translation: Dr. med. Sammy Bedoui, Hannover
Editorial staff at Elsevier: Dr. med. Dorothea Hennessen
                     Alexander Gattnarzik
                     Dr. rer. nat. Andrea Richarz
Illustrators: Ulrike Brugger, Munich; Rüdiger Himmelhan, Heidelberg; Horst Ruß, Munich; Henriette Rintelen, Velbern
Book production: Renate Hausdorf, Munich
Composed by: Typodata, Munich
Printed and bound by: Appl, Wemding
Cover design: Carsten Tschirner, Munich
Printed on Nopacoat 115 g

Printed in Germany
ISBN-13: 978-0-443-10349-0
ISBN-10: 0-443-10349-6

This atlas was founded by Johannes Sobotta†, former Professor of Anatomy and Director of the Anatomical Institute of the University of Bonn, Germany.

German Editions:
1st Edition: 1904–1907 J. F. Lehmanns Verlag, Munich
2nd–11th Edition: 1913–1944 J. F. Lehmanns Verlag, Munich
12th–20th Edition: 1948–1993 Urban & Schwarzenberg, Munich
13th Edition: 1953, editor H. Becher
14th Edition: 1956, editor H. Becher
15th Edition: 1957, editor H. Becher
16th Edition: 1967, editor H. Becher
17th Edition: 1972, editors H. Ferner and J. Staubesand
18th Edition: 1982, editors H. Ferner and J. Staubesand
19th Edition: 1988, editor J. Staubesand
20th Edition: 1993, editors R. Putz and R. Pabst
21st Edition: 2000, editors R. Putz and R. Pabst, Urban & Fischer Verlag, Munich
22nd Edition: 2006, editors R. Putz and R. Pabst, Elsevier GmbH, Munich

Foreign Editions:
Arabic Edition
Modern Technical Center, Damascus
Chinese Edition (complex characters)
Ho-Chi Book Publishing Co, Taiwan
Chinese Edition (simplified Chinese edition)
Elsevier, Health Sciences Asia, Singapore
Croatian Edition
Naklada Slap, Jastrebarsko
Dutch Edition
Bohn Stafleu van Loghum, Houten
English Edition (with nomenclature in English)
Atlas of Human Anatomy
Lippincott Williams & Wilkins
English Edition (with nomenclature in Latin)
Atlas of Human Anatomy
Elsevier GmbH, Urban & Fischer
French Edition
Atlas d'Anatomie Humaine
Tec & Doc Lavoisier, Paris
Greek Edition (with nomenclature in Greek)
Maria G. Parissianos, Athens
Greek Edition (with nomenclature in Latin)
Maria G. Parissianos, Athens
Hungarian Edition
az ember anatómiájának atlasza
Alliter Kiadái, Budapest
Indonesian Edition
Atlas Anatomi Manusia
Penerbit Buku Kedokteran EGC, Jakarta
Italian Edition
Atlante di Anatomia Umana
UTET, Torino
Japanese Edition
Igaku Shoin Ltd., Tokyo
Korean Edition
ShingHeung MedScience, Seoul
Polish Edition
Atlas anatomii cztowieka
Urban & Partner, Wroclaw
Portuguese Edition (with nomenclature in English)
Atlas de Anatomia Humana
Editora Guanabara Koogan, Rio de Janeiro
Portuguese Edition (with nomenclature in Latin)
Atlas de Anatomia Humana
Editora Guanabara Koogan, Rio de Janeiro
Spanish Edition
Atlas de Anatomia Humana
Editorial Medica Panamericana, Buenos Aires/Madrid
Turkish Edition
Insan Anatomisi Atlasi
Beta Basim Yayim Dagitim, Istanbul

Current information by www.elsevier.com and www.elsevier.de

Contents

Preface

It was just over a hundred years ago that Johannes Sobotta set out to publish the first edition of his Atlas of Human Anatomy. Since then, this piece of work has evolved step by step as a result of the constant interaction between students, lecturers and editors. It has not only been the most modern basis for the complex subject of macroscopic anatomy throughout many generations of doctors, but has also developed into a lasting work of reference for both clinical training and advanced medical education. All in all, it has become a book for a medical doctor's life. Once again, in this new edition the additional figures have been drawn strictly on the basis of original specimens.

The 14ᵗʰ edition has been particularly designed to meet the demands of a reformed medical curriculum, emphasizing the integration of clinical medicine into the preclinical curriculum. For this purpose, the new edition has been extended to include the following features:
- Surface anatomy including projection of internal organs (45 colour photos)
- Anatomical diagrams next to imaging figures
- Integration of imaging techniques to a greater extent (ultrasound, X-ray, CT, MRI; 119 figures)
- Endoscopic, intraoperative colour images and figures exemplifying techniques of puncture and examination (54 figures)
- Images of patients presenting with typical palsies
- Diagrams of the most important arterial variations (93 figures)
- Frequent variations in the location of internal organs (24 figures)
- Integration of histology at low magnification of important internal organs (intestine, liver, kidney, etc.)

In order to improve the presentation of the knowledge, the following features have been introduced:
- Clear-cut arrangement of the chapters according to the different regions of the body
- Thematically corresponding figures presented on double pages
- A concise, separate booklet (included in Volume 1) contains tables of muscles, joints and nerves, enabling the reader to place it next to any figure in the atlas

One particular aim of the new edition is to facilitate finding of specific structures. The SOBOTTA depicts anatomical structures precisely without the reader loosing the greater picture. Therefore, specific didactic tools have been improved and new aspects included:
- Each chapter has been allocated to a particular colour
- A "menu bar" on each double page ensures precise orientation within a given chapter
- The number of outlines depicting spatial orientation has been significantly increased (270 figures)
- Overviews of total body regions ensure general orientation
- New diagrams of particular muscles clarify their location and course (24 figures)

- Confusion is kept to a minimum by only depicting limbs of the right side of the body
- "Compass roses" point to adjacent figures, thus facilitating following a given structure over several pages
- Continuous leader lines facilitate finding of structures
- Coloured dots at the end of leader lines in topographic diagrams mark arteries, veins, nerves, and muscles
- The figures in the booklet relate directly to the figures in the atlas
- The larger dimensions of the book improve clarity

With the exception of discussions about the general concept of the atlas and mutual correction, the editors have worked separately on individual chapters, with the work divided as follows:

R. Putz: General anatomy, upper limb, brain, eye, ear, back, lower limb;

R. Pabst: Head, neck, thoracic and abdominal walls, thoracic, abdominal and pelvic viscera.

The inclusion of a large number of new figures is the result of the extraordinary capability of the following medical illustrators: Ulrike Brugger, Rüdiger Himmelhan and Horst Ruß. It is to their credit that the classic "SOBOTTA style" has been retained. Several of the diagrams have been generated on the computer by Henriette Rintelen. We also gratefully acknowledge our clinical colleagues for making clinical illustrations available to us (see picture credits). We owe a debt of gratitude to our colleagues from the institutes for their understanding and helpful suggestions. Dr. N. Sokolov and A. Buchhorn have put meticulous efforts into generating the specimen preparations. S. Fryk and G. Hoppmann have supported us in text processing.

The staff of the editorial office of Elsevier publishers, in particular Dr. D. Hennessen and A. Gattnarzik, has our sincere thanks. Some of the creative development of the work is a result of very fruitful discussions. We would also like to thank R. Hausdorf for tremendous efforts in the production of the atlas. R. Putz together with G. Meier were responsible for the proofreading and simplification of page design and legends. Our special thanks go to Dr. U. Osterkamp-Baust for generating the index, and all others involved in the corrections. With our joint efforts, the SOBOTTA has been once more modernized both in contents and design.

We have included many of the helpful suggestions made over the years by students and colleagues, and would therefore ask all readers of this edition to pass on to us any criticism or suggestions on the new format of this atlas.

Munich and Hannover, September 2005
R. Putz and R. Pabst

Univ.-Prof. Dr. med. Reinhard Putz

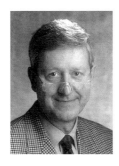

Born in Innsbruck/Austria
1962–1968	Studied medicine at the Leopold-Franzens-University of Innsbruck
1968	Received a doctorate
1968–1982	University assistant at the Institute of Anatomy at the University of Innsbruck
1978	Lecturer in anatomy
1979	Consultant for anatomy
1982–1989	Chair of the Anatomical Institute at the Albert-Ludwigs-University of Freiburg
since 1989	Chair of the Anatomical Institute at the Ludwig-Maximilians-University of Munich
1992–1994	President of the European Association of Clinical Anatomists
1993	Registration to practise medicine
1998–1999	Chairman of the Anatomical Society
1999	Member of the Akademie der Naturforscher und Ärzte (Leopoldina)
2002	Dr. h.c. of the University of Constanta, Romania
2003	Prorector I of the Ludwig-Maximilians-University of Munich

Research and fields of interest

- Functional anatomy of the passive locomotor system
- Evolution and functional anatomy of the vertebral column
- Form-function-relations of joints
- Applied anatomy (anatomical basics of orthopaedics, surgery, radiology)
- Questions about the contents and organisation of the medical curriculum
- Development of didactic training programmes at universities

Univ.-Prof. Dr. med. Reinhard Pabst

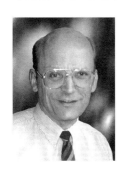

Born in Posen, grown up in Lüneburg
1965–1970	Studied medicine at the Hannover Medical School, and in Glasgow/Scotland
1970	University degree and doctorate
1971	Registration to practise medicine
1971–76	Scientific associate in the Department of Clinical Physiology, University of Ulm
1976	Lecturer for Clinical Physiology, University of Ulm, and new lectureship at the Hannover Medical School
1976–80	Senior assistant in the Department of Functional and Applied Anatomy, Hannover Medical School
1978	Extension of the Venia legendi to include anatomy
1980–1992	Head of the Department of Topographic Anatomy and Biomechanics
since 1992	Head of the Department of Functional and Applied Anatomy, Hannover Medical School
1986–1990	Prorector for studies and education, Hannover Medical School
1993–1997	Dean of the Hannover Medical School
1997–1998	Chairman of the Anatomical Society
1999–2003	Prorector of Research of the Hannover Medical School
2001	Member of the Akademie der Naturforscher und Ärzte (Leopoldina)

Research and fields of interest

- Functional anatomy of lymphatic organs
- Proliferation and migration of lymphocytes
- Development of the intestinal immune system
- Function of the pulmonary immune system
- Questions of a clinically orientated anatomy in the medical curriculum
- Evaluation of teaching

Picture credits

The editors sincerely thank all clinical colleagues that made ultrasound, computed tomographic and magnetic resonance images as well as endoscopic and intraoperative pictures available:

Prof. Altaras, Centre for Radiology, University of Gießen (Fig. 1009, 1031, 1032)

Dr. Baumeister, Department of Radiology, University of Freiburg (Fig. 1157)

PD Dr. Burgkardt, Orthopaedic Clinic, Technical University of Munich (Fig. 1431)

Prof. Brückmann & Dr. Linn, Neuroradiology, Institute for Diagnostic Radiology, University of Munich (Fig. 662, 726 a, b, 727 a, b)

Prof. Daniel, Department of Cardiology, University of Erlangen (Fig. 899, 900, 901, 973)

Prof. Degenhardt, Bielefeld (Fig. 1133, 1135)

Prof. Galanski & Dr. Kirchhoff, Department of Diagnostic Radiology, Hannover Medical School (Fig. 962, 964, 1212, 1213)

Prof. Galanski & Dr. Schäfer, Department of Diagnostic Radiology, Hannover Medical School (Fig. 871a, b, 927, 971, 991, 1194, 1204, 1207, 1209)

Prof. Gebel, Department of Gastroenterology, Hepatology and Endocrinology, Hannover Medical School (Fig. 242, 1011, 1026, 1027, 1038, 1039, 1074, 1092)

Dr. Goei, Radiology, Heerlen, The Netherlands (Fig. 1150, 1151) (with permission from Radiology 173; 137–141: 1989)

Dr. Greeven, St.-Elizabeth-Hospital, Neuwied (Fig. 150, 1238)

Prof. Hoffmann & PD Dr. Bektas, Clinic for Abdominal and Transplantation Surgery, Hannover Medical School (Fig. 1028, 1040)

Prof. Hohlfeld, Clinic for Pneumology, Hannover Medical School (Fig. 929, 930)

Prof. Jonas, Urology, Hannover Medical School (Fig. 1102 a, b, 1103)

Prof. Kampik & Prof. Müller, Ophthalmology, University of Munich (Fig. 657)

Dr. Kirchhoff & Dr. Weidemann, Department of Diagnostic Radiology, Hannover Medical School (Fig. 1041, 1093, 1102, 1196, 1198, 1200, 1202, 1205)

Prof. Kremers, Department for Restorative Dentistry and Periodontology, University of Munich (Fig. 169)

Prof. Kunze, von Haunersches Children's Hospital, University of Munich (Fig. 327–330)

Dr. Meyer, Department of Gastroenterology, Hepatology and Endocrinology, Hannover Medical School (Fig. 944, 987 a, b, 992, 1145, 1146)

Prof. Müller-Vahl, Neurology, Hannover Medical School (Fig. 128 a, b)

Prof. Pfeifer, Radiology, Institute for Diagnostic Radiology, University of Munich (Fig. 293, 294, 310, 312, 449, 451, 769–772, 807–810, 1255, 1286, 1287, 1317, 1318)

PD Dr. Rau, Department of Radiology, University of Freiburg (Fig. 912, 925, 926)

Prof. Ravelli †, formerly Institute of Anatomy, University of Innsbruck (Fig. 767)

PD Dr. Rieger, Radiology, Institute for Diagnostic Radiology, University of Munich (Fig. 1395)

Prof. Reich, Orofacial Surgery, University of Bonn (Fig. 113 a, b)

Prof. Reiser & Dr. Wagner, Institute for Diagnostic Radiology, University of Munich (Fig. 436, 449, 451, 453, 571, 572, 573, 576, 577, 792)

Prof. Rudzki-Janson, Department of Orthodontics, University of Munich (Fig. 72, 73)

Dr. Scheibe, Department of Surgery, Rosman Hospital, Breisach (Fig. 1289 a–c)

Prof. Scheumann, Clinic for Abdominal and Transplantation Surgery, Hannover Medical School (Fig. 243, 244, 245)

Prof. Schillinger, Department of Gynaecology, University of Freiburg (Fig. 1134)

Prof. Schliephake, Orofacial Surgery, Göttingen (Fig. 152, 196, 197)

Prof. Schlösser, Centre for Gynaecology, Hannover Medical School (Fig. 1132a, b, 1140, 1141, 1178)

Prof. Schumacher, Neuroradiology, Department of Radiology, University of Freiburg (Fig. 461 a, b)

Dr. Sommer & PD Dr. Bauer, Radiologists, Munich (Fig. 662, 1290–1292)

Prof. Stotz, Paediatrics, University of Munich (Fig. 1239, 1240)

PD Dr. Vogl, Radiology, University of Munich (Fig. 436, 453, 644, 645)

Prof. Vollrath, Ear-Nose-Throat Department, Mönchengladbach (Fig. 229, 230, 231)

Prof. Wagner †, Diagnostic Radiology II, Hannover Medical School (Fig. 952, 1064, 1065, 1069, 1072, 1152)

Prof. Wenz, formerly Department of Radiology, University of Freiburg (Fig. 768)

Prof. Witt, Department of Neurosurgery, University of Munich (Fig. 405)

Dr. Willführ, formerly Clinic for Abdominal and Transplantation Surgery, Hannover Medical School (Fig. 1051)

PD Dr. Wimmer, Department of Radiology, University of Freiburg (Fig. 799)

Additional illustrations were obtained from the following textbooks:

Benninghoff-Drenckhahn: Anatomie, Band 1 (Drenckhahn D., Hrsg.), 16. Aufl., Urban & Fischer, München 2003 (Fig. 823, 824, 848, 849, 850)

Welsch, U.: Lehrbuch Histologie, Urban & Fischer, München 2003 (Fig. 922, 1020, 1097, 1122, 1123)

Welsch, U. (Hrsg.): Sobotta, Atlas Histologie, 6. Aufl., Urban & Fischer, München 2002 (Fig. 1037, 1085, 1125 a, b)

Wicke, L.: Atlas der Röntgenanatomie, 3. Aufl., Urban & Schwarzenberg, München–Wien–Baltimore 1985 (Fig. 943 a)

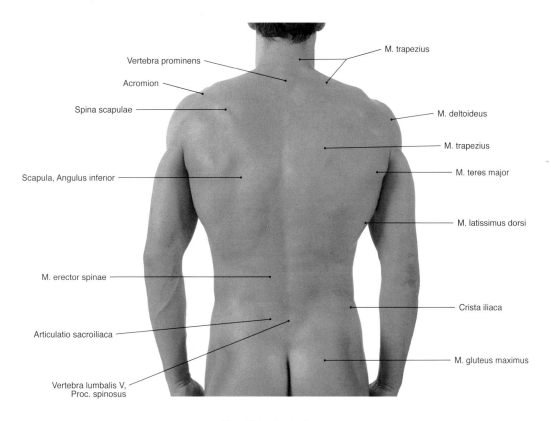

Vertebra prominens

Acromion

Spina scapulae

Scapula, Angulus inferior

M. erector spinae

Articulatio sacroiliaca

Vertebra lumbalis V, Proc. spinosus

M. trapezius

M. deltoideus

M. trapezius

M. teres major

M. latissimus dorsi

Crista iliaca

M. gluteus maximus

Fig. 728   Back, Dorsum; surface anatomy.

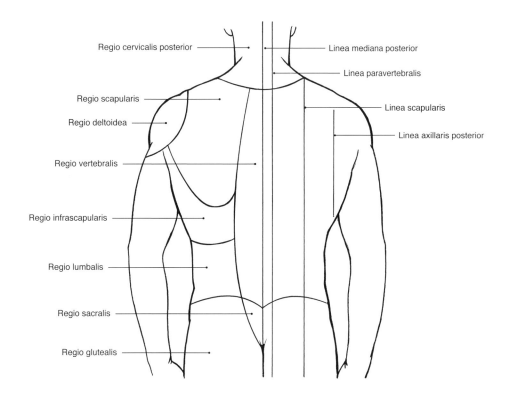

Regio cervicalis posterior

Regio scapularis

Regio deltoidea

Regio vertebralis

Regio infrascapularis

Regio lumbalis

Regio sacralis

Regio glutealis

Linea mediana posterior

Linea paravertebralis

Linea scapularis

Linea axillaris posterior

Fig. 729   Regions and orientation lines of the back.

Skeleton of the trunk

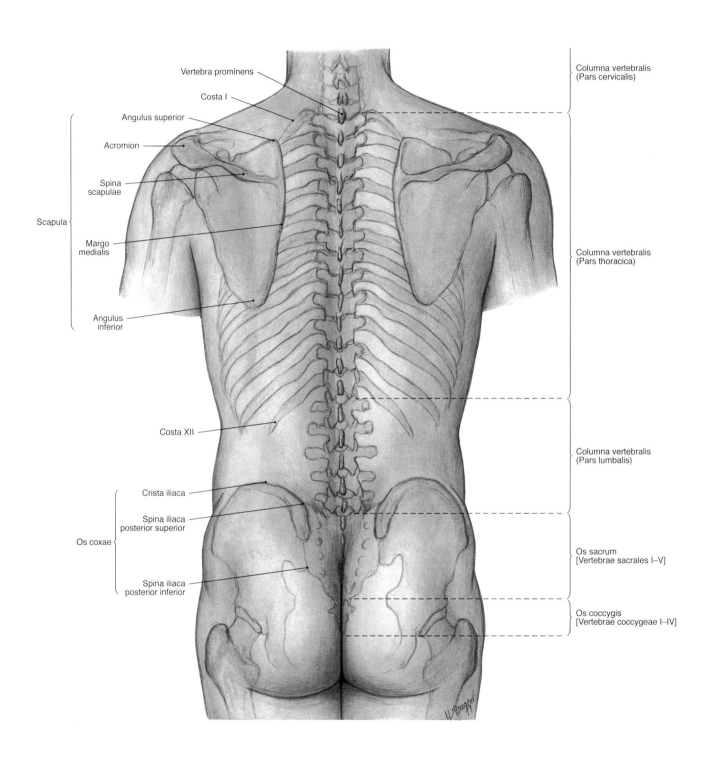

Fig. 730   Skeletal system, Systema skeletale, of the trunk.

Skeleton of the trunk

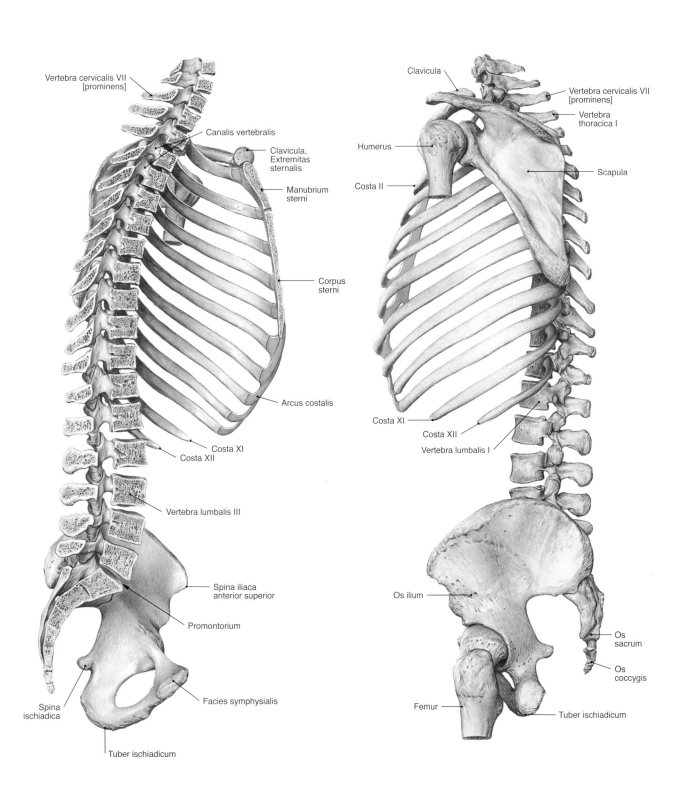

Vertebra cervicalis VII
[prominens]

Canalis vertebralis

Clavicula,
Extremitas
sternalis

Manubrium
sterni

Corpus
sterni

Arcus costalis

Costa XI
Costa XII

Vertebra lumbalis III

Spina iliaca
anterior superior

Promontorium

Facies symphysialis

Spina
ischiadica

Tuber ischiadicum

Clavicula

Vertebra cervicalis VII
[prominens]

Vertebra
thoracica I

Humerus

Scapula

Costa II

Costa XI

Costa XII

Vertebra lumbalis I

Os ilium

Os
sacrum

Os
coccygis

Femur

Tuber ischiadicum

Fig. 731 Vertebral column, Columna vertebralis;
pectoral girdle, Cingulum pectorale, and pelvic girdle,
Cingulum pelvicum;
median section through the vertebral column;
medial view.

Fig. 732 Vertebral column, Columna vertebralis;
pectoral girdle, Cingulum pectorale, and pelvic girdle,
Cingulum pelvicum;
median section through the vertebral column;
viewed from the left.

Vertebral column

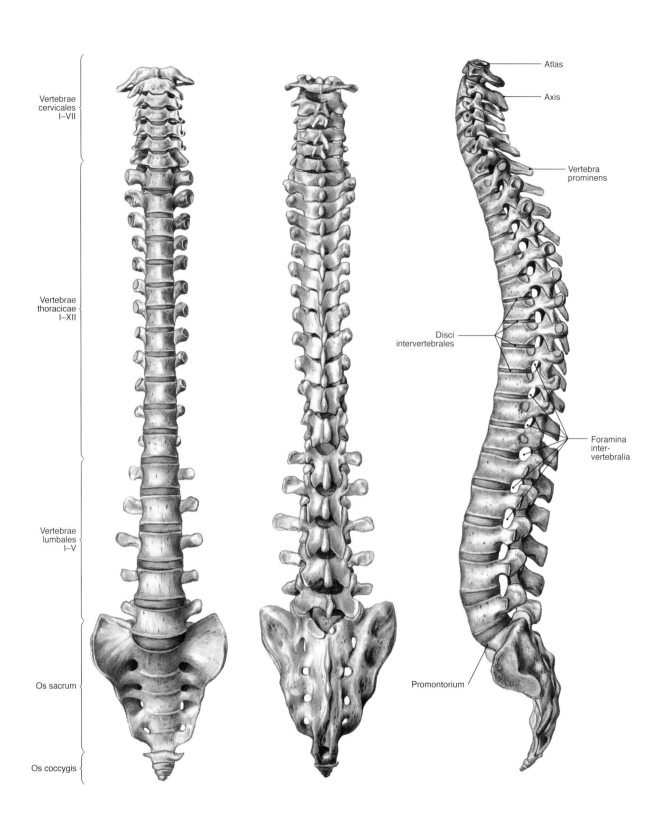

Vertebrae
cervicales
I–VII

Vertebrae
thoracicae
I–XII

Vertebrae
lumbales
I–V

Os sacrum

Os coccygis

Atlas

Axis

Vertebra
prominens

Disci
intervertebrales

Foramina
inter-
vertebralia

Promontorium

Fig. 733 Vertebral column,
Columna vertebralis;
ventral view.

Fig. 734 Vertebral column,
Columna vertebralis;
dorsal view.

Fig. 735 Vertebral column,
Columna vertebralis;
viewed from the left.

Vertebral column, development

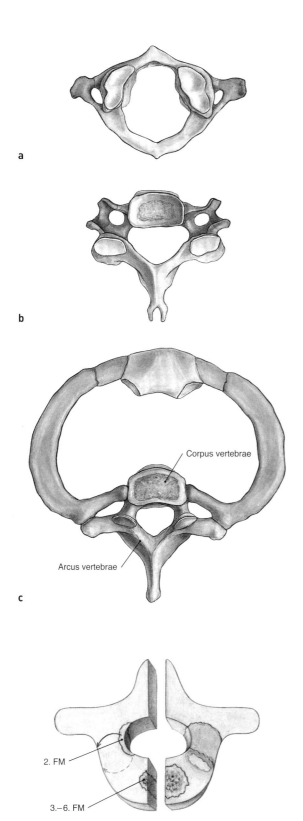

Corpus vertebrae

Arcus vertebrae

c

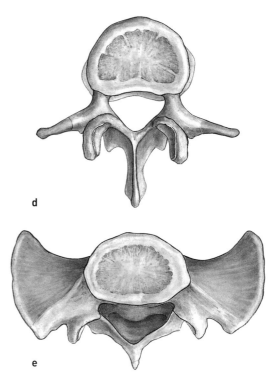

d

e

Fig. 736 a–e Regional characteristics of the vertebrae.
Only in the thoracic region of the vertebral column do
the lateral parts (labelled in red) remain separated and
form ribs.

a First cervical vertebra, Atlas
b Fourth cervical vertebra, Vertebra cervicalis IV
c First thoracic vertebra, Vertebra thoracica I, with
   corresponding ribs, Costae, and sternum, Sternum
d Third lumbar vertebra, Vertebra lumbalis III
e Sacrum, Os sacrum

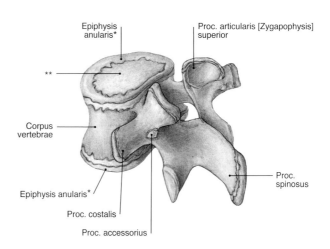

Epiphysis anularis*

Proc. articularis [Zygapophysis] superior

**

Corpus vertebrae

Epiphysis anularis*

Proc. costalis

Proc. accessorius

Proc. spinosus

2. FM

3.–6. FM

Fig. 737 Vertebral development.
Demonstration of the appearance of primary ossification
centres in a lumbar vertebra (pedicle: second foetal month;
corpus: third to sixth foetal month).
Synostosis of the ossification centres of the vertebral arch
with those of the corpus occurs between the third and the
sixth year of life.

Fig. 738 Vertebral development.
Circular ossification centres (= rims*) appear in the
epiphyses of the vertebrae during the eighth year of life and
fuse with the vertebral bodies until the eighteenth year of
life.
The central portions of the epiphyses remain as hyaline
cartilaginous laminae ** throughout life.
Secondary ossification centres (apophyses) develop at the
processes.

Atlas and axis

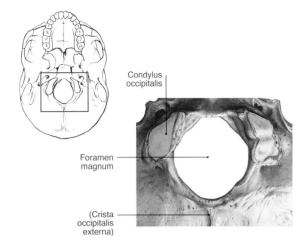

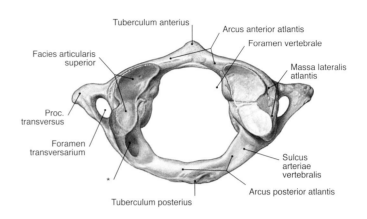

Fig. 739 Occipital bone, Os occipitale; section illustrating the foramen magnum and the articular surfaces of the atlanto-occipital joint; inferior view.

Fig. 740 First cervical vertebra, Atlas; superior view.
The superior articular surfaces of the atlas are frequently divided.
* Canalis arteriae vertebralis as a variation

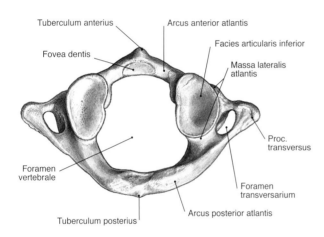

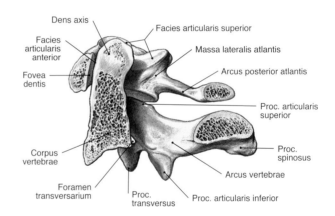

Fig. 741 First cervical vertebra, Atlas; inferior view.

Fig. 742 First and second cervical vertebrae, Atlas et Axis; median section.

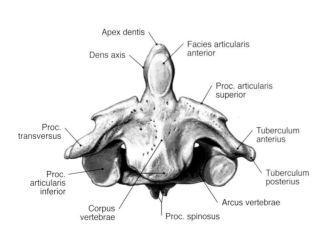

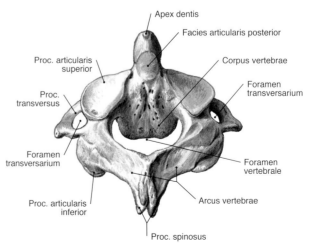

Fig. 743 Second cervical vertebra, Axis; ventral view.

Fig. 744 Second cervical vertebra, Axis; dorsosuperior view.

Cervical vertebrae

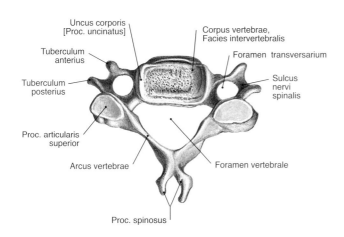

Fig. 745 Fifth cervical vertebra, Vertebra cervicalis V; superior view.
The tips of the spinous processes of the cervical vertebrae II–VI are frequently divided.

Fig. 746 Seventh cervical vertebra, Vertebra cervicalis VII; superior view.
In general the seventh cervical vertebra can be easily identified by its protruding spinous process and is referred to as vertebra prominens. In fact, the spinous process of the first thoracic vertebra often protrudes even further.

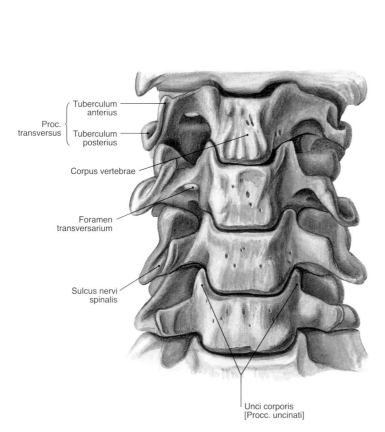

Fig. 747 Second to seventh cervical vertebrae, Vertebrae cervicales II–VII; ventral view.

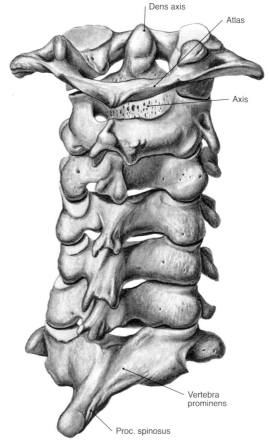

Fig. 748 First to seventh cervical vertebrae, Vertebrae cervicales I–VII; dorsolateral view.

Thoracic and lumbar vertebrae

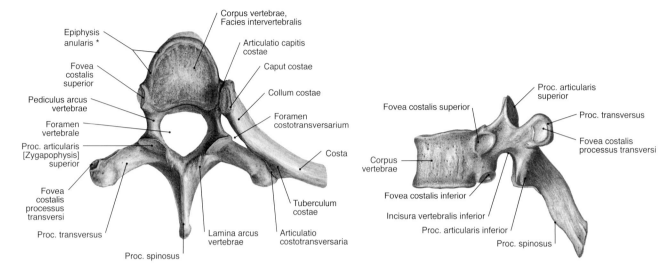

Fig. 749 Vertebra, Vertebra;
typical structural features exemplified by the
fifth thoracic vertebra;
superior view.
* Also: rim of vertebral body

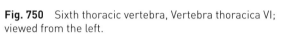

Fig. 750 Sixth thoracic vertebra, Vertebra thoracica VI;
viewed from the left.

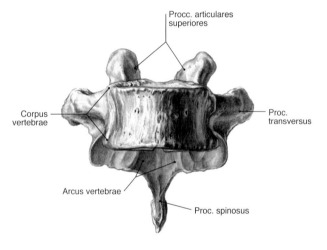

Fig. 751 Tenth thoracic vertebra, Vertebra thoracica X;
ventral view.

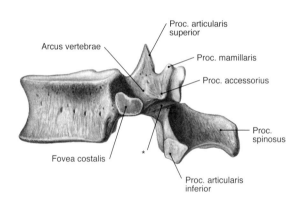

Fig. 752 Twelfth thoracic vertebra, Vertebra thoracica XII;
viewed from the left.
* Region of the vertebral arch between the superior and
inferior articular processes
("isthmus" = interarticular portion)

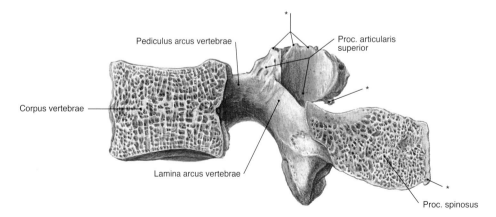

Fig. 753 Third lumbar vertebra, Vertebra lumbalis III;
median section; specimen of an older individual.
* Ossification of the ligamentous insertions

Thoracic and lumbar vertebrae

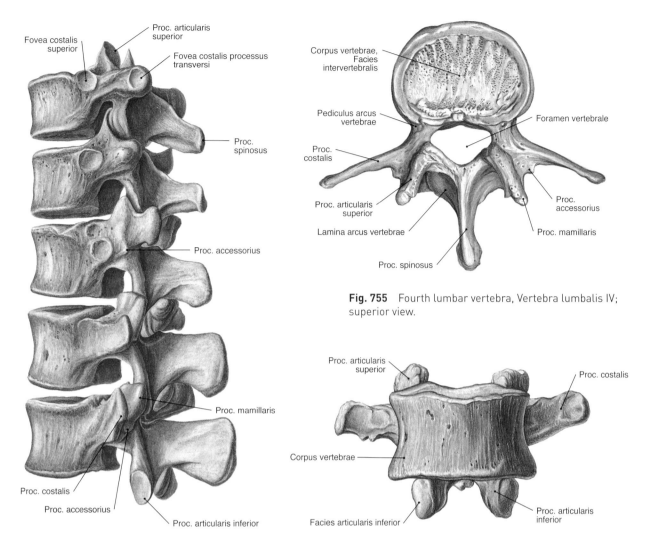

Fovea costalis superior

Proc. articularis superior

Fovea costalis processus transversi

Proc. spinosus

Proc. accessorius

Proc. mamillaris

Proc. costalis

Proc. accessorius

Proc. articularis inferior

Fig. 754 Tenth to twelfth thoracic vertebrae, Vertebrae thoracicae X–XII, and first to second lumbar vertebrae, Vertebrae lumbales I–II; dorsal view from the left.

Corpus vertebrae, Facies intervertebralis

Pediculus arcus vertebrae

Proc. costalis

Proc. articularis superior

Lamina arcus vertebrae

Proc. spinosus

Foramen vertebrale

Proc. accessorius

Proc. mamillaris

Fig. 755 Fourth lumbar vertebra, Vertebra lumbalis IV; superior view.

Proc. articularis superior

Proc. costalis

Corpus vertebrae

Facies articularis inferior

Proc. articularis inferior

Fig. 756 Fourth lumbar vertebra, Vertebra lumbalis IV; ventral view.

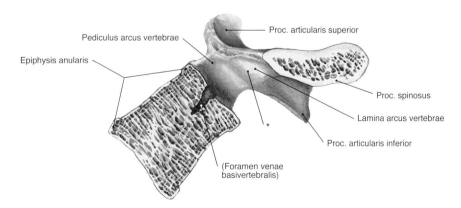

Pediculus arcus vertebrae

Epiphysis anularis

Proc. articularis superior

Proc. spinosus

Lamina arcus vertebrae

*

Proc. articularis inferior

(Foramen venae basivertebralis)

Fig. 757 Fifth lumbar vertebra, Vertebra lumbalis V; median section.
Note the characteristic wedge-shape of the body of the fifth lumbar vertebra.

* Region of the vertebral arch between the superior and inferior articular process. Here in the fifth and less frequently in the fourth lumbar vertebra a cleft, bridged by connective tissue (spondylolysis) can be formed. This is probably caused by local bending stress. As a consequence, the superior vertebra may slip (olisthesis) onto the inferior vertebra (spondylolisthesis).

Sacrum

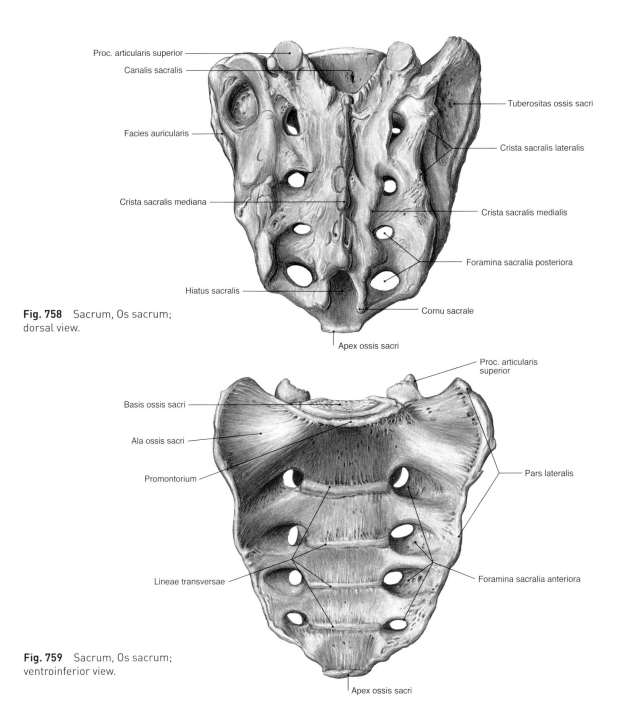

Proc. articularis superior
Canalis sacralis
Facies auricularis
Crista sacralis mediana
Hiatus sacralis
Tuberositas ossis sacri
Crista sacralis lateralis
Crista sacralis medialis
Foramina sacralia posteriora
Cornu sacrale
Apex ossis sacri

Fig. 758   Sacrum, Os sacrum;
dorsal view.

Basis ossis sacri
Ala ossis sacri
Promontorium
Lineae transversae
Proc. articularis superior
Pars lateralis
Foramina sacralia anteriora
Apex ossis sacri

Fig. 759   Sacrum, Os sacrum;
ventroinferior view.

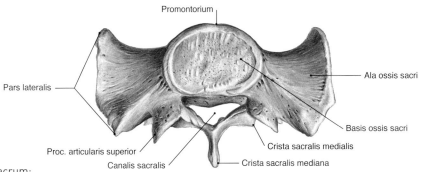

Promontorium
Pars lateralis
Proc. articularis superior
Canalis sacralis
Ala ossis sacri
Basis ossis sacri
Crista sacralis medialis
Crista sacralis mediana

Fig. 760   Sacrum, Os sacrum;
the bone has been sectioned at the
level of the second sacral vertebra;
superior view.

Sacrum and coccyx

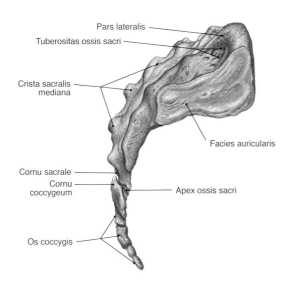

Pars lateralis
Tuberositas ossis sacri
Crista sacralis mediana
Facies auricularis
Cornu sacrale
Cornu coccygeum
Apex ossis sacri
Os coccygis

Fig. 761   Sacrum, Os sacrum; viewed from the right.

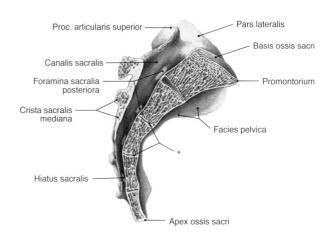

Proc. articularis superior
Canalis sacralis
Foramina sacralia posteriora
Crista sacralis mediana
Hiatus sacralis
Pars lateralis
Basis ossis sacri
Promontorium
Facies pelvica
*
Apex ossis sacri

Fig. 762   Sacrum, Os sacrum; median section.
* Remnants of intervertebral disc tissue persist even in the adult.

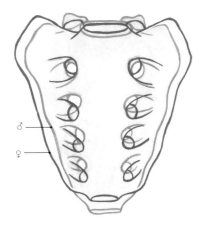

♂
♀

Fig. 763   Sacrum, Os sacrum; gender differences.

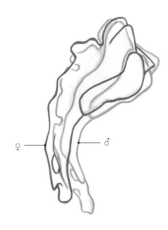

♀   ♂

Fig. 764   Sacrum, Os sacrum; gender differences.

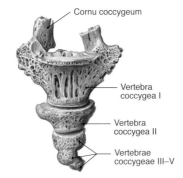

Cornu coccygeum
Vertebra coccygea I
Vertebra coccygea II
Vertebrae coccygeae III–V

Fig. 765   Coccyx, Os coccygis; ventrosuperior view.

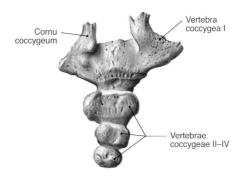

Cornu coccygeum
Vertebra coccygea I
Vertebrae coccygeae II–IV

Fig. 766   Coccyx, Os coccygis; dorsoinferior view.

Cervical part of the vertebral column, radiography

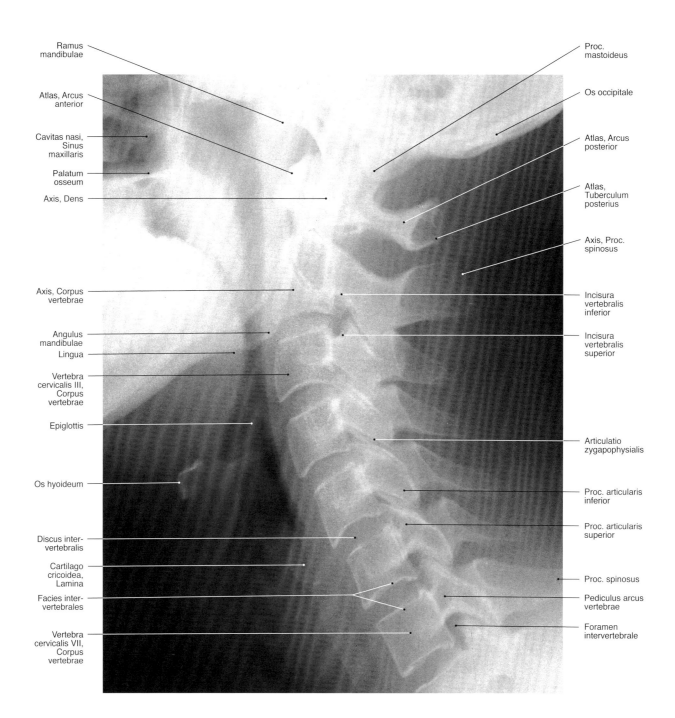

Ramus mandibulae

Atlas, Arcus anterior

Cavitas nasi, Sinus maxillaris

Palatum osseum

Axis, Dens

Axis, Corpus vertebrae

Angulus mandibulae

Lingua

Vertebra cervicalis III, Corpus vertebrae

Epiglottis

Os hyoideum

Discus intervertebralis

Cartilago cricoidea, Lamina

Facies intervertebrales

Vertebra cervicalis VII, Corpus vertebrae

Proc. mastoideus

Os occipitale

Atlas, Arcus posterior

Atlas, Tuberculum posterius

Axis, Proc. spinosus

Incisura vertebralis inferior

Incisura vertebralis superior

Articulatio zygapophysialis

Proc. articularis inferior

Proc. articularis superior

Proc. spinosus

Pediculus arcus vertebrae

Foramen intervertebrale

Fig. 767 Cervical vertebrae, Vertebrae cervicales;
lateral radiograph of the cervical part of the vertebral column;
upright position; the central beam is directed
onto the third cervical vertebra;
shoulders are pulled downwards.

Cervical part of the vertebral column, radiography

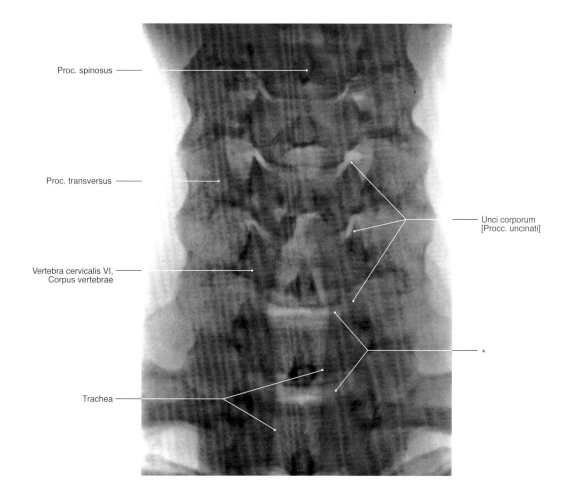

Proc. spinosus

Proc. transversus

Vertebra cervicalis VI,
Corpus vertebrae

Trachea

Unci corporum
[Procc. uncinati]

*

Fig. 768 Cervical vertebrae, Vertebrae cervicales;
AP-radiograph of the cervical part of the vertebral column;
upright position; the central beam is directed
onto the third cervical vertebra.
* Intervertebral disc spaces

Thoracic part of the vertebral column, radiography

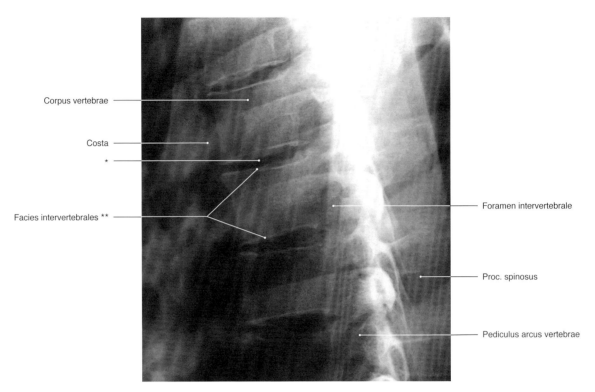

Corpus vertebrae

Costa

*

Facies intervertebrales **

Foramen intervertebrale

Proc. spinosus

Pediculus arcus vertebrae

Fig. 769 Thoracic vertebrae, Vertebrae thoracicae;
lateral radiograph of the thoracic part of the vertebral column;
upright position with the thorax in inspiration;
the central beam is directed onto the sixth thoracic vertebra.

* Intervertebral disc space
** Clinical term: end-plates

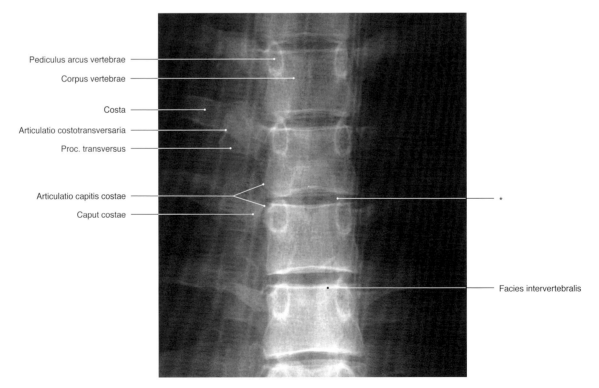

Pediculus arcus vertebrae

Corpus vertebrae

Costa

Articulatio costotransversaria

Proc. transversus

Articulatio capitis costae

Caput costae

*

Facies intervertebralis

Fig. 770 Thoracic vertebrae, Vertebrae thoracicae;
AP-radiograph of the thoracic part of the vertebral column;
upright position with the thorax in inspiration;
the central beam is directed onto the sixth thoracic vertebra.

* Intervertebral disc space

Lumbar part of the vertebral column, radiography

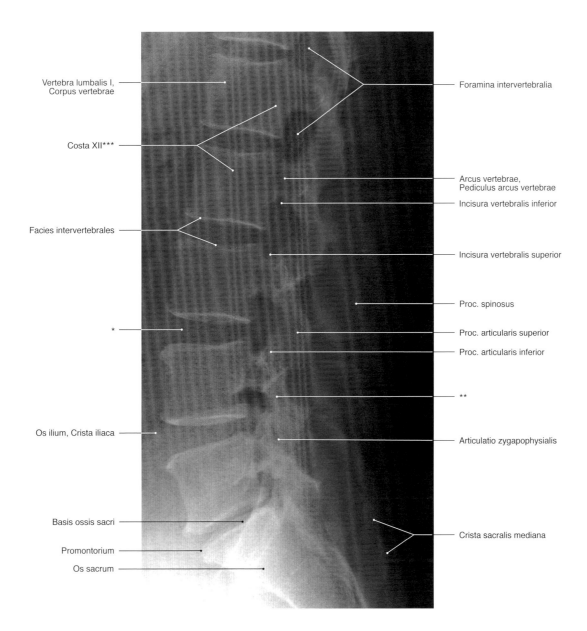

Vertebra lumbalis I,
Corpus vertebrae

Costa XII***

Facies intervertebrales

*

Os ilium, Crista iliaca

Basis ossis sacri

Promontorium

Os sacrum

Foramina intervertebralia

Arcus vertebrae,
Pediculus arcus vertebrae

Incisura vertebralis inferior

Incisura vertebralis superior

Proc. spinosus

Proc. articularis superior

Proc. articularis inferior

**

Articulatio zygapophysialis

Crista sacralis mediana

Fig. 771 Lumbar vertebrae, Vertebrae lumbales;
lateral radiograph of the lumbar part of the vertebral column;
upright position;
the central beam is directed onto the second lumbar vertebra.
In this case, the anterior edges of the lower lumbar vertebrae
are oblique due to pathological alterations.

* Intervertebral disc space
** Region of the vertebral arch between the superior and inferior
articular processes ("isthmus" = interarticular portion)
*** The marks indicate the position of the twelfth rib, which is poorly
visible in this copy of the radiograph.

Lumbar part of the vertebral column, radiography

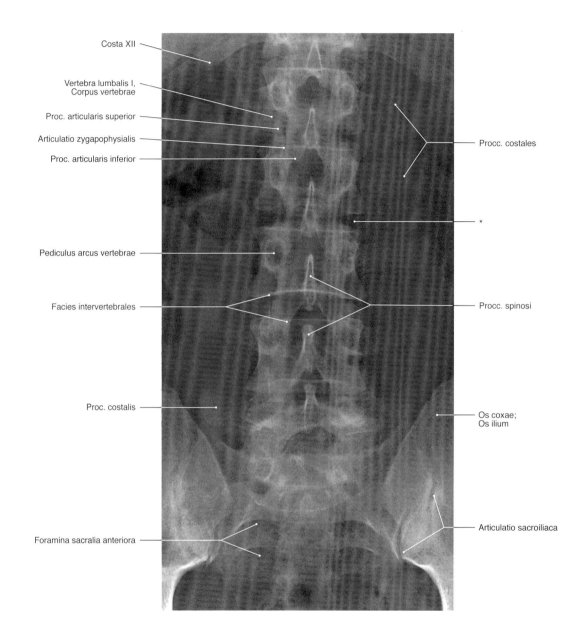

Costa XII

Vertebra lumbalis I,
Corpus vertebrae

Proc. articularis superior

Articulatio zygapophysialis

Proc. articularis inferior

Pediculus arcus vertebrae

Facies intervertebrales

Proc. costalis

Foramina sacralia anteriora

Procc. costales

*

Procc. spinosi

Os coxae;
Os ilium

Articulatio sacroiliaca

Fig. 772 Lumbar vertebrae, Vertebrae lumbales;
AP-radiograph of the lumbar part of the vertebral column
and the sacrum;
upright position; the central beam is directed onto the second
lumbar vertebra.
* Intervertebral disc space

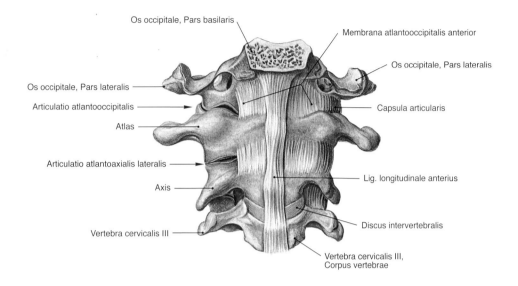

Os occipitale, Pars basilaris

Membrana atlantooccipitalis anterior

Os occipitale, Pars lateralis

Os occipitale, Pars lateralis

Capsula articularis

Articulatio atlantooccipitalis

Atlas

Articulatio atlantoaxialis lateralis

Axis

Lig. longitudinale anterius

Vertebra cervicalis III

Discus intervertebralis

Vertebra cervicalis III, Corpus vertebrae

Fig. 773 Craniocervical junctions and the upper cervical part of the vertebral column; ventral view.

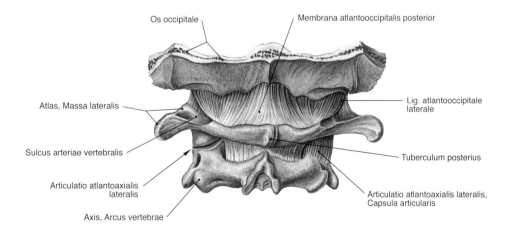

Os occipitale

Membrana atlantooccipitalis posterior

Atlas, Massa lateralis

Lig. atlantooccipitale laterale

Sulcus arteriae vertebralis

Tuberculum posterius

Articulatio atlantoaxialis lateralis

Articulatio atlantoaxialis lateralis, Capsula articularis

Axis, Arcus vertebrae

Fig. 774 Craniocervical junctions; dorsal view.

Craniocervical junctions

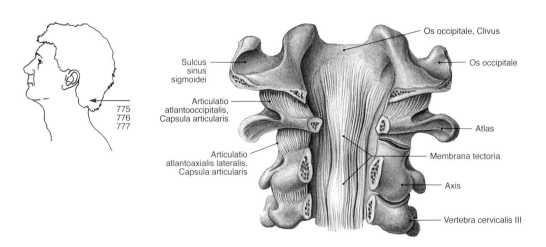

Fig. 775 Craniocervical junctions,
deep ligaments;
dorsal view.

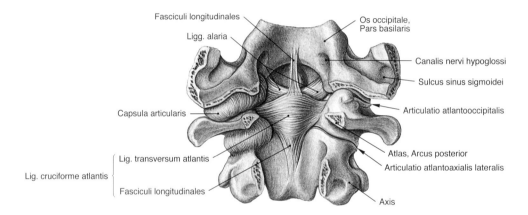

Fig. 776 Craniocervical junctions,
deep ligaments;
dorsal view.

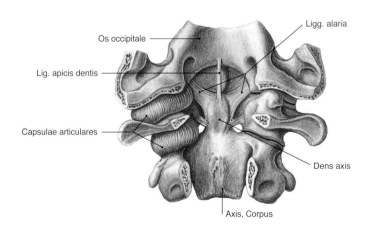

Fig. 777 Craniocervical junctions,
deep ligaments;
dorsal view.
The alar ligaments frequently extend to the lateral
masses of the atlas.

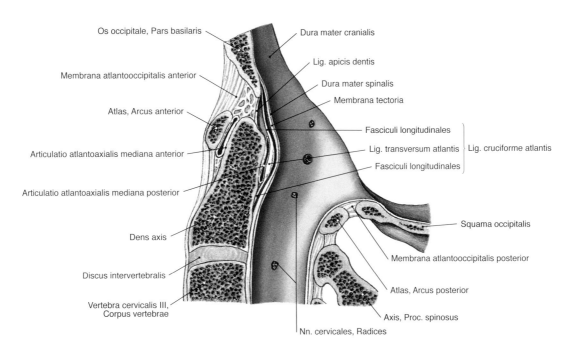

Os occipitale, Pars basilaris

Membrana atlantooccipitalis anterior

Atlas, Arcus anterior

Articulatio atlantoaxialis mediana anterior

Articulatio atlantoaxialis mediana posterior

Dens axis

Discus intervertebralis

Vertebra cervicalis III,
Corpus vertebrae

Nn. cervicales, Radices

Dura mater cranialis

Lig. apicis dentis

Dura mater spinalis

Membrana tectoria

Fasciculi longitudinales

Lig. transversum atlantis } Lig. cruciforme atlantis

Fasciculi longitudinales

Squama occipitalis

Membrana atlantooccipitalis posterior

Atlas, Arcus posterior

Axis, Proc. spinosus

Fig. 778 Craniocervical junctions;
median section.

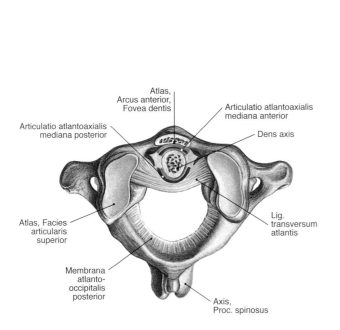

Atlas,
Arcus anterior,
Fovea dentis

Articulatio atlantoaxialis
mediana posterior

Articulatio atlantoaxialis
mediana anterior

Dens axis

Atlas, Facies
articularis
superior

Lig.
transversum
atlantis

Membrana
atlanto-
occipitalis
posterior

Axis,
Proc. spinosus

Fig. 779 Craniocervical junctions;
superior view.

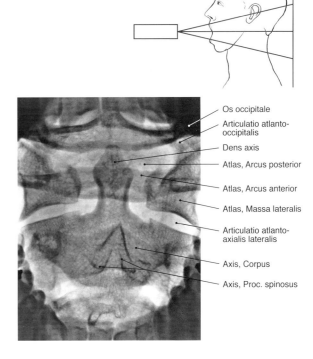

Os occipitale

Articulatio atlanto-
occipitalis

Dens axis

Atlas, Arcus posterior

Atlas, Arcus anterior

Atlas, Massa lateralis

Articulatio atlanto-
axialis lateralis

Axis, Corpus

Axis, Proc. spinosus

Fig. 780 Craniocervical junctions;
AP-radiograph.

Ligaments of the vertebral column

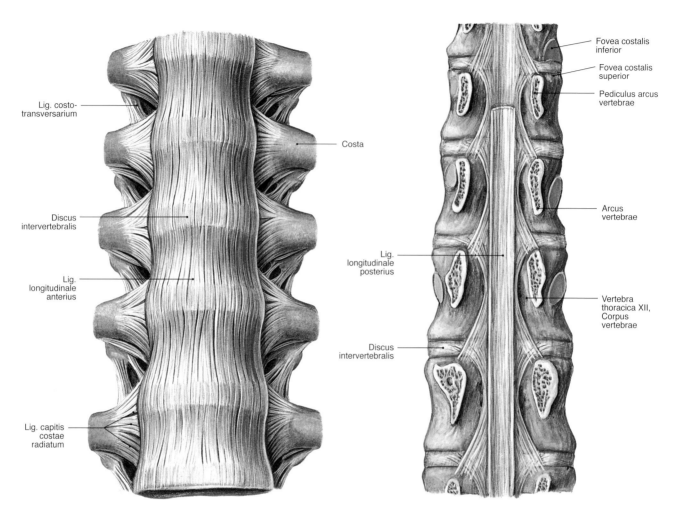

Lig. costo-transversarium

Costa

Discus intervertebralis

Lig. longitudinale anterius

Lig. capitis costae radiatum

Fovea costalis inferior

Fovea costalis superior

Pediculus arcus vertebrae

Lig. longitudinale posterius

Arcus vertebrae

Vertebra thoracica XII, Corpus vertebrae

Discus intervertebralis

Fig. 781   Ligaments of the vertebral column; exemplified by the lower thoracic part of the vertebral column; ventral view.

Fig. 782   Ligaments of the vertebral column; exemplified by the lower thoracic and the upper lumbar part of the vertebral column; dorsal view.

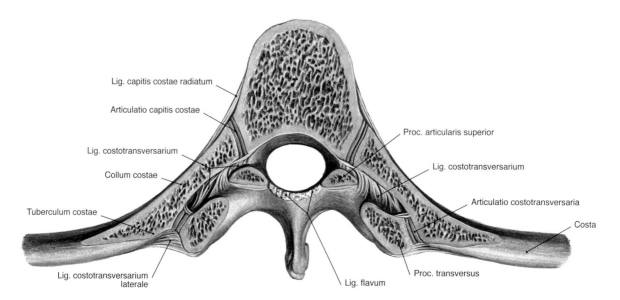

Lig. capitis costae radiatum

Articulatio capitis costae

Lig. costotransversarium

Collum costae

Tuberculum costae

Proc. articularis superior

Lig. costotransversarium

Articulatio costotransversaria

Costa

Lig. costotransversarium laterale

Lig. flavum

Proc. transversus

Fig. 783   Costovertebral joints, Articulationes costovertebrales; cross-section at the level of the lower part of the joint at a head of a rib; superior view.

Ligaments of the vertebral column

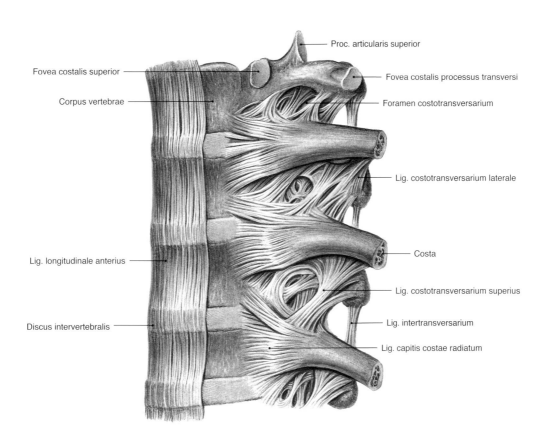

Proc. articularis superior

Fovea costalis superior

Fovea costalis processus transversi

Corpus vertebrae

Foramen costotransversarium

Lig. costotransversarium laterale

Costa

Lig. longitudinale anterius

Lig. costotransversarium superius

Lig. intertransversarium

Discus intervertebralis

Lig. capitis costae radiatum

Fig. 784 Ligaments of the vertebral column and the costovertebral joints, Articulationes costovertebrales; lateral parts of the anterior longitudinal ligament have been removed; viewed from the left.

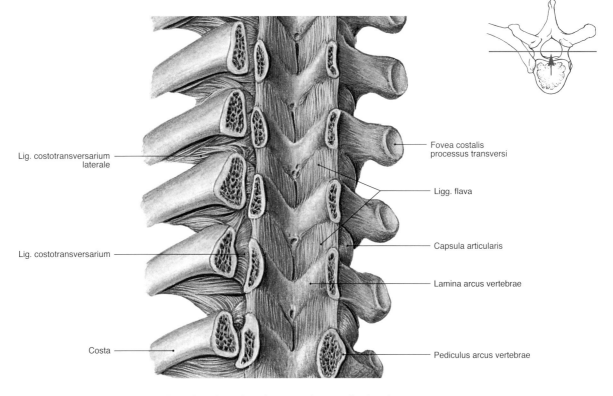

Lig. costotransversarium laterale

Fovea costalis processus transversi

Ligg. flava

Lig. costotransversarium

Capsula articularis

Lamina arcus vertebrae

Costa

Pediculus arcus vertebrae

Fig. 785 Junctions between the vertebral arches; ventral view.

Costovertebral joints

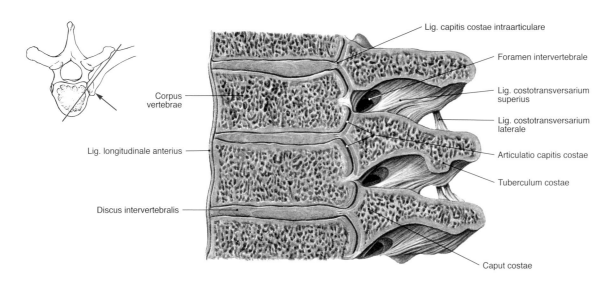

Lig. capitis costae intraarticulare

Foramen intervertebrale

Lig. costotransversarium superius

Lig. costotransversarium laterale

Articulatio capitis costae

Tuberculum costae

Corpus vertebrae

Lig. longitudinale anterius

Discus intervertebralis

Caput costae

Fig. 786 Costovertebral joints, Articulationes costovertebrales;
ventral view from the left.

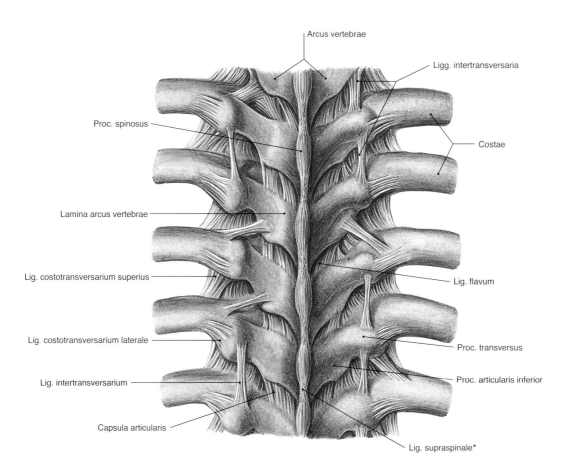

Arcus vertebrae

Ligg. intertransversaria

Proc. spinosus

Costae

Lamina arcus vertebrae

Lig. costotransversarium superius

Lig. flavum

Lig. costotransversarium laterale

Proc. transversus

Lig. intertransversarium

Proc. articularis inferior

Capsula articularis

Lig. supraspinale*

Fig. 787 Ligaments of the vertebral arches and the costovertebral joints, Articulationes costovertebrales;
dorsal view.
* The median portion of the thoracolumbar fascia is referred
  to as supraspinous ligament.

Ligaments of the lumbar part of the vertebral column

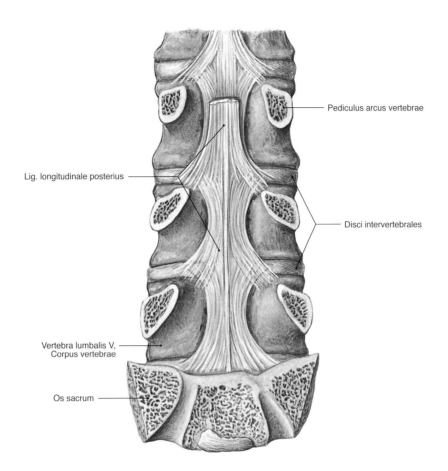

Pediculus arcus vertebrae

Lig. longitudinale posterius

Disci intervertebrales

Vertebra lumbalis V,
Corpus vertebrae

Os sacrum

Fig. 788 Ligaments of the lumbar part
of the vertebral column.

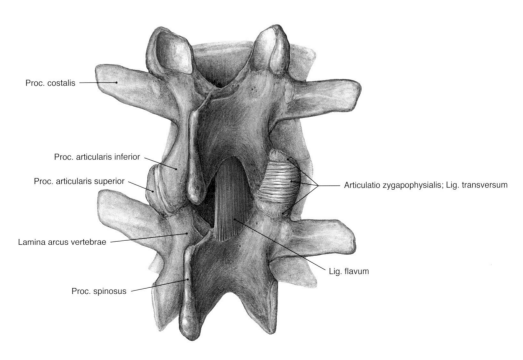

Proc. costalis

Proc. articularis inferior

Proc. articularis superior

Articulatio zygapophysialis; Lig. transversum

Lamina arcus vertebrae

Lig. flavum

Proc. spinosus

Fig. 789 Vertebral joints of the lumbar part of the vertebral
column, Articulationes zygapophysiales lumbales;
dorsal view from the right.

Reinforcement of the interarticular joints by strong and
transverse fibres (Ligg. transversa) is restricted to the lumbar
part of the vertebral column.

Intervertebral discs

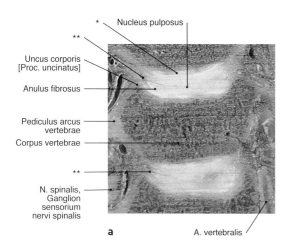

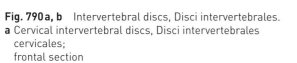

- Nucleus pulposus
- Uncus corporis [Proc. uncinatus]
- Anulus fibrosus
- Pediculus arcus vertebrae
- Corpus vertebrae
- N. spinalis, Ganglion sensorium nervi spinalis
- A. vertebralis

a

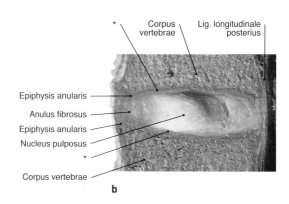

- Corpus vertebrae
- Lig. longitudinale posterius
- Epiphysis anularis
- Anulus fibrosus
- Epiphysis anularis
- Nucleus pulposus
- Corpus vertebrae

b

Fig. 790 a, b Intervertebral discs, Disci intervertebrales.
a Cervical intervertebral discs, Disci intervertebrales cervicales;
frontal section
b Lumbar intervertebral disc, Discus intervertebralis lumbalis;
median section

* Hyaline cartilaginous covering of the end-plates of the vertebral bodies reflecting the non-ossified portion of the epiphyses

** In the first decade of life, so-called uncovertebral clefts develop in the lateral zones of the cervical intervertebral discs, which can progress further towards the middle in the following decades.

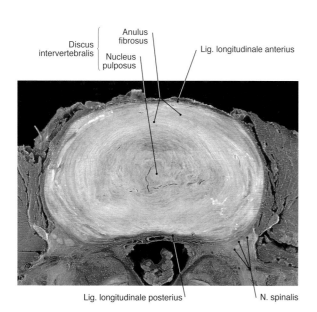

- Discus intervertebralis
  - Anulus fibrosus
  - Nucleus pulposus
- Lig. longitudinale anterius
- Lig. longitudinale posterius
- N. spinalis

Fig. 791 Lumbar intervertebral disc,
Discus intervertebralis lumbalis;
superior view.

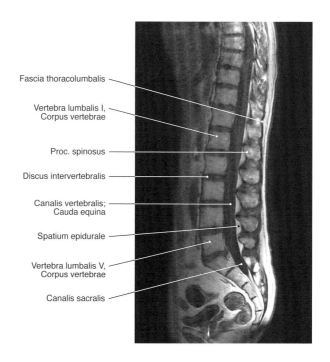

- Fascia thoracolumbalis
- Vertebra lumbalis I, Corpus vertebrae
- Proc. spinosus
- Discus intervertebralis
- Canalis vertebralis; Cauda equina
- Spatium epidurale
- Vertebra lumbalis V, Corpus vertebrae
- Canalis sacralis

Fig. 792 Lumbar parts of the vertebral column;
magnetic resonance tomographic image (MRI);
median section.

Motion segments

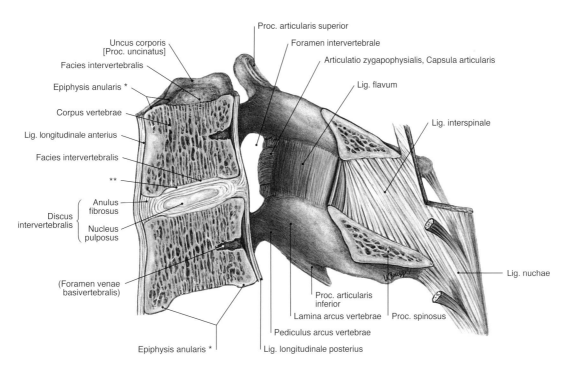

Proc. articularis superior
Uncus corporis [Proc. uncinatus]
Foramen intervertebrale
Facies intervertebralis
Articulatio zygapophysialis, Capsula articularis
Epiphysis anularis *
Lig. flavum
Corpus vertebrae
Lig. longitudinale anterius
Lig. interspinale
Facies intervertebralis
**
Anulus fibrosus
Discus intervertebralis
Nucleus pulposus
Lig. nuchae
(Foramen venae basivertebralis)
Proc. articularis inferior
Lamina arcus vertebrae
Proc. spinosus
Epiphysis anularis *
Lig. longitudinale posterius
Pediculus arcus vertebrae

Fig. 793 Cervical motion segment; schematic median section.

* Also: rim of vertebral body
** Hyaline cartilaginous covering of the end-plate of the vertebral body reflecting the non-ossified portion of the epiphysis

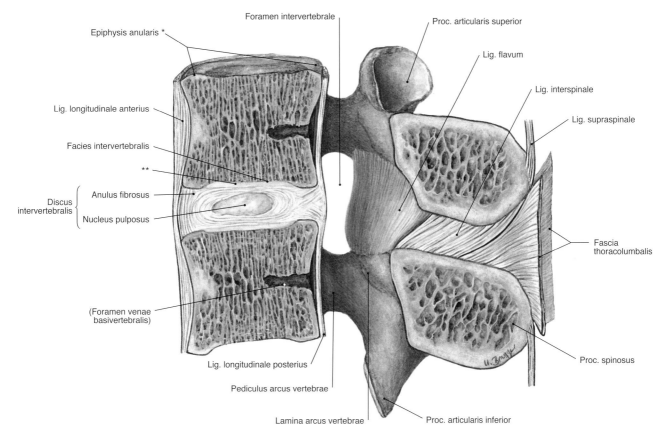

Foramen intervertebrale
Proc. articularis superior
Epiphysis anularis *
Lig. flavum
Lig. interspinale
Lig. longitudinale anterius
Lig. supraspinale
Facies intervertebralis
**
Anulus fibrosus
Discus intervertebralis
Nucleus pulposus
Fascia thoracolumbalis
(Foramen venae basivertebralis)
Lig. longitudinale posterius
Proc. spinosus
Pediculus arcus vertebrae
Lamina arcus vertebrae
Proc. articularis inferior

Fig. 794 Lumbar motion segment; schematic median section.

* Also: rim of vertebral body
** Hyaline cartilaginous covering of the end-plate of the vertebral body reflecting the non-ossified portion of the epiphysis

Superficial muscles of the back

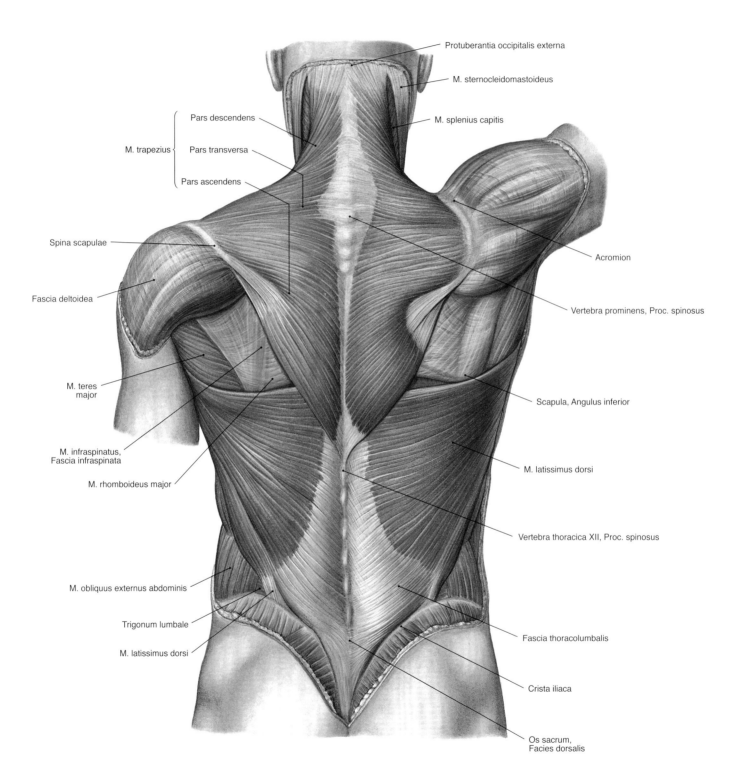

Protuberantia occipitalis externa

M. sternocleidomastoideus

Pars descendens

M. trapezius { Pars transversa

Pars ascendens

M. splenius capitis

Spina scapulae

Fascia deltoidea

Acromion

Vertebra prominens, Proc. spinosus

M. teres major

M. infraspinatus, Fascia infraspinata

M. rhomboideus major

Scapula, Angulus inferior

M. latissimus dorsi

M. obliquus externus abdominis

Trigonum lumbale

M. latissimus dorsi

Vertebra thoracica XII, Proc. spinosus

Fascia thoracolumbalis

Crista iliaca

Os sacrum, Facies dorsalis

→ T 17, T 18

Fig. 795   Muscles of the back, Mm. dorsi; superficial layer of the trunk-arm and trunk-shoulder girdle muscles.

Superficial muscles of the back

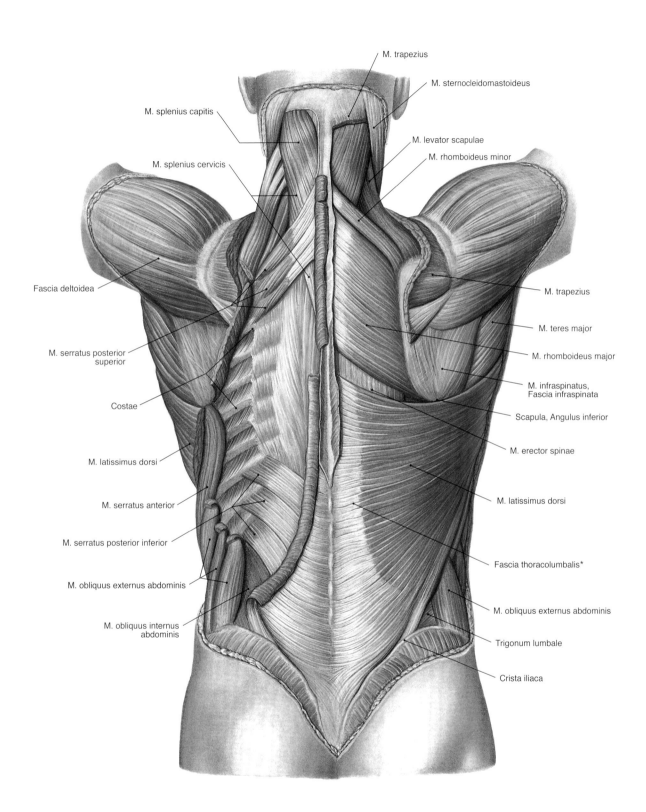

M. trapezius

M. sternocleidomastoideus

M. splenius capitis

M. levator scapulae

M. rhomboideus minor

M. splenius cervicis

Fascia deltoidea

M. trapezius

M. teres major

M. serratus posterior superior

M. rhomboideus major

M. infraspinatus, Fascia infraspinata

Costae

Scapula, Angulus inferior

M. erector spinae

M. latissimus dorsi

M. latissimus dorsi

M. serratus anterior

M. serratus posterior inferior

Fascia thoracolumbalis*

M. obliquus externus abdominis

M. obliquus externus abdominis

M. obliquus internus abdominis

Trigonum lumbale

Crista iliaca

Fig. 796 Muscles of the back, Mm. dorsi; deep layer of the trunk-arm and trunk-shoulder girdle muscles.

* The so-called thoracolumbar fascia forms a dense aponeurosis.

→ T 17–T 19

Deep muscles of the back

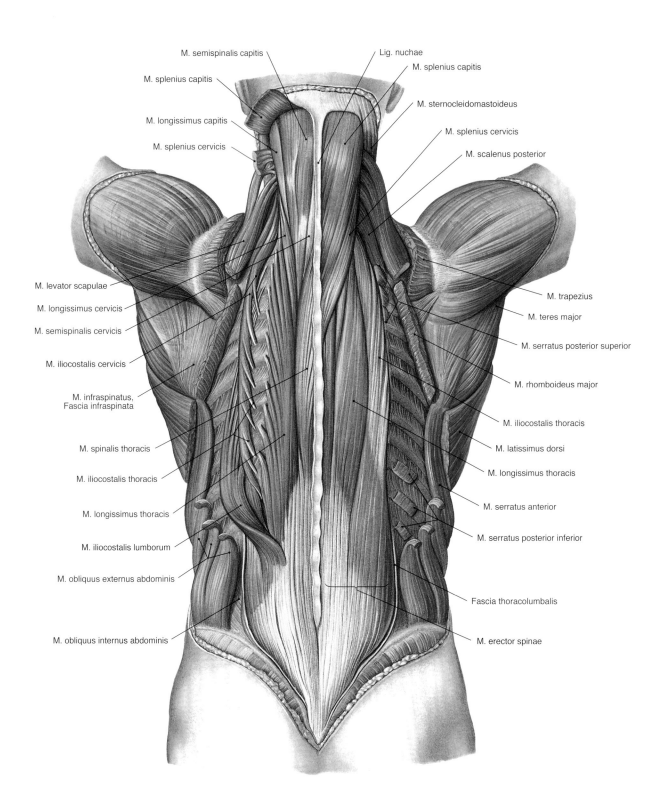

M. semispinalis capitis

M. splenius capitis

M. longissimus capitis

M. splenius cervicis

Lig. nuchae

M. splenius capitis

M. sternocleidomastoideus

M. splenius cervicis

M. scalenus posterior

M. levator scapulae

M. longissimus cervicis

M. semispinalis cervicis

M. iliocostalis cervicis

M. infraspinatus,
Fascia infraspinata

M. spinalis thoracis

M. iliocostalis thoracis

M. longissimus thoracis

M. iliocostalis lumborum

M. obliquus externus abdominis

M. obliquus internus abdominis

M. trapezius

M. teres major

M. serratus posterior superior

M. rhomboideus major

M. iliocostalis thoracis

M. latissimus dorsi

M. longissimus thoracis

M. serratus anterior

M. serratus posterior inferior

Fascia thoracolumbalis

M. erector spinae

→ T 20 a, b

Fig. 797 Muscles of the back, Mm. dorsi;
superficial layer of the deep (autochthonous) muscles.

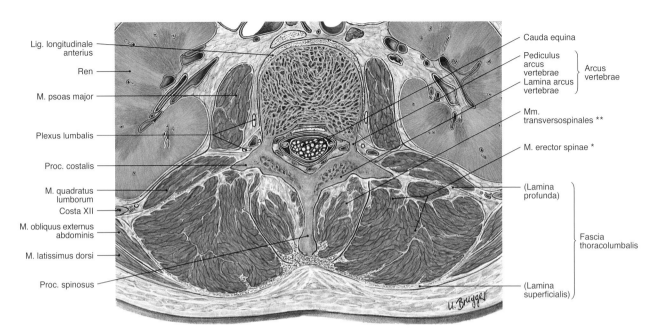

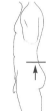

Fig. 798 Muscles of the back, Mm. dorsi;
cross-section at the level of the second lumbar vertebra;
inferior view.

The deep (autochthonous) muscles of the back lie within an osteofibrous
tube formed by dorsal parts of the vertebrae and the surrounding
aponeurotic thoracolumbar fascia. The muscles are divided into a lateral *
and a medial ** tract.

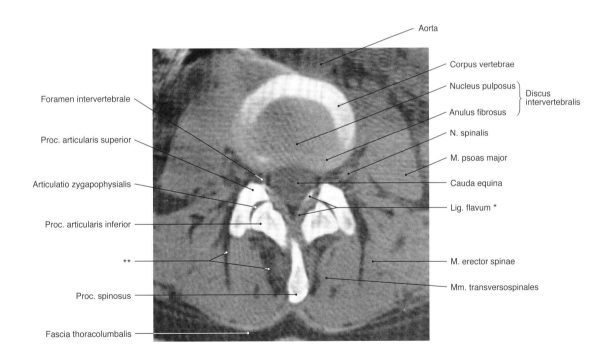

Fig. 799 Muscles of the back, Mm. dorsi;
computed tomographic cross-section (CT) at the level of the
intervertebral disc between the third and the fourth lumbar
vertebra;
inferior view.

* Calcification or ossification frequently occurs at the sites of insertion
  of the ligamenta flava, even in younger individuals.
** Adipose tissue deposits

Deep muscles of the back

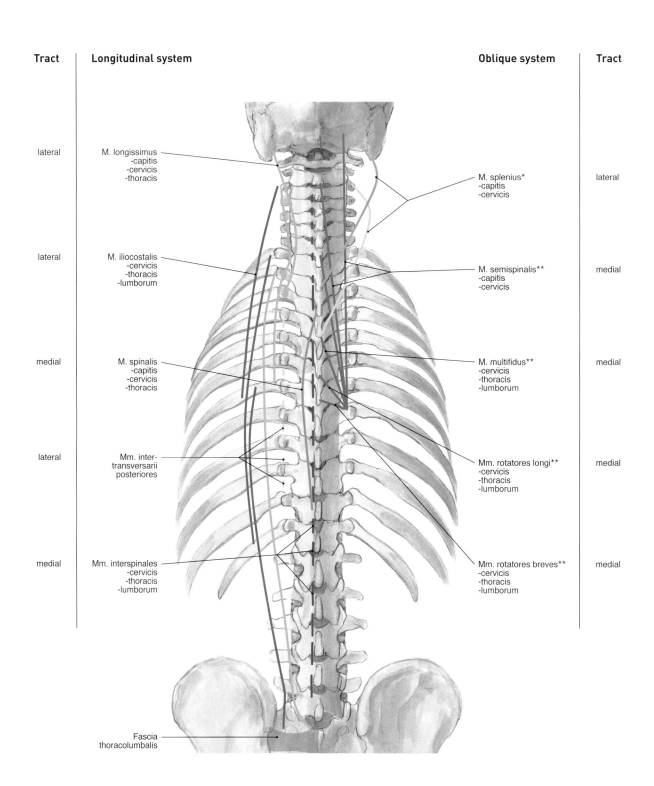

Tract	Longitudinal system		Oblique system	Tract
lateral	M. longissimus -capitis -cervicis -thoracis		M. splenius* -capitis -cervicis	lateral
lateral	M. iliocostalis -cervicis -thoracis -lumborum		M. semispinalis** -capitis -cervicis	medial
medial	M. spinalis -capitis -cervicis -thoracis		M. multifidus** -cervicis -thoracis -lumborum	medial
lateral	Mm. inter- transversarii posteriores		Mm. rotatores longi** -cervicis -thoracis -lumborum	medial
medial	Mm. interspinales -cervicis -thoracis -lumborum		Mm. rotatores breves** -cervicis -thoracis -lumborum	medial
	Fascia thoracolumbalis			

Fig. 800   Deep (autochthonous) muscles of the back;
diagram of the different groups of muscles.
The deep (autochthonous) muscles of the back can be
divided into a longitudinal and an oblique system, as
well as into a medial and a lateral tract.
* Spinotransverse
** Transversospinal

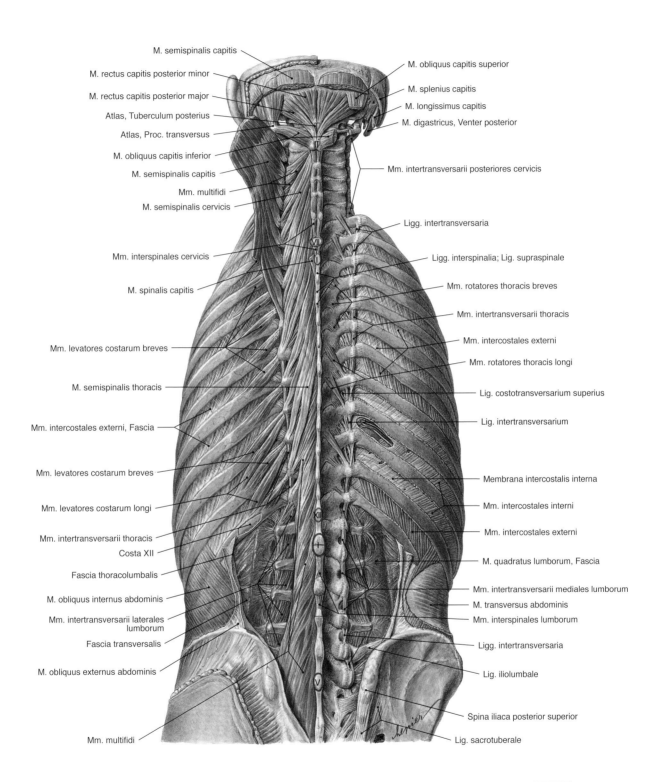

M. semispinalis capitis

M. rectus capitis posterior minor

M. rectus capitis posterior major

Atlas, Tuberculum posterius

Atlas, Proc. transversus

M. obliquus capitis inferior

M. semispinalis capitis

Mm. multifidi

M. semispinalis cervicis

Mm. interspinales cervicis

M. spinalis capitis

Mm. levatores costarum breves

M. semispinalis thoracis

Mm. intercostales externi, Fascia

Mm. levatores costarum breves

Mm. levatores costarum longi

Mm. intertransversarii thoracis

Costa XII

Fascia thoracolumbalis

M. obliquus internus abdominis

Mm. intertransversarii laterales lumborum

Fascia transversalis

M. obliquus externus abdominis

Mm. multifidi

M. obliquus capitis superior

M. splenius capitis

M. longissimus capitis

M. digastricus, Venter posterior

Mm. intertransversarii posteriores cervicis

Ligg. intertransversaria

Ligg. interspinalia; Lig. supraspinale

Mm. rotatores thoracis breves

Mm. intertransversarii thoracis

Mm. intercostales externi

Mm. rotatores thoracis longi

Lig. costotransversarium superius

Lig. intertransversarium

Membrana intercostalis interna

Mm. intercostales interni

Mm. intercostales externi

M. quadratus lumborum, Fascia

Mm. intertransversarii mediales lumborum

M. transversus abdominis

Mm. interspinales lumborum

Ligg. intertransversaria

Lig. iliolumbale

Spina iliaca posterior superior

Lig. sacrotuberale

Fig. 801 Muscles of the back, Mm. dorsi, and suboccipital muscles, Mm. suboccipitales.

→ T 20 b, c

Deep muscles of the back

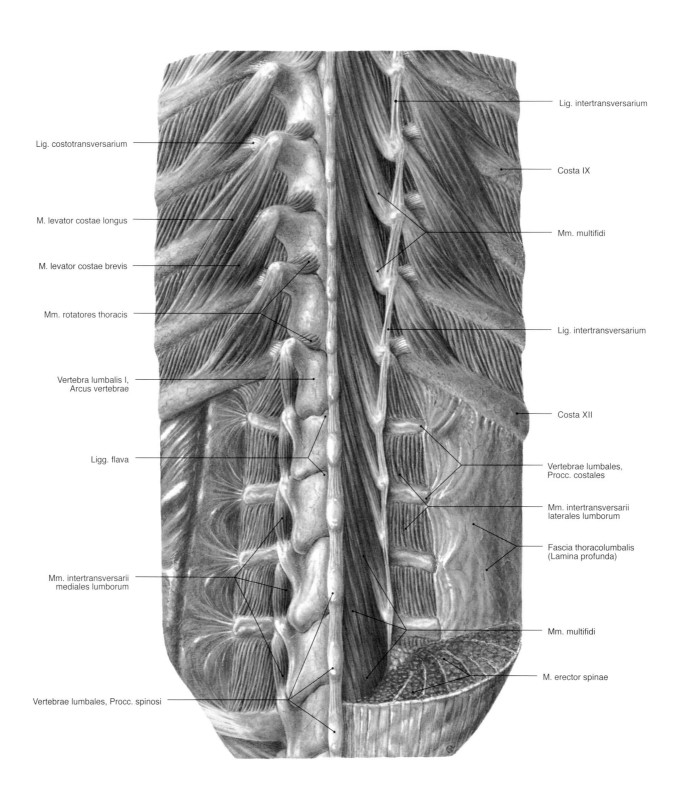

Lig. costotransversarium

M. levator costae longus

M. levator costae brevis

Mm. rotatores thoracis

Vertebra lumbalis I, Arcus vertebrae

Ligg. flava

Mm. intertransversarii mediales lumborum

Vertebrae lumbales, Procc. spinosi

Lig. intertransversarium

Costa IX

Mm. multifidi

Lig. intertransversarium

Costa XII

Vertebrae lumbales, Procc. costales

Mm. intertransversarii laterales lumborum

Fascia thoracolumbalis (Lamina profunda)

Mm. multifidi

M. erector spinae

→ T 20 a, b

Fig. 802 Muscles of the back, Mm. dorsi; deepest layer in the region of the lower thoracic and the lumbar part of the vertebral column.

Suboccipital muscles

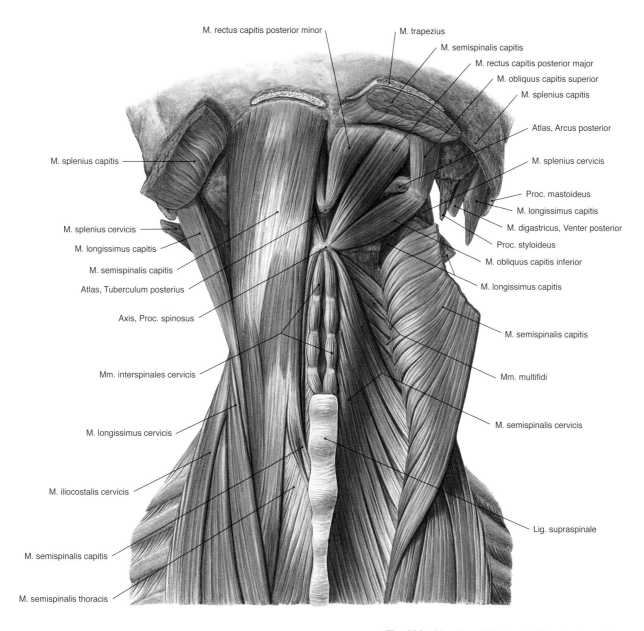

M. rectus capitis posterior minor

M. trapezius

M. semispinalis capitis

M. rectus capitis posterior major

M. obliquus capitis superior

M. splenius capitis

Atlas, Arcus posterior

M. splenius capitis

M. splenius cervicis

Proc. mastoideus

M. longissimus capitis

M. digastricus, Venter posterior

Proc. styloideus

M. obliquus capitis inferior

M. longissimus capitis

M. splenius cervicis

M. longissimus capitis

M. semispinalis capitis

Atlas, Tuberculum posterius

Axis, Proc. spinosus

M. semispinalis capitis

Mm. interspinales cervicis

Mm. multifidi

M. longissimus cervicis

M. semispinalis cervicis

M. iliocostalis cervicis

Lig. supraspinale

M. semispinalis capitis

M. semispinalis thoracis

Fig. 803 Muscles of the back, Mm. dorsi, and suboccipital muscles, Mm. suboccipitales.

→ T 20 b, c

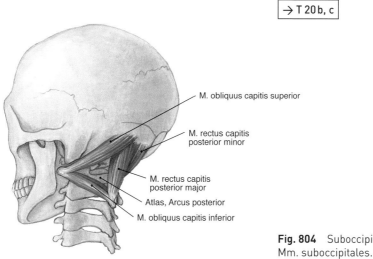

M. obliquus capitis superior

M. rectus capitis posterior minor

M. rectus capitis posterior major

Atlas, Arcus posterior

M. obliquus capitis inferior

Fig. 804 Suboccipital muscles, Mm. suboccipitales.

→ T 20 c

Suboccipital muscles

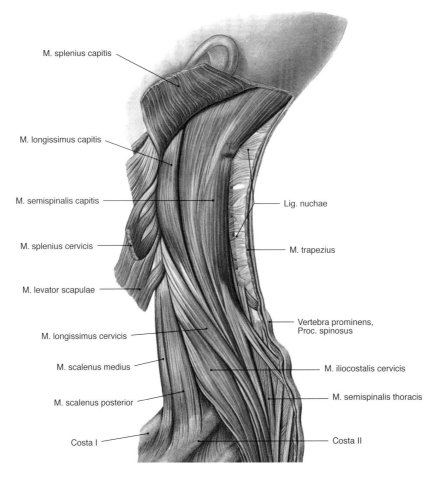

M. splenius capitis

M. longissimus capitis

M. semispinalis capitis

M. splenius cervicis

M. levator scapulae

M. longissimus cervicis

M. scalenus medius

M. scalenus posterior

Costa I

Lig. nuchae

M. trapezius

Vertebra prominens, Proc. spinosus

M. iliocostalis cervicis

M. semispinalis thoracis

Costa II

→ T 20 a, b

Fig. 805   Muscles of the back, Mm. dorsi, and muscles of the neck, Mm. colli.

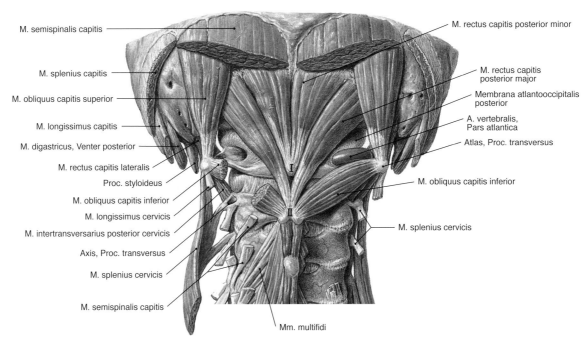

M. semispinalis capitis

M. splenius capitis

M. obliquus capitis superior

M. longissimus capitis

M. digastricus, Venter posterior

M. rectus capitis lateralis

Proc. styloideus

M. obliquus capitis inferior

M. longissimus cervicis

M. intertransversarius posterior cervicis

Axis, Proc. transversus

M. splenius cervicis

M. semispinalis capitis

Mm. multifidi

M. rectus capitis posterior minor

M. rectus capitis posterior major

Membrana atlantooccipitalis posterior

A. vertebralis, Pars atlantica

Atlas, Proc. transversus

M. obliquus capitis inferior

M. splenius cervicis

→ T 20 c

Fig. 806   Suboccipital muscles, Mm. suboccipitales.

I = Posterior tubercle of the atlas
II = Spinous process of the axis

Vertebral column, sections

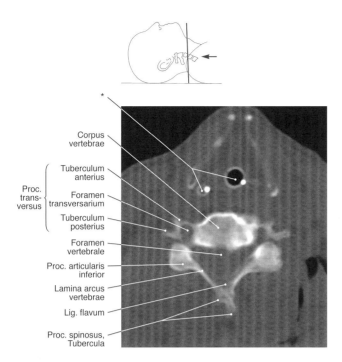

Corpus
vertebrae

Proc. trans-versus {
Tuberculum
anterius

Foramen
transversarium

Tuberculum
posterius

Foramen
vertebrale

Proc. articularis
inferior

Lamina arcus
vertebrae

Lig. flavum

Proc. spinosus,
Tubercula

Fig. 807 Cervical part of the vertebral column;
computed tomographic cross-section (CT) at the level
of the intervertebral disc between the fourth and the fifth
cervical vertebra.

* Endotracheal tube and endoscope

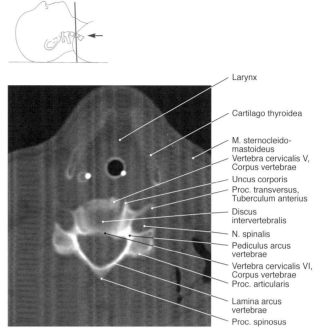

Larynx

Cartilago thyroidea

M. sternocleido-
mastoideus

Vertebra cervicalis V,
Corpus vertebrae

Uncus corporis

Proc. transversus,
Tuberculum anterius

Discus
intervertebralis

N. spinalis

Pediculus arcus
vertebrae

Vertebra cervicalis VI,
Corpus vertebrae

Proc. articularis

Lamina arcus
vertebrae

Proc. spinosus

Fig. 808 Cervical part of the vertebral column;
computed tomographic cross-section (CT) at the level
of the fifth and the sixth cervical vertebra.

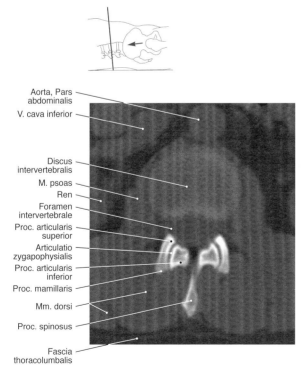

Aorta, Pars
abdominalis

V. cava inferior

Discus
intervertebralis

M. psoas

Ren

Foramen
intervertebrale

Proc. articularis
superior

Articulatio
zygapophysialis

Proc. articularis
inferior

Proc. mamillaris

Mm. dorsi

Proc. spinosus

Fascia
thoracolumbalis

Fig. 809 Lumbar part of the vertebral column;
computed tomographic cross-section (CT) at the level
of the intervertebral disc between the second and
the third lumbar vertebra.

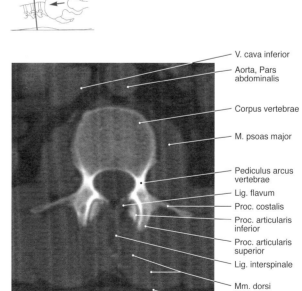

V. cava inferior

Aorta, Pars
abdominalis

Corpus vertebrae

M. psoas major

Pediculus arcus
vertebrae

Lig. flavum

Proc. costalis

Proc. articularis
inferior

Proc. articularis
superior

Lig. interspinale

Mm. dorsi

Fascia
thoracolumbalis

Fig. 810 Lumbar part of the vertebral column;
computed tomographic cross-section (CT) at the level
of the pedicles of the third lumbar vertebra.

Cutaneous innervation

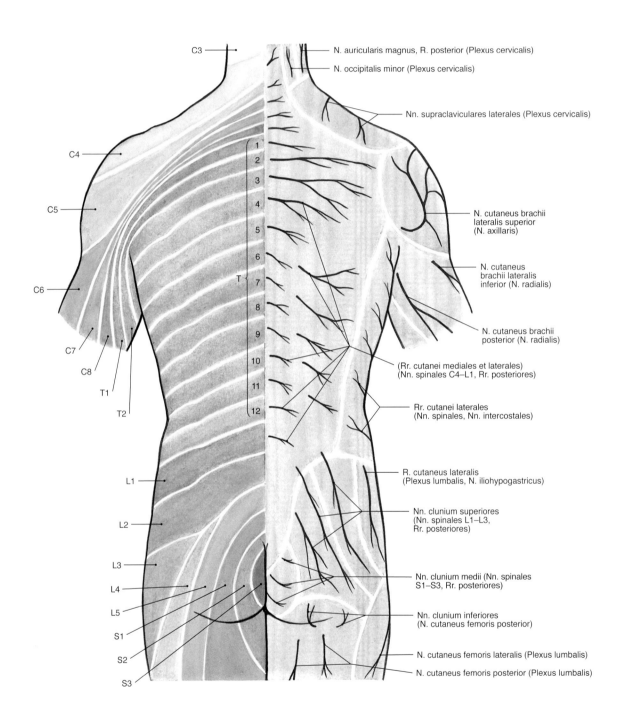

C3

C4

C5

C6

C7

C8

T1

T2

L1

L2

L3

L4

L5

S1

S2

S3

N. auricularis magnus, R. posterior (Plexus cervicalis)

N. occipitalis minor (Plexus cervicalis)

Nn. supraclaviculares laterales (Plexus cervicalis)

N. cutaneus brachii lateralis superior (N. axillaris)

N. cutaneus brachii lateralis inferior (N. radialis)

N. cutaneus brachii posterior (N. radialis)

(Rr. cutanei mediales et laterales) (Nn. spinales C4–L1, Rr. posteriores)

Rr. cutanei laterales (Nn. spinales, Nn. intercostales)

R. cutaneus lateralis (Plexus lumbalis, N. iliohypogastricus)

Nn. clunium superiores (Nn. spinales L1–L3, Rr. posteriores)

Nn. clunium medii (Nn. spinales S1–S3, Rr. posteriores)

Nn. clunium inferiores (N. cutaneus femoris posterior)

N. cutaneus femoris lateralis (Plexus lumbalis)

N. cutaneus femoris posterior (Plexus lumbalis)

Fig. 811   Segmental cutaneous innervation (dermatomes) and cutaneous nerves of the back.

Vessels and nerves of the back

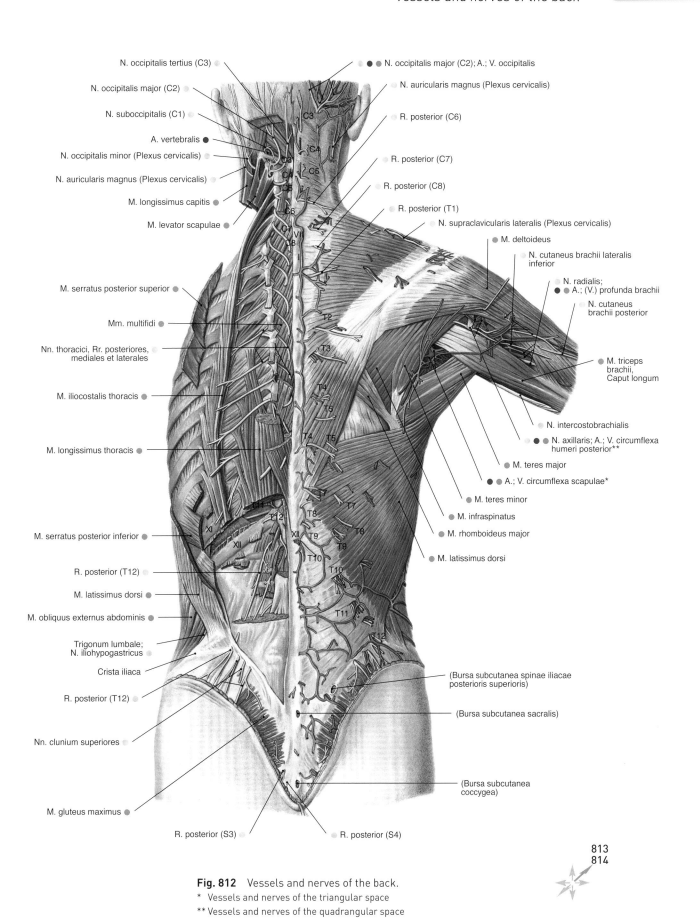

N. occipitalis tertius (C3)

N. occipitalis major (C2)

N. suboccipitalis (C1)

A. vertebralis ●

N. occipitalis minor (Plexus cervicalis)

N. auricularis magnus (Plexus cervicalis)

M. longissimus capitis ●

M. levator scapulae ●

M. serratus posterior superior ●

Mm. multifidi ●

Nn. thoracici, Rr. posteriores, mediales et laterales

M. iliocostalis thoracis ●

M. longissimus thoracis ●

M. serratus posterior inferior ●

R. posterior (T12) ●

M. latissimus dorsi ●

M. obliquus externus abdominis ●

Trigonum lumbale; N. iliohypogastricus

Crista iliaca

R. posterior (T12) ●

Nn. clunium superiores ●

M. gluteus maximus ●

R. posterior (S3)

N. occipitalis major (C2); A.; V. occipitalis ● ●

N. auricularis magnus (Plexus cervicalis)

R. posterior (C6)

R. posterior (C7)

R. posterior (C8)

R. posterior (T1)

N. supraclavicularis lateralis (Plexus cervicalis)

M. deltoideus ●

N. cutaneus brachii lateralis inferior

N. radialis; ● ● A.; (V.) profunda brachii

N. cutaneus brachii posterior

M. triceps brachii, Caput longum ●

N. intercostobrachialis

N. axillaris; A.; V. circumflexa ● ● ● humeri posterior**

M. teres major ●

A.; V. circumflexa scapulae* ● ●

M. teres minor ●

M. infraspinatus ●

M. rhomboideus major ●

M. latissimus dorsi ●

(Bursa subcutanea spinae iliacae posterioris superioris)

(Bursa subcutanea sacralis)

(Bursa subcutanea coccygea)

R. posterior (S4)

C3
C4
C5
C4
C5
C6
C7
VII
C8
T2
T3
T4
T5
T4 T5
T11
T12
XI
XII
XII
T7
T8
T9
T8
T9
T10
T10
T11
T12

813
814

Fig. 812   Vessels and nerves of the back.
*   Vessels and nerves of the triangular space
** Vessels and nerves of the quadrangular space

Vessels and nerves of the posterior cervical region

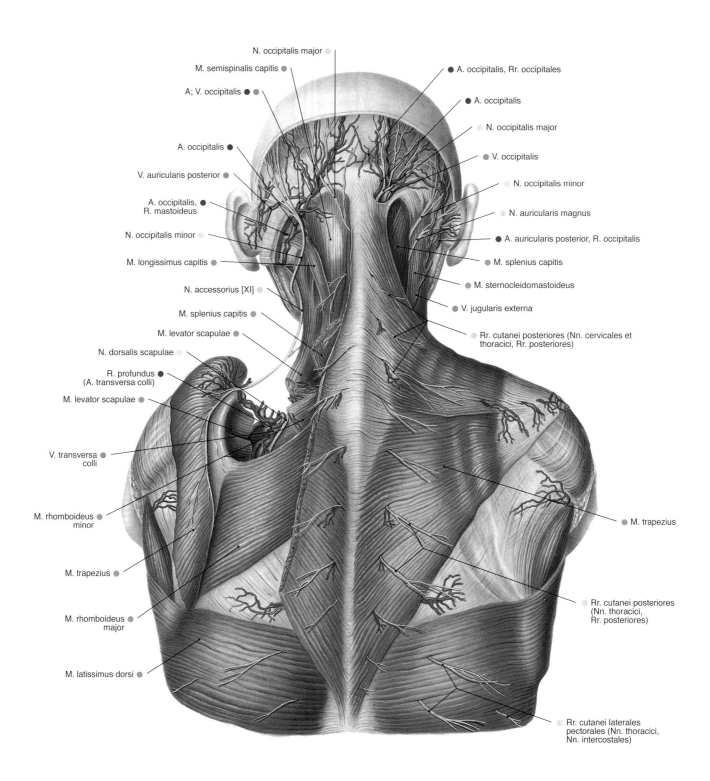

N. occipitalis major

M. semispinalis capitis

A; V. occipitalis

A. occipitalis

V. auricularis posterior

A. occipitalis,
R. mastoideus

N. occipitalis minor

M. longissimus capitis

N. accessorius [XI]

M. splenius capitis

M. levator scapulae

N. dorsalis scapulae

R. profundus
(A. transversa colli)

M. levator scapulae

V. transversa
colli

M. rhomboideus
minor

M. trapezius

M. rhomboideus
major

M. latissimus dorsi

A. occipitalis, Rr. occipitales

A. occipitalis

N. occipitalis major

V. occipitalis

N. occipitalis minor

N. auricularis magnus

A. auricularis posterior, R. occipitalis

M. splenius capitis

M. sternocleidomastoideus

V. jugularis externa

Rr. cutanei posteriores (Nn. cervicales et
thoracici, Rr. posteriores)

M. trapezius

Rr. cutanei posteriores
(Nn. thoracici,
Rr. posteriores)

Rr. cutanei laterales
pectorales (Nn. thoracici,
Nn. intercostales)

814

812

Fig. 813 Vessels and nerves of the occipital region,
Regio occipitalis, the posterior cervical region,
Regio cervicalis posterior, and the upper back.

Vessels and nerves of the posterior cervical region

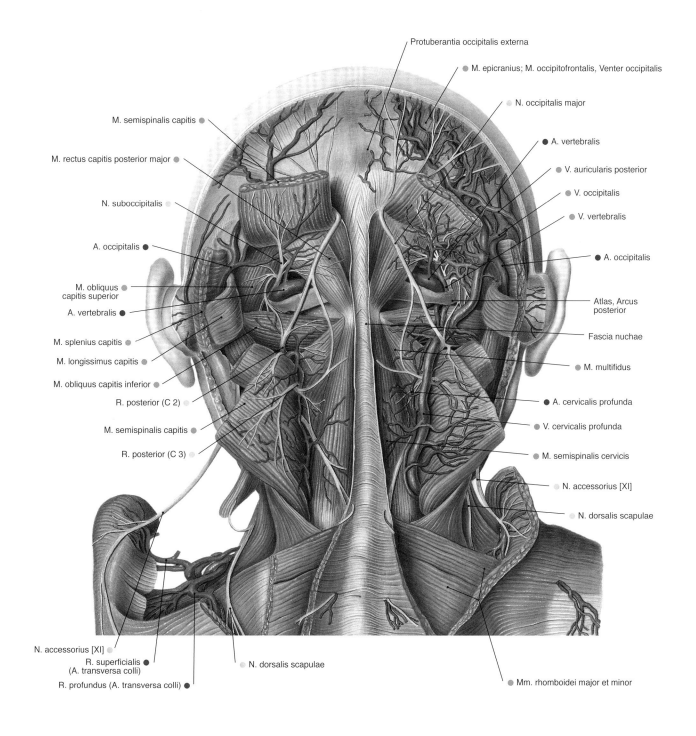

Protuberantia occipitalis externa

● M. epicranius; M. occipitofrontalis, Venter occipitalis

● N. occipitalis major

● A. vertebralis

● V. auricularis posterior

● V. occipitalis

● V. vertebralis

● A. occipitalis

Atlas, Arcus posterior

Fascia nuchae

● M. multifidus

● A. cervicalis profunda

● V. cervicalis profunda

● M. semispinalis cervicis

● N. accessorius [XI]

● N. dorsalis scapulae

● Mm. rhomboidei major et minor

M. semispinalis capitis ●

M. rectus capitis posterior major ●

N. suboccipitalis ●

A. occipitalis ●

M. obliquus ● capitis superior

A. vertebralis ●

M. splenius capitis ●

M. longissimus capitis ●

M. obliquus capitis inferior ●

R. posterior (C 2) ●

M. semispinalis capitis ●

R. posterior (C 3) ●

N. accessorius [XI] ●

R. superficialis ● (A. transversa colli)

R. profundus (A. transversa colli) ●

● N. dorsalis scapulae

Fig. 814   Vessels and nerves of the occipital region, Regio occipitalis, and the posterior cervical region, Regio cervicalis posterior.

815

813

Cervical part of the vertebral canal

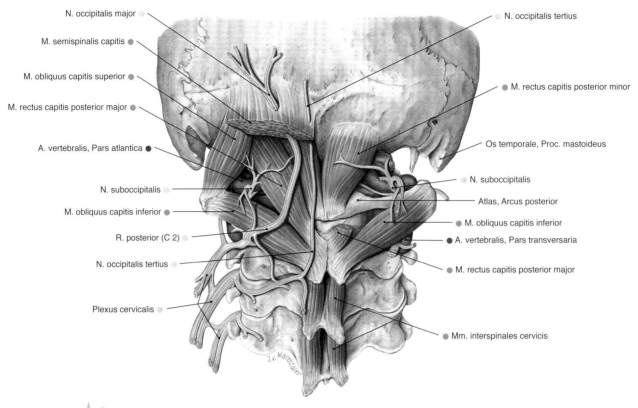

N. occipitalis major

M. semispinalis capitis

M. obliquus capitis superior

M. rectus capitis posterior major

A. vertebralis, Pars atlantica ●

N. suboccipitalis

M. obliquus capitis inferior

R. posterior (C 2)

N. occipitalis tertius

Plexus cervicalis

N. occipitalis tertius

M. rectus capitis posterior minor

Os temporale, Proc. mastoideus

N. suboccipitalis

Atlas, Arcus posterior

M. obliquus capitis inferior

● A. vertebralis, Pars transversaria

M. rectus capitis posterior major

Mm. interspinales cervicis

Fig. 815   Nerves of the posterior cervical region, Regio cervicalis posterior, and the vertebral artery, A. vertebralis.

814

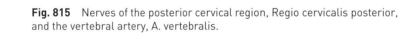

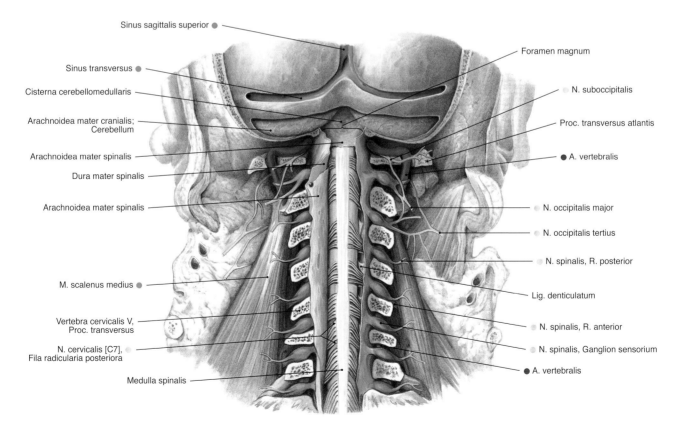

Sinus sagittalis superior

Sinus transversus

Cisterna cerebellomedullaris

Arachnoidea mater cranialis; Cerebellum

Arachnoidea mater spinalis

Dura mater spinalis

Arachnoidea mater spinalis

M. scalenus medius

Vertebra cervicalis V, Proc. transversus

N. cervicalis [C7], Fila radicularia posteriora

Medulla spinalis

Foramen magnum

N. suboccipitalis

Proc. transversus atlantis

● A. vertebralis

N. occipitalis major

N. occipitalis tertius

N. spinalis, R. posterior

Lig. denticulatum

N. spinalis, R. anterior

N. spinalis, Ganglion sensorium

● A. vertebralis

Fig. 816   Vessels and nerves of the deep posterior cervical region, Regio cervicalis posterior, and the content of the vertebral canal.

Lumbar part of the vertebral canal

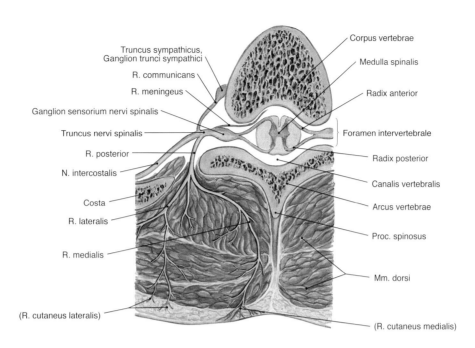

Truncus sympathicus, Ganglion trunci sympathici
R. communicans
R. meningeus
Ganglion sensorium nervi spinalis
Truncus nervi spinalis
R. posterior
N. intercostalis
Costa
R. lateralis
R. medialis
(R. cutaneus lateralis)

Corpus vertebrae
Medulla spinalis
Radix anterior
Foramen intervertebrale
Radix posterior
Canalis vertebralis
Arcus vertebrae
Proc. spinosus
Mm. dorsi
(R. cutaneus medialis)

Fig. 817   Spinal nerve, N. spinalis; in the thoracic region.

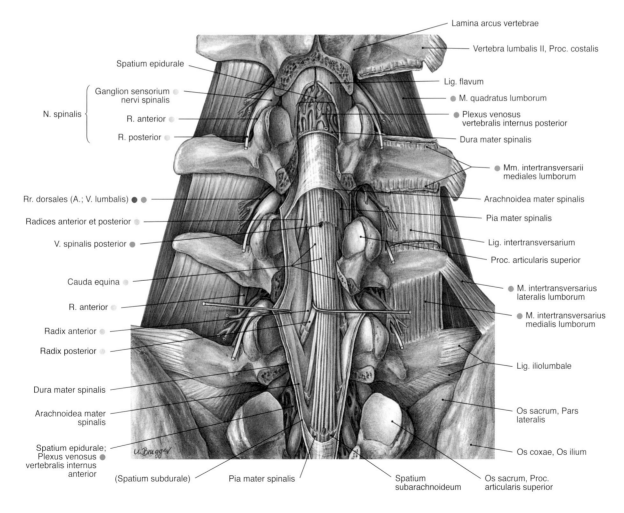

Spatium epidurale
Ganglion sensorium nervi spinalis
N. spinalis
R. anterior
R. posterior
Rr. dorsales (A.; V. lumbalis) ● ●
Radices anterior et posterior ●
V. spinalis posterior ●
Cauda equina ●
R. anterior ●
Radix anterior ●
Radix posterior ●
Dura mater spinalis
Arachnoidea mater spinalis
Spatium epidurale; Plexus venosus ● vertebralis internus anterior
(Spatium subdurale)
Pia mater spinalis
Spatium subarachnoideum

Lamina arcus vertebrae
Vertebra lumbalis II, Proc. costalis
Lig. flavum
● M. quadratus lumborum
● Plexus venosus vertebralis internus posterior
Dura mater spinalis
● Mm. intertransversarii mediales lumborum
Arachnoidea mater spinalis
Pia mater spinalis
Lig. intertransversarium
Proc. articularis superior
● M. intertransversarius lateralis lumborum
● M. intertransversarius medialis lumborum
Lig. iliolumbale
Os sacrum, Pars lateralis
Os coxae, Os ilium
Os sacrum, Proc. articularis superior

Fig. 818   Vessels and nerves of the lumbar part of the vertebral canal, Regio lumbalis.

Veins and nerves of the lumbar part of the vertebral column

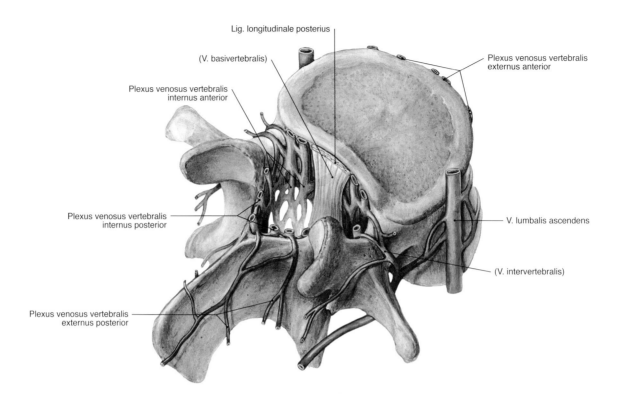

Lig. longitudinale posterius

(V. basivertebralis)

Plexus venosus vertebralis
internus anterior

Plexus venosus vertebralis
internus posterior

Plexus venosus vertebralis
externus posterior

Plexus venosus vertebralis
externus anterior

V. lumbalis ascendens

(V. intervertebralis)

Fig. 819 Veins of the vertebral canal, Canalis vertebralis;
venous plexus.

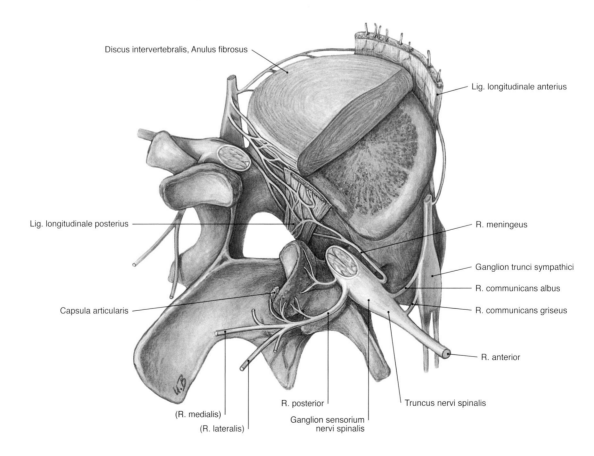

Discus intervertebralis, Anulus fibrosus

Lig. longitudinale anterius

Lig. longitudinale posterius

Capsula articularis

R. meningeus

Ganglion trunci sympathici

R. communicans albus

R. communicans griseus

R. anterior

Truncus nervi spinalis

(R. medialis)

(R. lateralis)

R. posterior

Ganglion sensorium
nervi spinalis

Fig. 820 Nerves of the vertebral column, Columna vertebralis;
somatic and autonomous innervation.

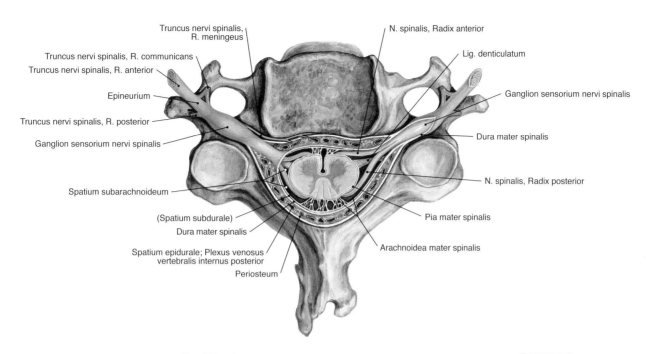

Truncus nervi spinalis, R. meningeus
Truncus nervi spinalis, R. communicans
Truncus nervi spinalis, R. anterior
Epineurium
Truncus nervi spinalis, R. posterior
Ganglion sensorium nervi spinalis
Spatium subarachnoideum
(Spatium subdurale)
Dura mater spinalis
Spatium epidurale; Plexus venosus vertebralis internus posterior
Periosteum

N. spinalis, Radix anterior
Lig. denticulatum
Ganglion sensorium nervi spinalis
Dura mater spinalis
N. spinalis, Radix posterior
Pia mater spinalis
Arachnoidea mater spinalis

Fig. 821 Content of the vertebral canal, Canalis vertebralis; cross-section at the level of the fifth cervical vertebra.

→ 599 ff

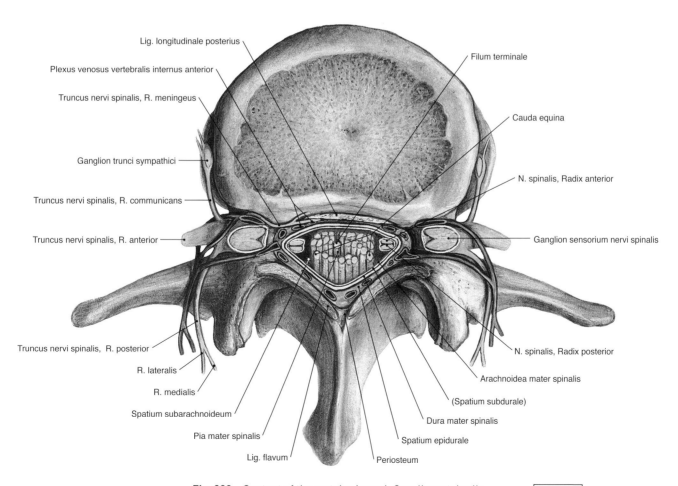

Lig. longitudinale posterius
Plexus venosus vertebralis internus anterior
Truncus nervi spinalis, R. meningeus
Ganglion trunci sympathici
Truncus nervi spinalis, R. communicans
Truncus nervi spinalis, R. anterior
Truncus nervi spinalis, R. posterior
R. lateralis
R. medialis
Spatium subarachnoideum
Pia mater spinalis
Lig. flavum

Filum terminale
Cauda equina
N. spinalis, Radix anterior
Ganglion sensorium nervi spinalis
N. spinalis, Radix posterior
Arachnoidea mater spinalis
(Spatium subdurale)
Dura mater spinalis
Spatium epidurale
Periosteum

Fig. 822 Content of the vertebral canal, Canalis vertebralis; cross-section at the level of the third lumbar vertebra.

→ 599 ff

Lumbar and sacral puncture

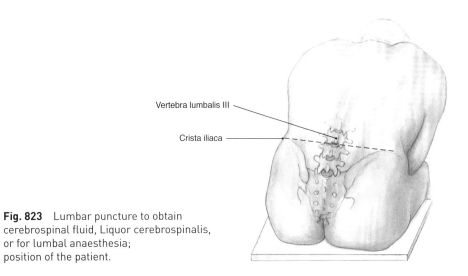

Vertebra lumbalis III

Crista iliaca

Fig. 823 Lumbar puncture to obtain cerebrospinal fluid, Liquor cerebrospinalis, or for lumbal anaesthesia; position of the patient.

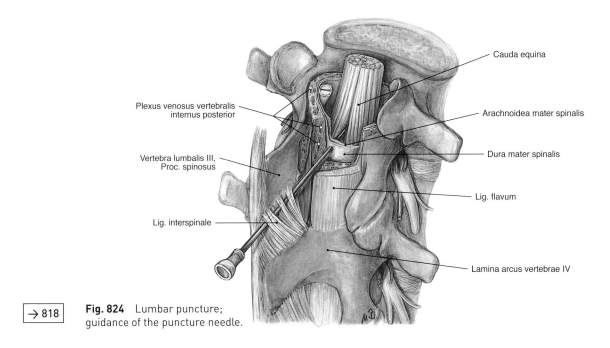

Cauda equina

Plexus venosus vertebralis internus posterior

Arachnoidea mater spinalis

Vertebra lumbalis III, Proc. spinosus

Dura mater spinalis

Lig. flavum

Lig. interspinale

Lamina arcus vertebrae IV

→ 818 **Fig. 824** Lumbar puncture; guidance of the puncture needle.

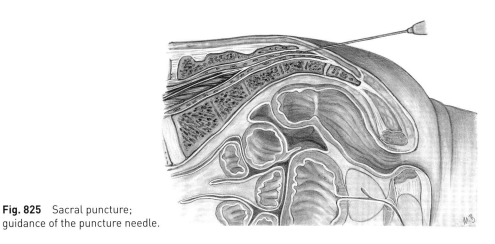

Fig. 825 Sacral puncture; guidance of the puncture needle.

Vessels and nerves of the vertebral canal

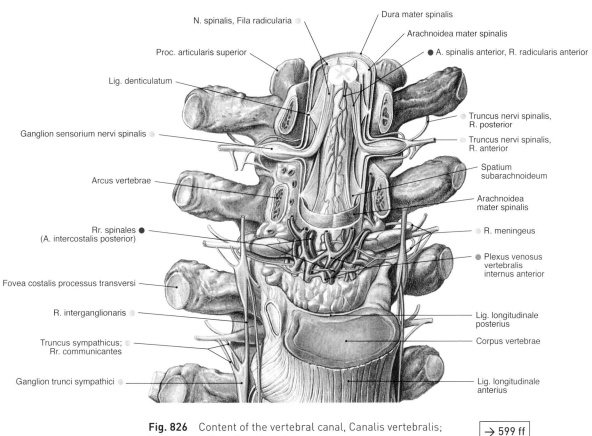

N. spinalis, Fila radicularia

Proc. articularis superior

Lig. denticulatum

Ganglion sensorium nervi spinalis

Arcus vertebrae

Rr. spinales ●
(A. intercostalis posterior)

Fovea costalis processus transversi

R. interganglionaris

Truncus sympathicus;
Rr. communicantes

Ganglion trunci sympathici ●

Dura mater spinalis

Arachnoidea mater spinalis

● A. spinalis anterior, R. radicularis anterior

Truncus nervi spinalis,
R. posterior

Truncus nervi spinalis,
R. anterior

Spatium
subarachnoideum

Arachnoidea
mater spinalis

R. meningeus

● Plexus venosus
vertebralis
internus anterior

Lig. longitudinale
posterius

Corpus vertebrae

Lig. longitudinale
anterius

Fig. 826   Content of the vertebral canal, Canalis vertebralis;
thoracic portion after stepwise exposure;
ventral view.

→ 599 ff

R. communicans

R. meningeus

Truncus nervi spinalis (L3)

R. posterior

R. anterior

Radix anterior

Radix posterior

Spatium subarachnoideum

Lig. flavum

Discus intervertebralis,
Anulus fibrosus

a

b

Fig. 827 a, b   Intervertebral foramina, Foramina intervertebralia;
lumbar part of the vertebral column.

a Viewed from the left
b Sagittal section

Surface anatomy

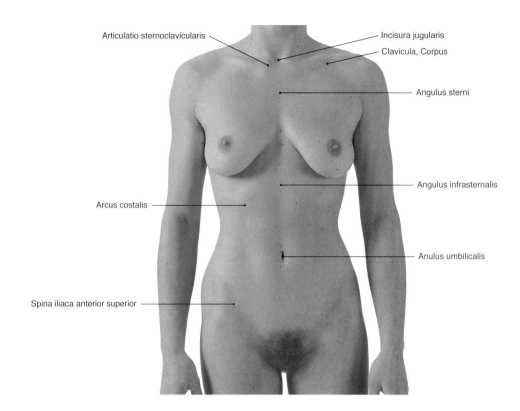

Fig. 828   Surface anatomy of the thoracic and abdominal wall of a young woman.

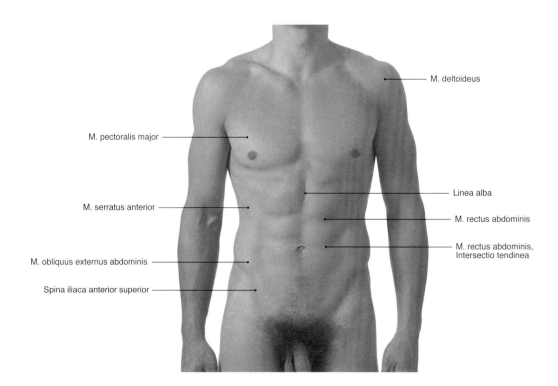

Fig. 829   Surface anatomy of the thoracic and abdominal wall of a young man.

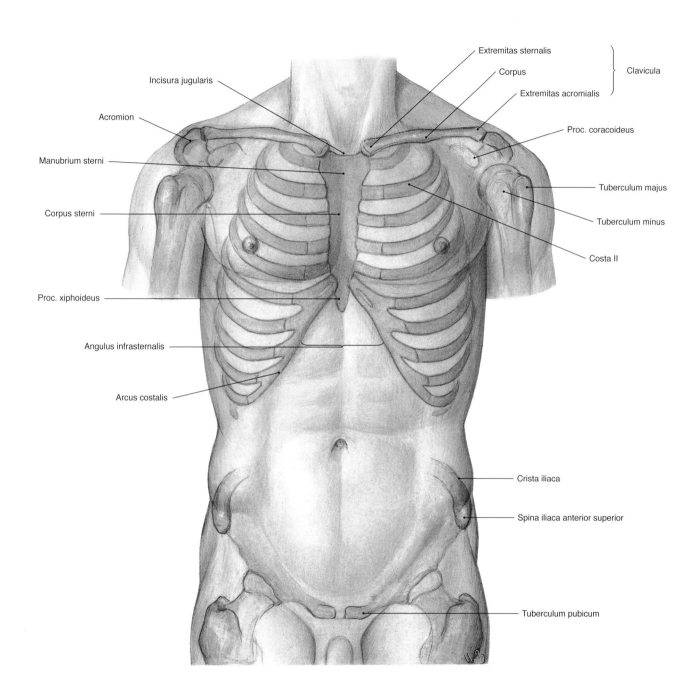

Incisura jugularis

Extremitas sternalis

Corpus

Extremitas acromialis

Clavicula

Acromion

Proc. coracoideus

Manubrium sterni

Tuberculum majus

Corpus sterni

Tuberculum minus

Costa II

Proc. xiphoideus

Angulus infrasternalis

Arcus costalis

Crista iliaca

Spina iliaca anterior superior

Tuberculum pubicum

Fig. 830   Projection of the skeleton
onto the thoracic and abdominal wall.

Skeleton of the trunk

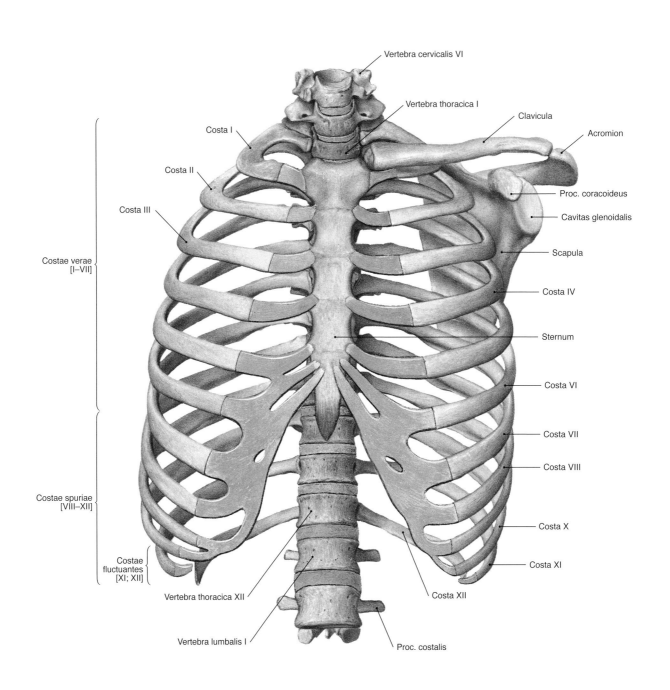

Fig. 831   Thoracic cage, Cavea thoracis, and left shoulder girdle, Cingulum pectorale.

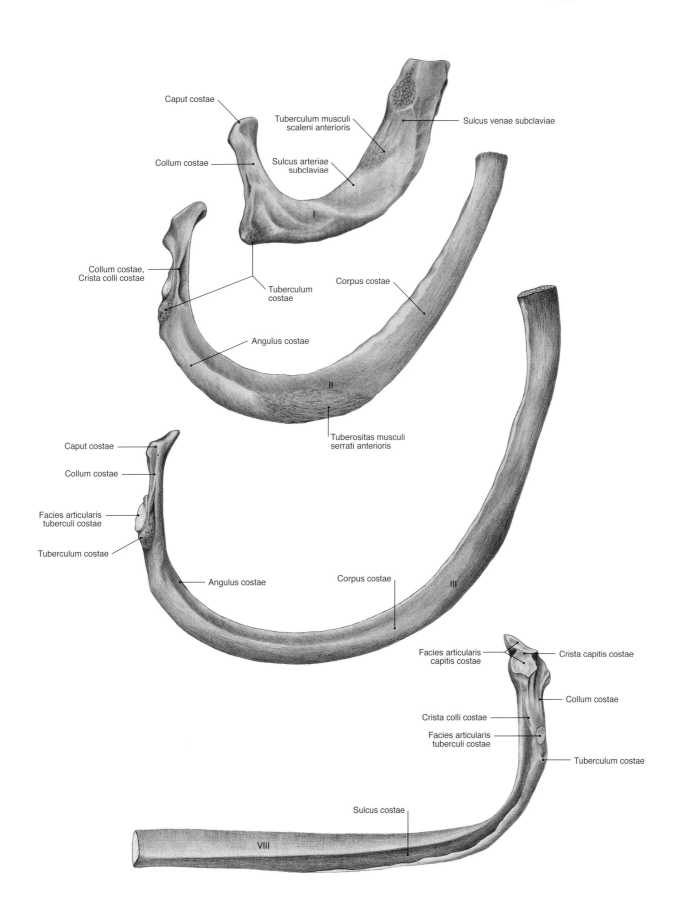

Caput costae

Tuberculum musculi scaleni anterioris

Sulcus venae subclaviae

Collum costae

Sulcus arteriae subclaviae

Collum costae, Crista colli costae

Corpus costae

Tuberculum costae

Angulus costae

Tuberositas musculi serrati anterioris

Caput costae

Collum costae

Facies articularis tuberculi costae

Tuberculum costae

Angulus costae

Corpus costae

Facies articularis capitis costae

Crista capitis costae

Collum costae

Crista colli costae

Facies articularis tuberculi costae

Tuberculum costae

Sulcus costae

Fig. 832 Ribs, Costae;
I.–III. rib, superior view;
VIII. rib, inferior view.

Sternum

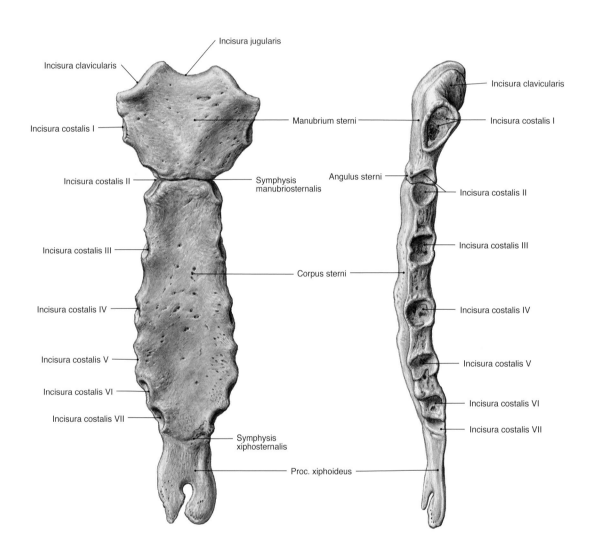

Fig. 833 Sternum, Sternum.　　**Fig. 834** Sternum, Sternum.

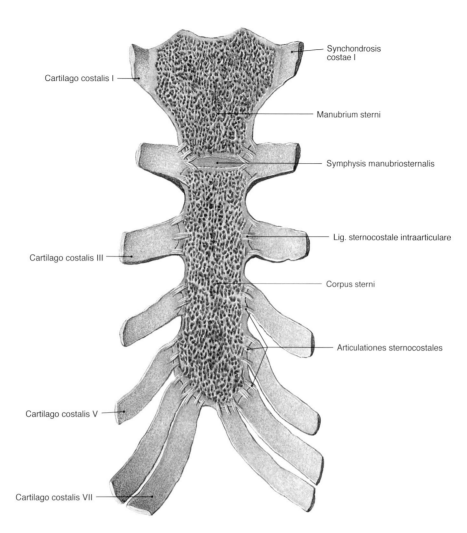

Cartilago costalis I

Synchondrosis costae I

Manubrium sterni

Symphysis manubriosternalis

Lig. sternocostale intraarticulare

Cartilago costalis III

Corpus sterni

Articulationes sternocostales

Cartilago costalis V

Cartilago costalis VII

Fig. 835 Sternum, Sternum, and costal cartilages, Cartilagines costales; section.

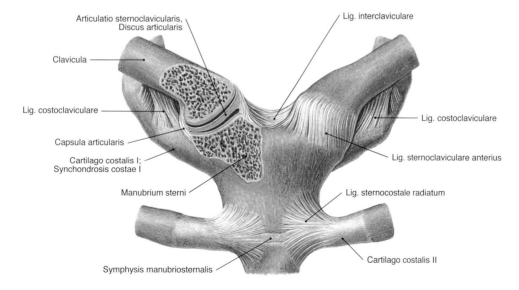

Articulatio sternoclavicularis, Discus articularis

Lig. interclaviculare

Clavicula

Lig. costoclaviculare

Lig. costoclaviculare

Capsula articularis

Cartilago costalis I; Synchondrosis costae I

Lig. sternoclaviculare anterius

Manubrium sterni

Lig. sternocostale radiatum

Symphysis manubriosternalis

Cartilago costalis II

Fig. 836 Sternoclavicular joint, Articulatio sternoclavicularis.

Muscles of the thoracic and the abdominal wall

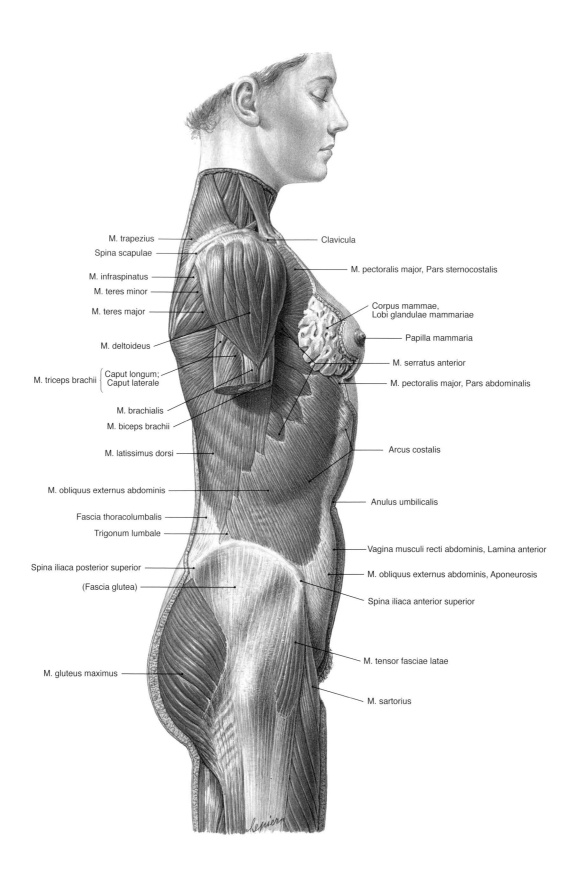

M. trapezius — Clavicula

Spina scapulae

M. infraspinatus

M. teres minor

M. teres major

M. deltoideus

M. triceps brachii { Caput longum; Caput laterale

M. brachialis

M. biceps brachii

M. latissimus dorsi

M. obliquus externus abdominis

Fascia thoracolumbalis

Trigonum lumbale

Spina iliaca posterior superior

(Fascia glutea)

M. gluteus maximus

M. pectoralis major, Pars sternocostalis

Corpus mammae, Lobi glandulae mammariae

Papilla mammaria

M. serratus anterior

M. pectoralis major, Pars abdominalis

Arcus costalis

Anulus umbilicalis

Vagina musculi recti abdominis, Lamina anterior

M. obliquus externus abdominis, Aponeurosis

Spina iliaca anterior superior

M. tensor fasciae latae

M. sartorius

→ T 15, T 17, T 18, T 26

Fig. 837   Muscles of the thoracic and the abdominal wall, Mm. thoracis et abdominis.

Muscles of the thoracic and the abdominal wall

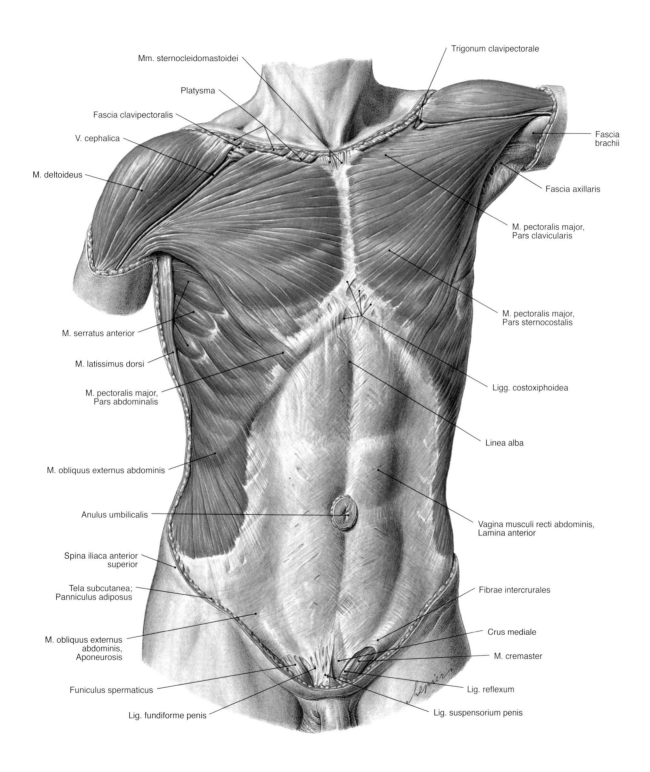

Mm. sternocleidomastoidei

Platysma

Fascia clavipectoralis

V. cephalica

M. deltoideus

M. serratus anterior

M. latissimus dorsi

M. pectoralis major,
Pars abdominalis

M. obliquus externus abdominis

Anulus umbilicalis

Spina iliaca anterior
superior

Tela subcutanea;
Panniculus adiposus

M. obliquus externus
abdominis,
Aponeurosis

Funiculus spermaticus

Lig. fundiforme penis

Trigonum clavipectorale

Fascia
brachii

Fascia axillaris

M. pectoralis major,
Pars clavicularis

M. pectoralis major,
Pars sternocostalis

Ligg. costoxiphoidea

Linea alba

Vagina musculi recti abdominis,
Lamina anterior

Fibrae intercrurales

Crus mediale

M. cremaster

Lig. reflexum

Lig. suspensorium penis

Fig. 838 Muscles of the thoracic and the abdominal wall;
superficial layer.

→ T 15, T 17, T 18, T 26

Muscles of the thoracic and the abdominal wall

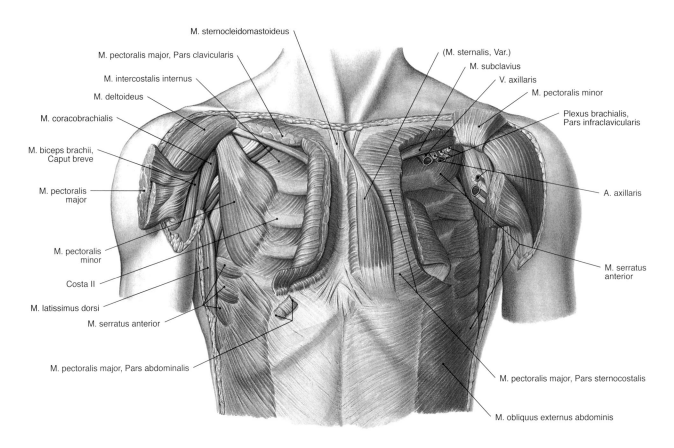

M. sternocleidomastoideus
M. pectoralis major, Pars clavicularis
M. intercostalis internus
M. deltoideus
M. coracobrachialis
M. biceps brachii, Caput breve
M. pectoralis major
M. pectoralis minor
Costa II
M. latissimus dorsi
M. serratus anterior
M. pectoralis major, Pars abdominalis

(M. sternalis, Var.)
M. subclavius
V. axillaris
M. pectoralis minor
Plexus brachialis, Pars infraclavicularis
A. axillaris
M. serratus anterior
M. pectoralis major, Pars sternocostalis
M. obliquus externus abdominis

→ T 13, T 15, T 26

Fig. 839   Muscles of the thoracic wall, Mm. thoracis.

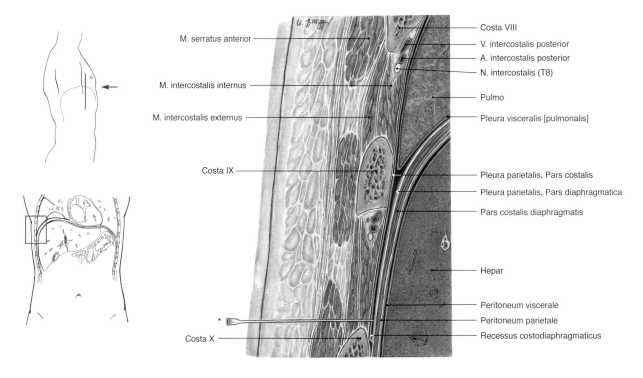

M. serratus anterior
M. intercostalis internus
M. intercostalis externus
Costa IX
Costa X

Costa VIII
V. intercostalis posterior
A. intercostalis posterior
N. intercostalis (T8)
Pulmo
Pleura visceralis [pulmonalis]
Pleura parietalis, Pars costalis
Pleura parietalis, Pars diaphragmatica
Pars costalis diaphragmatis
Hepar
Peritoneum viscerale
Peritoneum parietale
Recessus costodiaphragmaticus

→ T 13

Fig. 840   Muscles of the thoracic wall, Mm. thoracis;
frontal section.
* Position of the needle for puncture of the pleural cavity (pleurocentesis)

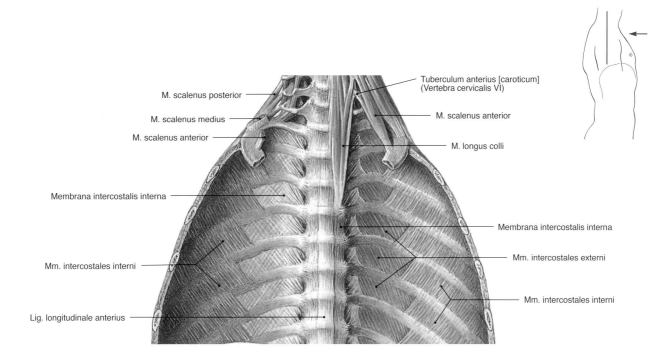

M. scalenus posterior

M. scalenus medius

M. scalenus anterior

Membrana intercostalis interna

Mm. intercostales interni

Lig. longitudinale anterius

Tuberculum anterius [caroticum]
(Vertebra cervicalis VI)

M. scalenus anterior

M. longus colli

Membrana intercostalis interna

Mm. intercostales externi

Mm. intercostales interni

Fig. 841   Thoracic cage, Cavea thoracis;
posterior wall.

→ T 11–T 13

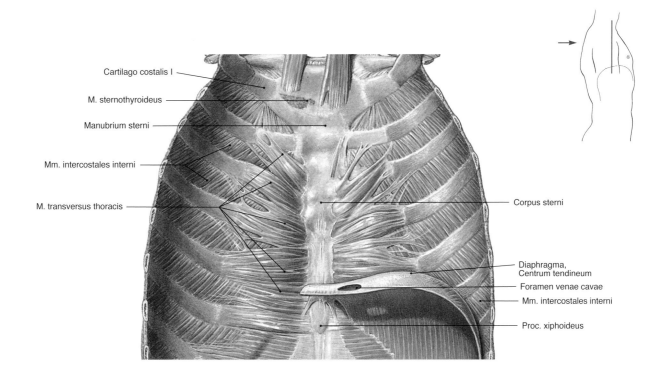

Cartilago costalis I

M. sternothyroideus

Manubrium sterni

Mm. intercostales interni

M. transversus thoracis

Corpus sterni

Diaphragma,
Centrum tendineum

Foramen venae cavae

Mm. intercostales interni

Proc. xiphoideus

Fig. 842   Thoracic cage, Cavea thoracis;
anterior wall.

→ T 13

Abdominal muscles

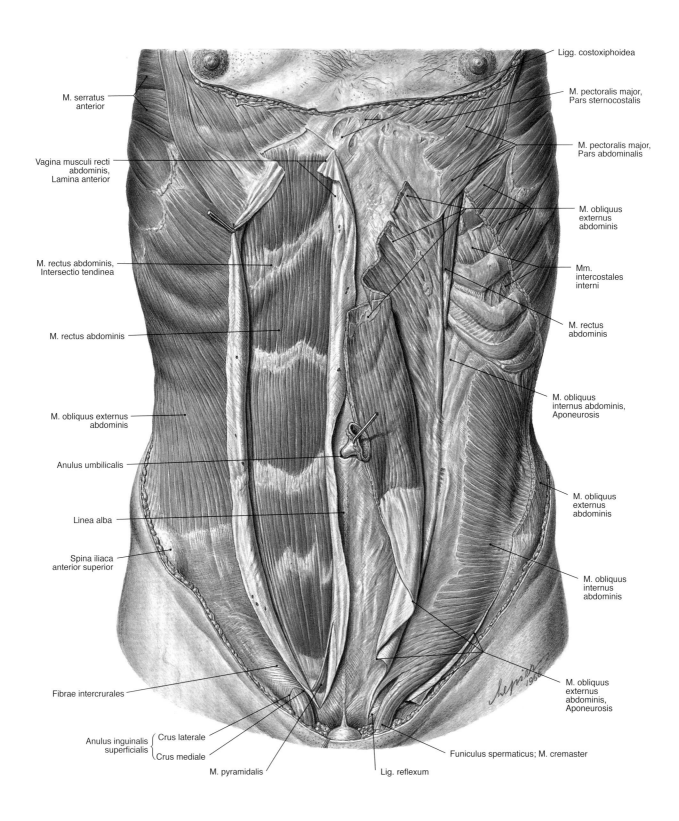

Ligg. costoxiphoidea

M. serratus anterior

M. pectoralis major, Pars sternocostalis

Vagina musculi recti abdominis, Lamina anterior

M. pectoralis major, Pars abdominalis

M. rectus abdominis, Intersectio tendinea

M. obliquus externus abdominis

M. rectus abdominis

Mm. intercostales interni

M. obliquus externus abdominis

M. rectus abdominis

Anulus umbilicalis

M. obliquus internus abdominis, Aponeurosis

Linea alba

M. obliquus externus abdominis

Spina iliaca anterior superior

M. obliquus internus abdominis

Fibrae intercrurales

M. obliquus externus abdominis, Aponeurosis

Anulus inguinalis superficialis { Crus laterale / Crus mediale }

Funiculus spermaticus; M. cremaster

M. pyramidalis

Lig. reflexum

→ T 13–T 15, T 17, T 26

Fig. 843   Muscles of the abdominal wall, Mm. abdominis; superficial and middle layer.

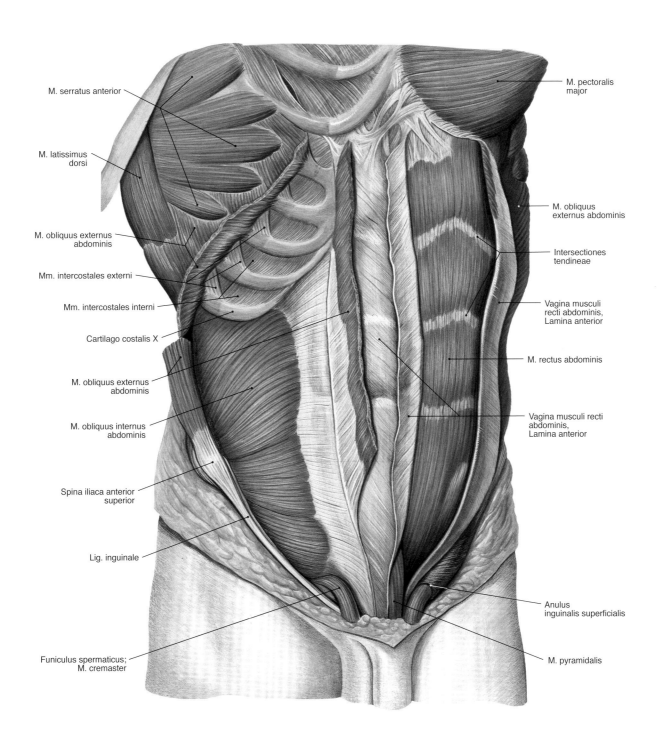

M. serratus anterior

M. latissimus dorsi

M. obliquus externus abdominis

Mm. intercostales externi

Mm. intercostales interni

Cartilago costalis X

M. obliquus externus abdominis

M. obliquus internus abdominis

Spina iliaca anterior superior

Lig. inguinale

Funiculus spermaticus; M. cremaster

M. pectoralis major

M. obliquus externus abdominis

Intersectiones tendineae

Vagina musculi recti abdominis, Lamina anterior

M. rectus abdominis

Vagina musculi recti abdominis, Lamina anterior

Anulus inguinalis superficialis

M. pyramidalis

Fig. 844 Muscles of the abdominal wall, Mm. abdominis; middle layer.

→ T 13–T 15, T 17

Abdominal muscles

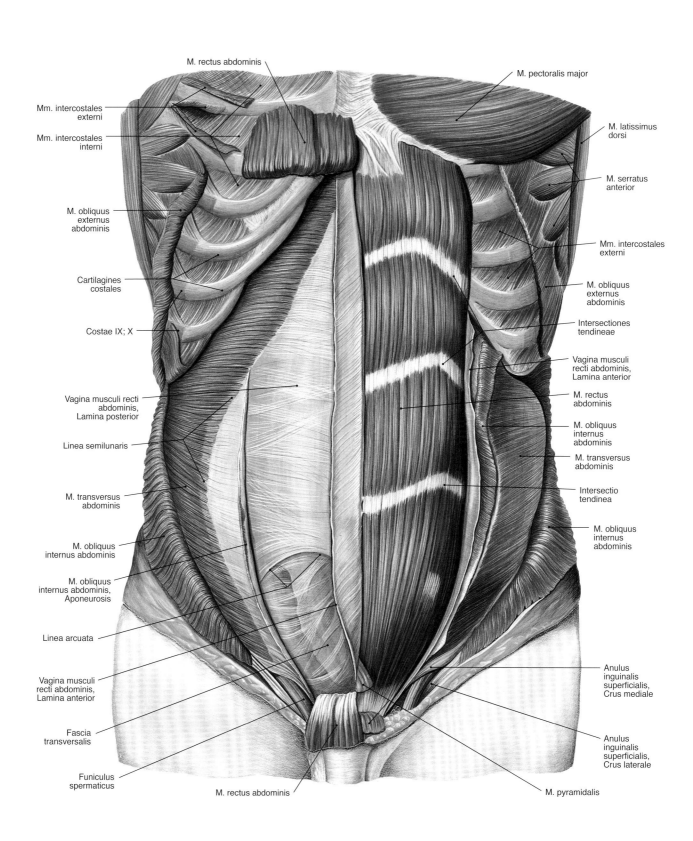

M. rectus abdominis

Mm. intercostales externi

Mm. intercostales interni

M. obliquus externus abdominis

Cartilagines costales

Costae IX; X

Vagina musculi recti abdominis, Lamina posterior

Linea semilunaris

M. transversus abdominis

M. obliquus internus abdominis

M. obliquus internus abdominis, Aponeurosis

Linea arcuata

Vagina musculi recti abdominis, Lamina anterior

Fascia transversalis

Funiculus spermaticus

M. rectus abdominis

M. pectoralis major

M. latissimus dorsi

M. serratus anterior

Mm. intercostales externi

M. obliquus externus abdominis

Intersectiones tendineae

Vagina musculi recti abdominis, Lamina anterior

M. rectus abdominis

M. obliquus internus abdominis

M. transversus abdominis

Intersectio tendinea

M. obliquus internus abdominis

Anulus inguinalis superficialis, Crus mediale

Anulus inguinalis superficialis, Crus laterale

M. pyramidalis

→ T 13–T 15

Fig. 845 Muscles of the abdominal wall, Mm. abdominis; deep layer.

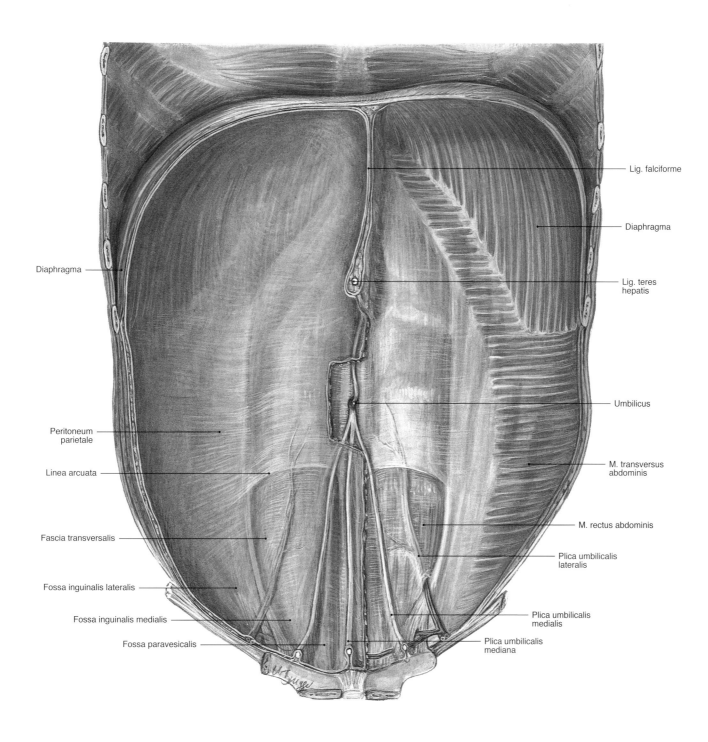

Lig. falciforme

Diaphragma

Lig. teres hepatis

Diaphragma

Umbilicus

Peritoneum parietale

M. transversus abdominis

Linea arcuata

M. rectus abdominis

Fascia transversalis

Plica umbilicalis lateralis

Fossa inguinalis lateralis

Plica umbilicalis medialis

Fossa inguinalis medialis

Plica umbilicalis mediana

Fossa paravesicalis

Fig. 846   Internal surface of the anterior abdominal wall.

→ T 14, T 15, T 21

Inguinal canal

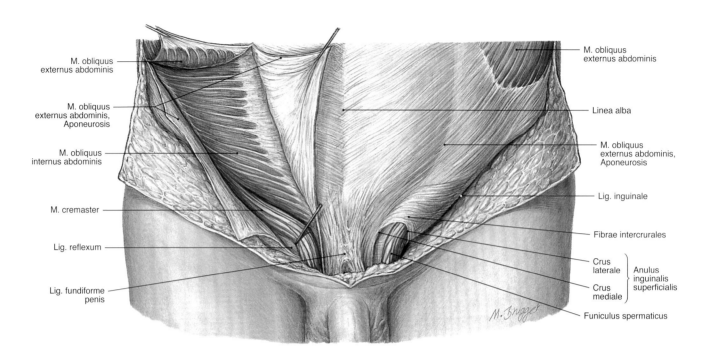

M. obliquus
externus abdominis

M. obliquus
externus abdominis,
Aponeurosis

M. obliquus
internus abdominis

M. cremaster

Lig. reflexum

Lig. fundiforme
penis

M. obliquus
externus abdominis

Linea alba

M. obliquus
externus abdominis,
Aponeurosis

Lig. inguinale

Fibrae intercrurales

Crus
laterale ⎫ Anulus
⎬ inguinalis
Crus ⎭ superficialis
mediale

Funiculus spermaticus

Fig. 847   Superficial inguinal ring, Anulus inguinalis superficialis.

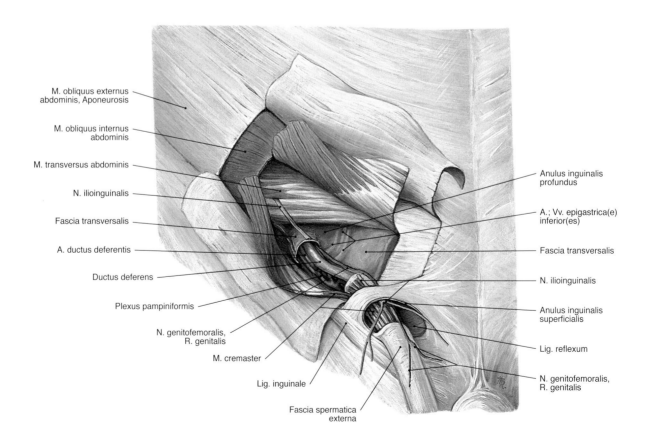

M. obliquus externus
abdominis, Aponeurosis

M. obliquus internus
abdominis

M. transversus abdominis

N. ilioinguinalis

Fascia transversalis

A. ductus deferentis

Ductus deferens

Plexus pampiniformis

N. genitofemoralis,
R. genitalis

M. cremaster

Lig. inguinale

Fascia spermatica
externa

Anulus inguinalis
profundus

A.; Vv. epigastrica(e)
inferior(es)

Fascia transversalis

N. ilioinguinalis

Anulus inguinalis
superficialis

Lig. reflexum

N. genitofemoralis,
R. genitalis

Fig. 848   Walls of the inguinal canal.

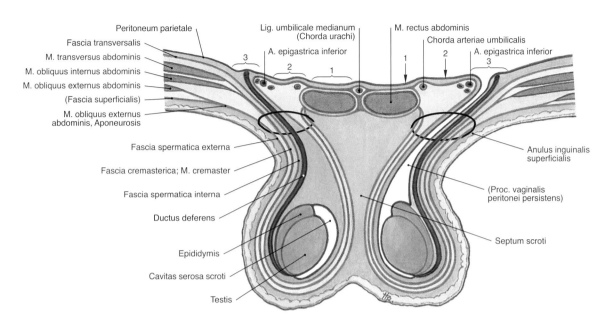

Peritoneum parietale
Fascia transversalis
M. transversus abdominis
M. obliquus internus abdominis
M. obliquus externus abdominis
(Fascia superficialis)
M. obliquus externus abdominis, Aponeurosis
Fascia spermatica externa
Fascia cremasterica; M. cremaster
Fascia spermatica interna
Ductus deferens
Epididymis
Cavitas serosa scroti
Testis

Lig. umbilicale medianum (Chorda urachi)
A. epigastrica inferior
M. rectus abdominis
Chorda arteriae umbilicalis
A. epigastrica inferior
Anulus inguinalis superficialis
(Proc. vaginalis peritonei persistens)
Septum scroti

Fig. 849 Diagram of the inguinal canal.
The inguinal canal, the spermatic cord and the scrotum are
illustrated in the same plane for didactical reasons.

1 Fossa supravesicalis
2 Fossa inguinalis medialis
3 Fossa inguinalis lateralis

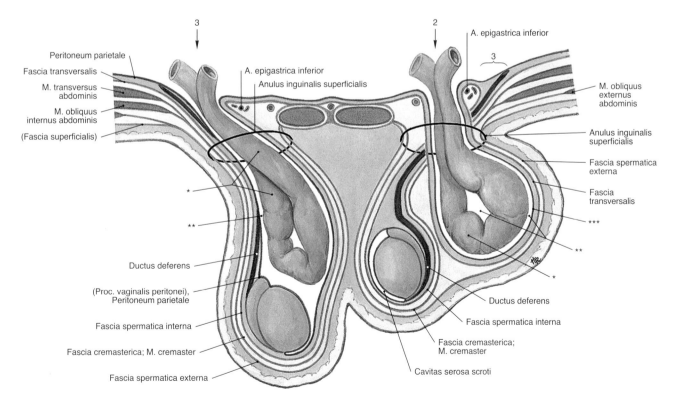

Peritoneum parietale
Fascia transversalis
M. transversus abdominis
M. obliquus internus abdominis
(Fascia superficialis)

A. epigastrica inferior
A. epigastrica inferior
Anulus inguinalis superficialis

M. obliquus externus abdominis
Anulus inguinalis superficialis
Fascia spermatica externa
Fascia transversalis

Ductus deferens
(Proc. vaginalis peritonei), Peritoneum parietale
Fascia spermatica interna
Fascia cremasterica; M. cremaster
Fascia spermatica externa

Ductus deferens
Fascia spermatica interna
Fascia cremasterica; M. cremaster
Cavitas serosa scroti

Fig. 850 Diagram of inguinal hernias;
left side: lateral, indirect hernia;
right side: medial, direct hernia.

* Hernial sac with an intestinal loop
** Peritoneal space
*** Newly formed peritoneal hernial sac

Diaphragm and posterior abdominal wall

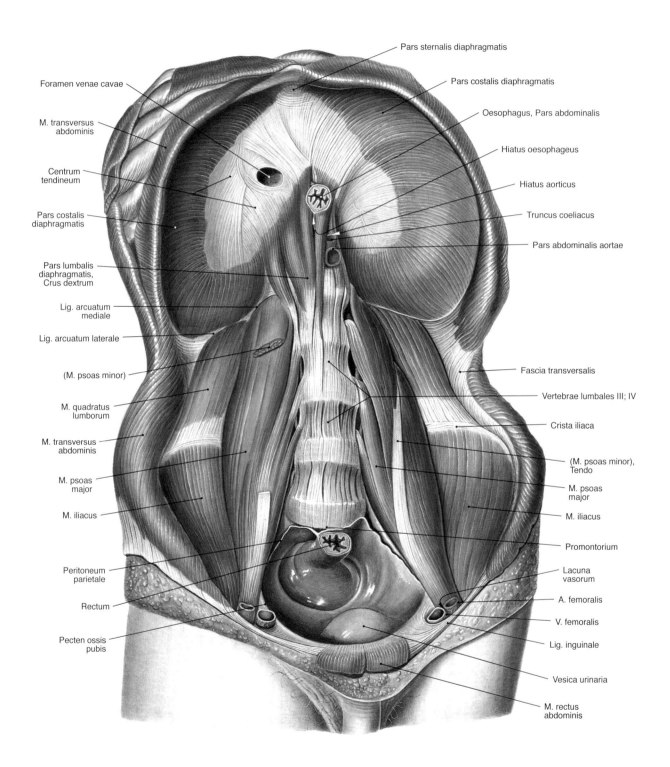

Pars sternalis diaphragmatis

Foramen venae cavae

Pars costalis diaphragmatis

M. transversus abdominis

Oesophagus, Pars abdominalis

Centrum tendineum

Hiatus oesophageus

Hiatus aorticus

Pars costalis diaphragmatis

Truncus coeliacus

Pars abdominalis aortae

Pars lumbalis diaphragmatis, Crus dextrum

Lig. arcuatum mediale

Lig. arcuatum laterale

Fascia transversalis

(M. psoas minor)

Vertebrae lumbales III; IV

M. quadratus lumborum

Crista iliaca

M. transversus abdominis

(M. psoas minor), Tendo

M. psoas major

M. psoas major

M. iliacus

M. iliacus

Promontorium

Peritoneum parietale

Lacuna vasorum

Rectum

A. femoralis

V. femoralis

Pecten ossis pubis

Lig. inguinale

Vesica urinaria

M. rectus abdominis

→ T 15, T 16, T 21, T 42

Fig. 851 Diaphragm, Diaphragma, and muscles of the abdominal wall, Mm. abdominis.

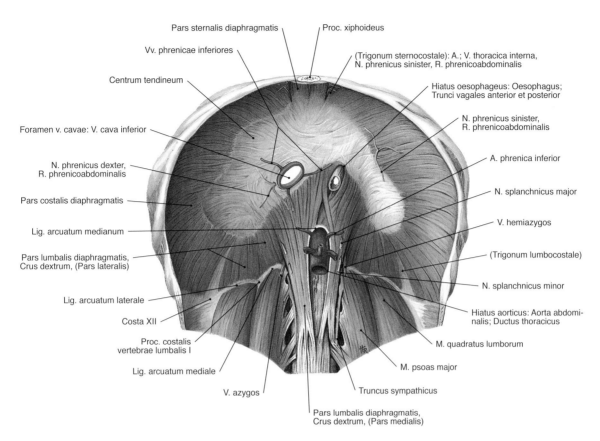

Pars sternalis diaphragmatis

Proc. xiphoideus

Vv. phrenicae inferiores

(Trigonum sternocostale): A.; V. thoracica interna, N. phrenicus sinister, R. phrenicoabdominalis

Centrum tendineum

Hiatus oesophageus: Oesophagus; Trunci vagales anterior et posterior

Foramen v. cavae: V. cava inferior

N. phrenicus sinister, R. phrenicoabdominalis

N. phrenicus dexter, R. phrenicoabdominalis

A. phrenica inferior

Pars costalis diaphragmatis

N. splanchnicus major

Lig. arcuatum medianum

V. hemiazygos

Pars lumbalis diaphragmatis, Crus dextrum, (Pars lateralis)

(Trigonum lumbocostale)

N. splanchnicus minor

Lig. arcuatum laterale

Hiatus aorticus: Aorta abdominalis; Ductus thoracicus

Costa XII

Proc. costalis vertebrae lumbalis I

M. quadratus lumborum

Lig. arcuatum mediale

M. psoas major

V. azygos

Truncus sympathicus

Pars lumbalis diaphragmatis, Crus dextrum, (Pars medialis)

Fig. 852   Diaphragm, Diaphragma.

→ T 21

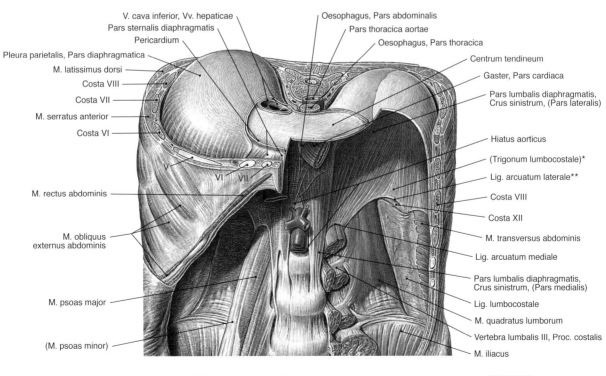

V. cava inferior, Vv. hepaticae

Oesophagus, Pars abdominalis

Pars sternalis diaphragmatis

Pars thoracica aortae

Pericardium

Oesophagus, Pars thoracica

Pleura parietalis, Pars diaphragmatica

Centrum tendineum

M. latissimus dorsi

Gaster, Pars cardiaca

Costa VIII

Pars lumbalis diaphragmatis, Crus sinistrum, (Pars lateralis)

Costa VII

M. serratus anterior

Hiatus aorticus

Costa VI

(Trigonum lumbocostale)*

Lig. arcuatum laterale**

M. rectus abdominis

Costa VIII

Costa XII

M. obliquus externus abdominis

M. transversus abdominis

Lig. arcuatum mediale

Pars lumbalis diaphragmatis, Crus sinistrum, (Pars medialis)

M. psoas major

Lig. lumbocostale

M. quadratus lumborum

Vertebra lumbalis III, Proc. costalis

(M. psoas minor)

M. iliacus

Fig. 853   Diaphragm, Diaphragma, with apertures and muscles of the posterior abdominal wall.

*   Clinical term: BOCHDALEK's triangle

** Psoas arcade

→ T 21

Breast

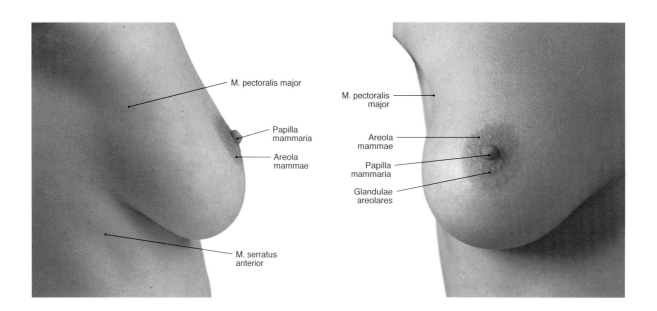

Fig. 854   Breast, Mamma.

Fig. 855   Breast, Mamma.

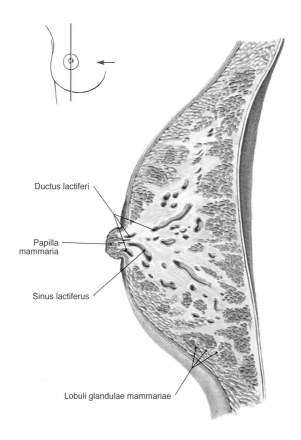

Fig. 856   Breast, Mamma, of a pregnant woman.

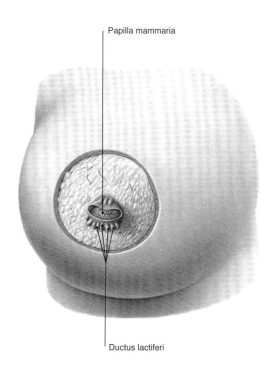

Fig. 857   Breast, Mamma, of a pregnant woman.

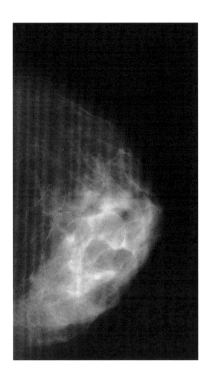

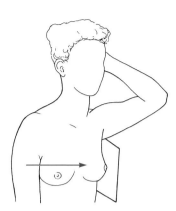

Fig. 858 Radiograph of the breast, mammography, of a 47-year-old woman.

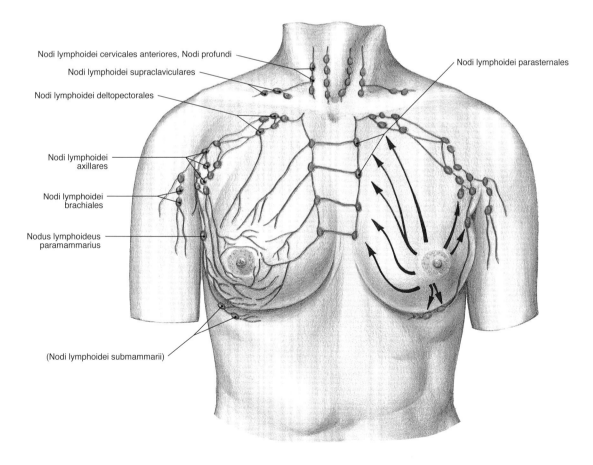

Nodi lymphoidei cervicales anteriores, Nodi profundi

Nodi lymphoidei supraclaviculares

Nodi lymphoidei deltopectorales

Nodi lymphoidei axillares

Nodi lymphoidei brachiales

Nodus lymphoideus paramammarius

(Nodi lymphoidei submammarii)

Nodi lymphoidei parasternales

Fig. 859 Lymphatic drainage of the breast and location of the regional lymph nodes.

Vessels and nerves of the wall of the trunk

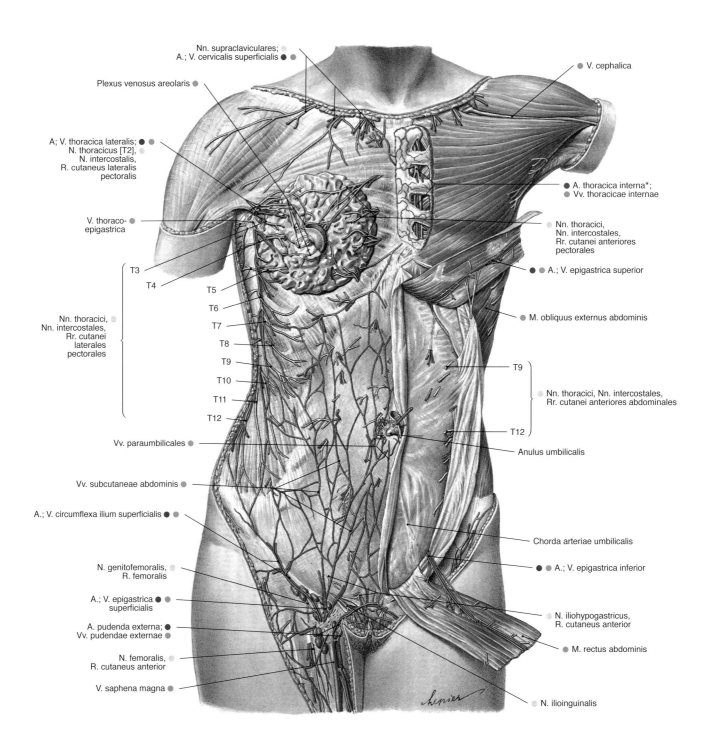

Nn. supraclaviculares; ●
A.; V. cervicalis superficialis ● ●

Plexus venosus areolaris ●

A; V. thoracica lateralis; ● ●
N. thoracicus [T2], ●
N. intercostalis,
R. cutaneus lateralis
pectoralis

V. thoraco- ●
epigastrica

T3
T4
T5
T6
T7
T8
T9
T10
T11
T12

Nn. thoracici, ●
Nn. intercostales,
Rr. cutanei
laterales
pectorales

Vv. paraumbilicales ●

Vv. subcutaneae abdominis ●

A.; V. circumflexa ilium superficialis ● ●

N. genitofemoralis, ●
R. femoralis

A.; V. epigastrica ● ●
superficialis

A. pudenda externa; ●
Vv. pudendae externae ●

N. femoralis, ●
R. cutaneus anterior

V. saphena magna ●

● V. cephalica

● A. thoracica interna*;
● Vv. thoracicae internae

● Nn. thoracici,
Nn. intercostales,
Rr. cutanei anteriores
pectorales

● ● A.; V. epigastrica superior

● M. obliquus externus abdominis

T9
T12

Nn. thoracici, Nn. intercostales,
Rr. cutanei anteriores abdominales

Anulus umbilicalis

Chorda arteriae umbilicalis

● ● A.; V. epigastrica inferior

N. iliohypogastricus,
R. cutaneus anterior

● M. rectus abdominis

N. ilioinguinalis

Fig. 860 Vessels and nerves of the thoracic and the abdominal wall.
* Clinical term: internal mammary artery

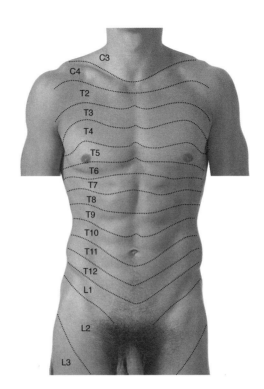

Fig. 861 Segmental sensory innervation of the anterior thoracic and abdominal wall (dermatomes).

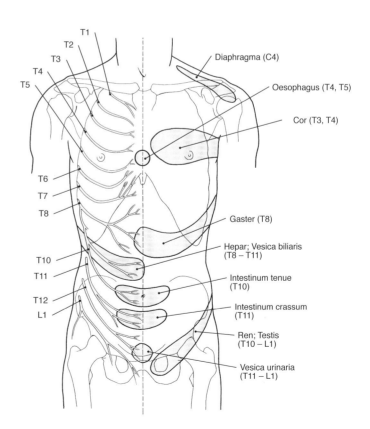

Fig. 862 Segmental sensory innervation of the anterior thoracic and abdominal wall. Regions to which pain from diseased viscera (zones of HEAD) is referred to are indicated in grey.

Lumbosacral plexus

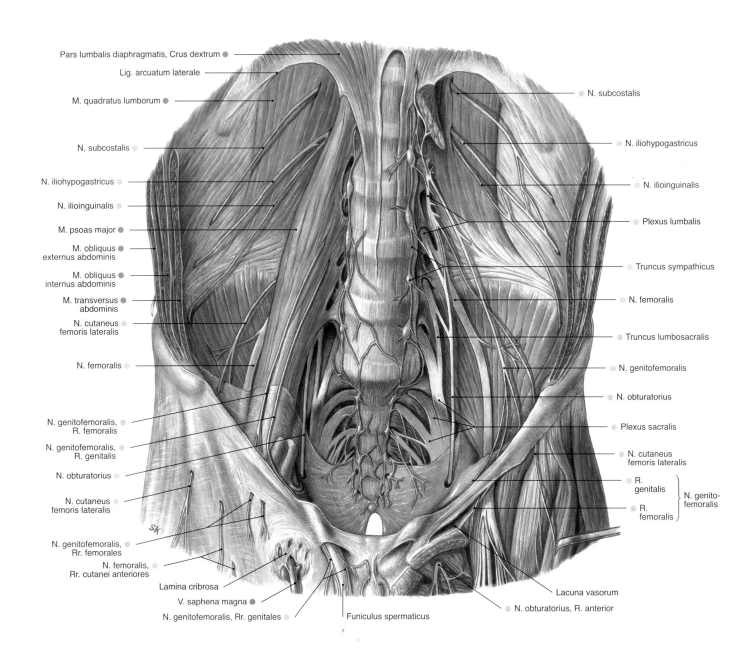

Pars lumbalis diaphragmatis, Crus dextrum

Lig. arcuatum laterale

M. quadratus lumborum

N. subcostalis

N. iliohypogastricus

N. ilioinguinalis

M. psoas major

M. obliquus externus abdominis

M. obliquus internus abdominis

M. transversus abdominis

N. cutaneus femoris lateralis

N. femoralis

N. genitofemoralis, R. femoralis

N. genitofemoralis, R. genitalis

N. obturatorius

N. cutaneus femoris lateralis

N. genitofemoralis, Rr. femorales

N. femoralis, Rr. cutanei anteriores

Lamina cribrosa

V. saphena magna

N. genitofemoralis, Rr. genitales

Funiculus spermaticus

N. subcostalis

N. iliohypogastricus

N. ilioinguinalis

Plexus lumbalis

Truncus sympathicus

N. femoralis

Truncus lumbosacralis

N. genitofemoralis

N. obturatorius

Plexus sacralis

N. cutaneus femoris lateralis

R. genitalis

R. femoralis

N. genitofemoralis

Lacuna vasorum

N. obturatorius, R. anterior

→ 47, T 40

Fig. 863 Lumbosacral plexus, Plexus lumbosacralis.

Vessels of the anterior wall of the trunk

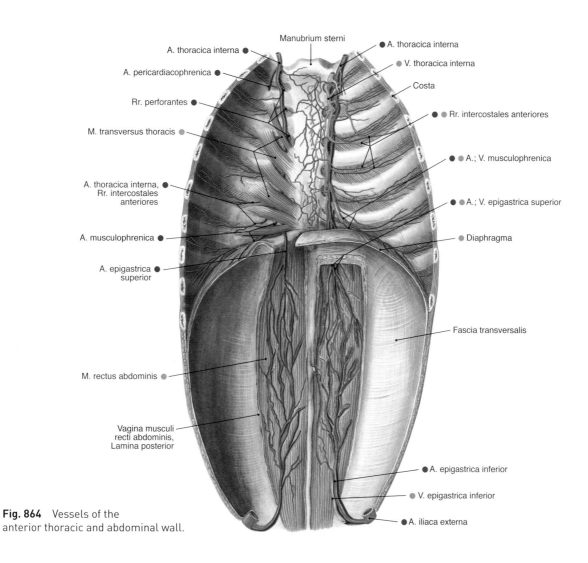

Manubrium sterni

A. thoracica interna ●
A. pericardiacophrenica ●
Rr. perforantes ●
M. transversus thoracis ●
A. thoracica interna, ●
Rr. intercostales anteriores
A. musculophrenica ●
A. epigastrica ● superior
M. rectus abdominis ●
Vagina musculi recti abdominis, Lamina posterior

● A. thoracica interna
● V. thoracica interna
Costa
● ● Rr. intercostales anteriores
● ● A.; V. musculophrenica
● ● A.; V. epigastrica superior
● Diaphragma
Fascia transversalis
● A. epigastrica inferior
● V. epigastrica inferior
● A. iliaca externa

Fig. 864 Vessels of the anterior thoracic and abdominal wall.

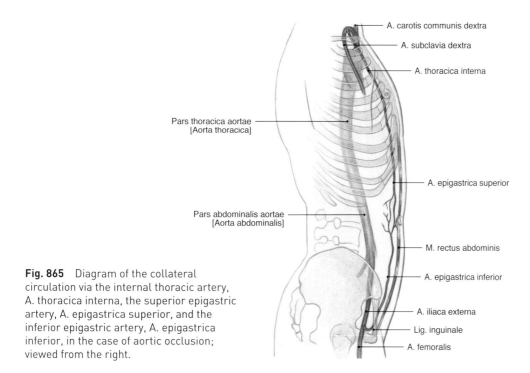

A. carotis communis dextra
A. subclavia dextra
A. thoracica interna
Pars thoracica aortae [Aorta thoracica]
A. epigastrica superior
Pars abdominalis aortae [Aorta abdominalis]
M. rectus abdominis
A. epigastrica inferior
A. iliaca externa
Lig. inguinale
A. femoralis

Fig. 865 Diagram of the collateral circulation via the internal thoracic artery, A. thoracica interna, the superior epigastric artery, A. epigastrica superior, and the inferior epigastric artery, A. epigastrica inferior, in the case of aortic occlusion; viewed from the right.

Abdominal wall of a neonate

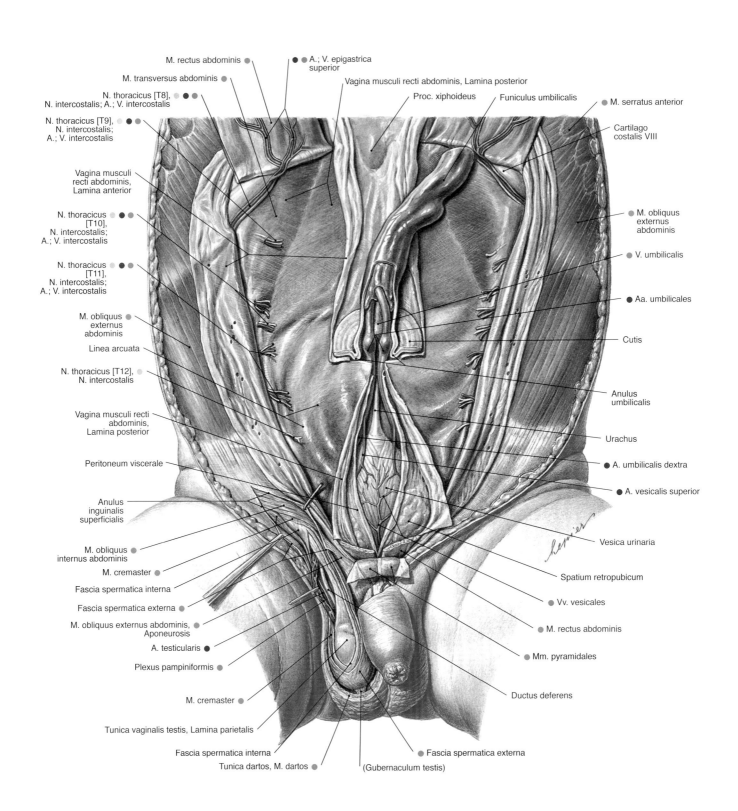

M. rectus abdominis ●

M. transversus abdominis ●

N. thoracicus [T8], ● ●
N. intercostalis; A.; V. intercostalis

N. thoracicus [T9], ● ●
N. intercostalis;
A.; V. intercostalis

Vagina musculi
recti abdominis,
Lamina anterior

N. thoracicus ● ● ●
[T10],
N. intercostalis;
A.; V. intercostalis

N. thoracicus ● ● ●
[T11],
N. intercostalis;
A.; V. intercostalis

M. obliquus ●
externus
abdominis

Linea arcuata

N. thoracicus [T12], ●
N. intercostalis

Vagina musculi recti
abdominis,
Lamina posterior

Peritoneum viscerale

Anulus
inguinalis
superficialis

M. obliquus ●
internus abdominis

M. cremaster ●

Fascia spermatica interna

Fascia spermatica externa ●

M. obliquus externus abdominis, ●
Aponeurosis

A. testicularis ●

Plexus pampiniformis ●

M. cremaster ●

Tunica vaginalis testis, Lamina parietalis

Fascia spermatica interna
Tunica dartos, M. dartos ●

● ● A.; V. epigastrica
superior

Vagina musculi recti abdominis, Lamina posterior

Proc. xiphoideus   Funiculus umbilicalis

● M. serratus anterior

Cartilago
costalis VIII

● M. obliquus
externus
abdominis

● V. umbilicalis

● Aa. umbilicales

Cutis

Anulus
umbilicalis

Urachus

● A. umbilicalis dextra

● A. vesicalis superior

Vesica urinaria

Spatium retropubicum

● Vv. vesicales

● M. rectus abdominis

● Mm. pyramidales

Ductus deferens

● Fascia spermatica externa

(Gubernaculum testis)

Fig. 866   Anterior abdominal wall of a neonate.

Inner contour of the anterior abdominal wall

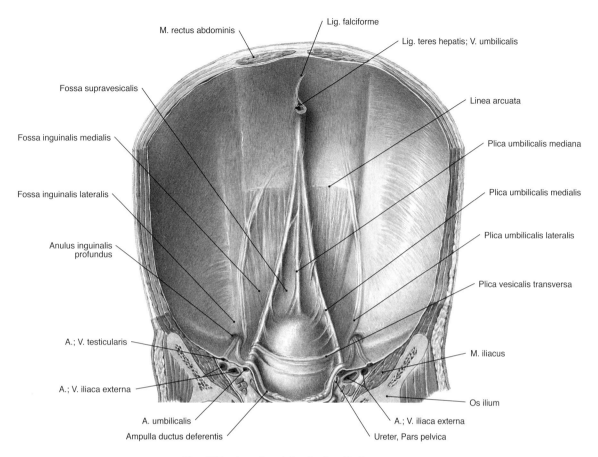

M. rectus abdominis

Lig. falciforme

Lig. teres hepatis; V. umbilicalis

Fossa supravesicalis

Fossa inguinalis medialis

Fossa inguinalis lateralis

Anulus inguinalis profundus

A.; V. testicularis

A.; V. iliaca externa

A. umbilicalis

Ampulla ductus deferentis

Linea arcuata

Plica umbilicalis mediana

Plica umbilicalis medialis

Plica umbilicalis lateralis

Plica vesicalis transversa

M. iliacus

Os ilium

A.; V. iliaca externa

Ureter, Pars pelvica

Fig. 867   Anterior abdominal wall of a neonate.

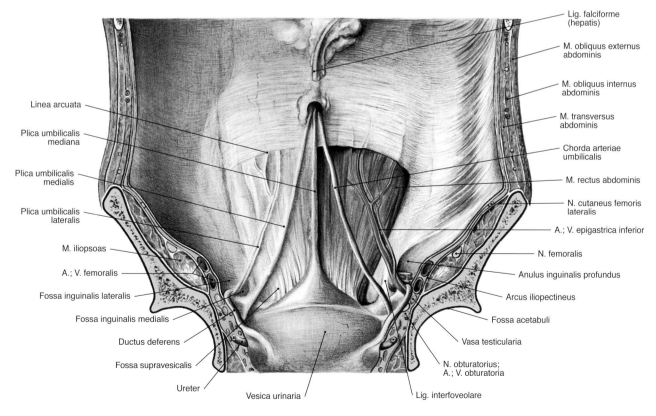

Linea arcuata

Plica umbilicalis mediana

Plica umbilicalis medialis

Plica umbilicalis lateralis

M. iliopsoas

A.; V. femoralis

Fossa inguinalis lateralis

Fossa inguinalis medialis

Ductus deferens

Fossa supravesicalis

Ureter

Vesica urinaria

Lig. falciforme (hepatis)

M. obliquus externus abdominis

M. obliquus internus abdominis

M. transversus abdominis

Chorda arteriae umbilicalis

M. rectus abdominis

N. cutaneus femoris lateralis

A.; V. epigastrica inferior

N. femoralis

Anulus inguinalis profundus

Arcus iliopectineus

Fossa acetabuli

Vasa testicularia

N. obturatorius; A.; V. obturatoria

Lig. interfoveolare

Fig. 868   Anterior abdominal wall, internal aspect.

Abdominal wall, sections

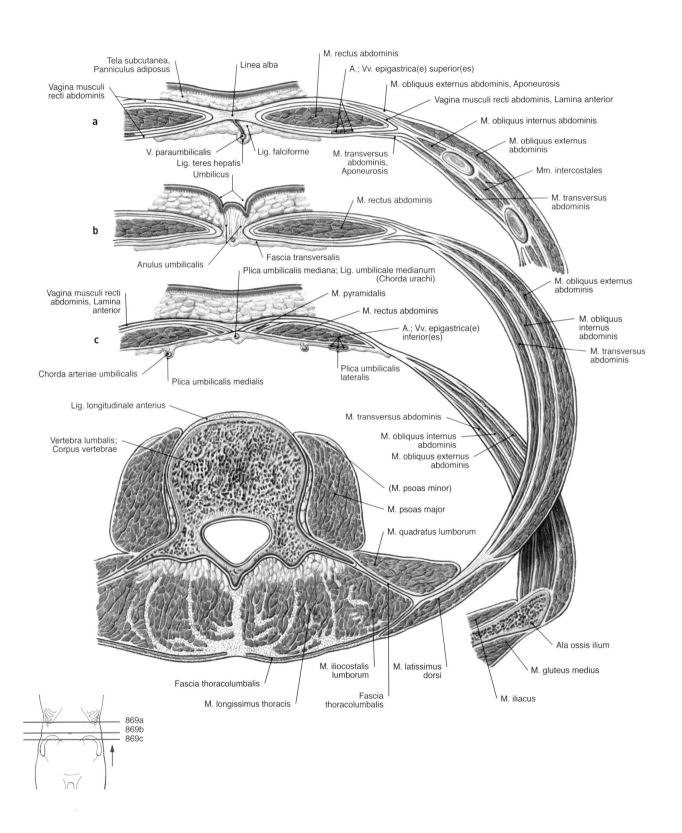

Tela subcutanea, Panniculus adiposus
Linea alba
M. rectus abdominis
A.; Vv. epigastrica(e) superior(es)
M. obliquus externus abdominis, Aponeurosis
Vagina musculi recti abdominis
Vagina musculi recti abdominis, Lamina anterior
M. obliquus internus abdominis
M. obliquus externus abdominis
Mm. intercostales
M. transversus abdominis
a
V. paraumbilicalis
Lig. falciforme
M. transversus abdominis, Aponeurosis
Lig. teres hepatis
Umbilicus

M. rectus abdominis
M. obliquus externus abdominis
M. obliquus internus abdominis
M. transversus abdominis
b
Anulus umbilicalis
Fascia transversalis
Plica umbilicalis mediana; Lig. umbilicale medianum (Chorda urachi)
M. pyramidalis

Vagina musculi recti abdominis, Lamina anterior
M. rectus abdominis
A.; Vv. epigastrica(e) inferior(es)
M. obliquus externus abdominis
M. obliquus internus abdominis
M. transversus abdominis
c
Chorda arteriae umbilicalis
Plica umbilicalis medialis
Plica umbilicalis lateralis

Lig. longitudinale anterius
M. transversus abdominis
M. obliquus internus abdominis
M. obliquus externus abdominis
Vertebra lumbalis; Corpus vertebrae
(M. psoas minor)
M. psoas major
M. quadratus lumborum
Ala ossis ilium
M. gluteus medius
M. iliacus
Fascia thoracolumbalis
M. iliocostalis lumborum
M. latissimus dorsi
M. longissimus thoracis
Fascia thoracolumbalis

869a
869b
869c

→ T 14–T 16, T 20 a, b, T 42

Fig. 869 a–c   Muscles of the abdominal wall, Mm. abdominis; horizontal sections.

Abdominal wall, sections

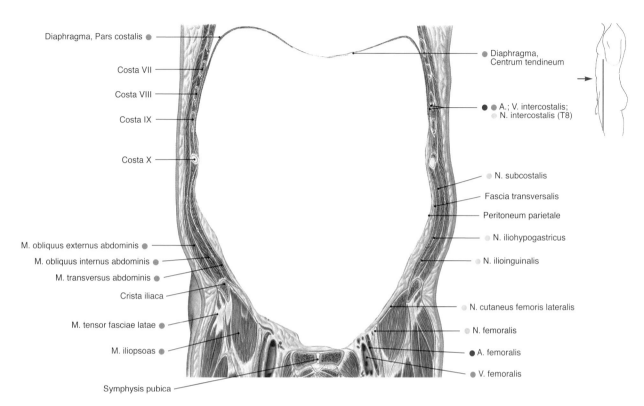

Diaphragma, Pars costalis ●

Costa VII

Costa VIII

Costa IX

Costa X

M. obliquus externus abdominis ●
M. obliquus internus abdominis ●
M. transversus abdominis ●

Crista iliaca

M. tensor fasciae latae ●

M. iliopsoas ●

Symphysis pubica

● Diaphragma, Centrum tendineum

● ● A.; V. intercostalis; N. intercostalis (T8)

● N. subcostalis

Fascia transversalis

Peritoneum parietale

● N. iliohypogastricus

● N. ilioinguinalis

● N. cutaneus femoris lateralis

● N. femoralis

● A. femoralis

● V. femoralis

Fig. 870 Muscles of the abdominal wall, Mm. abdominis; frontal section.

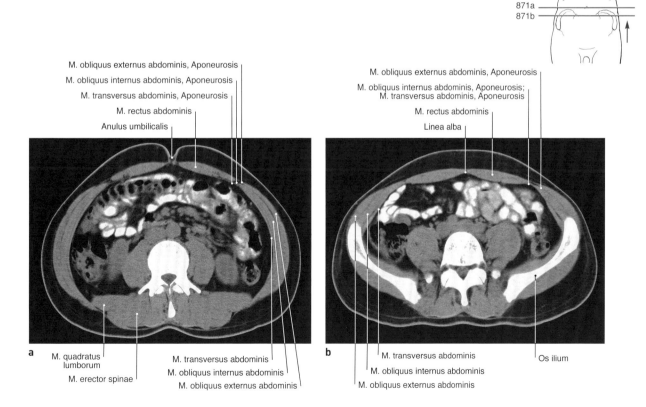

871a
871b

M. obliquus externus abdominis, Aponeurosis
M. obliquus internus abdominis, Aponeurosis
M. transversus abdominis, Aponeurosis
M. rectus abdominis
Anulus umbilicalis

M. obliquus externus abdominis, Aponeurosis
M. obliquus internus abdominis, Aponeurosis; M. transversus abdominis, Aponeurosis
M. rectus abdominis
Linea alba

a
M. quadratus lumborum
M. erector spinae
M. transversus abdominis
M. obliquus internus abdominis
M. obliquus externus abdominis

b
M. transversus abdominis
M. obliquus internus abdominis
M. obliquus externus abdominis
Os ilium

Fig. 871 a, b Muscles of the abdominal wall, Mm. abdominis; computed tomographic cross-sections (CT).

Heart

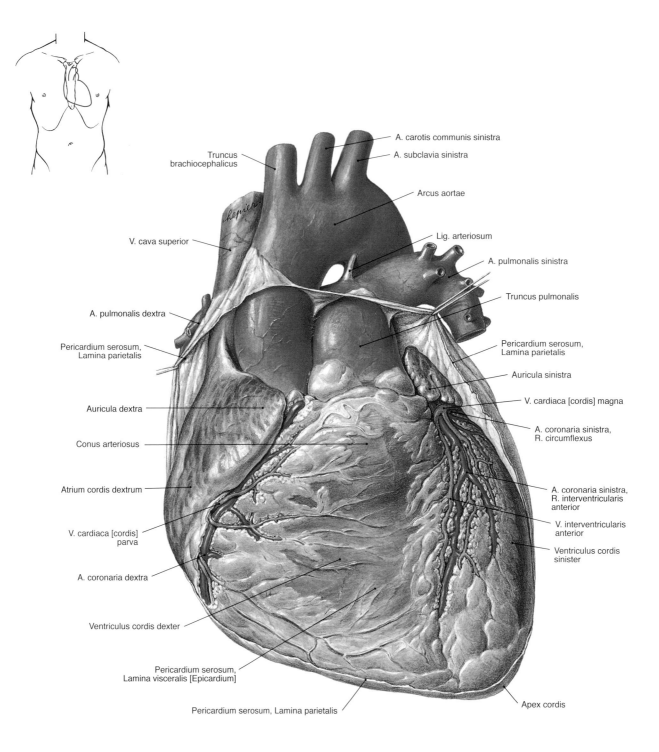

Truncus brachiocephalicus

A. carotis communis sinistra

A. subclavia sinistra

Arcus aortae

V. cava superior

Lig. arteriosum

A. pulmonalis sinistra

Truncus pulmonalis

A. pulmonalis dextra

Pericardium serosum, Lamina parietalis

Pericardium serosum, Lamina parietalis

Auricula sinistra

Auricula dextra

V. cardiaca [cordis] magna

A. coronaria sinistra, R. circumflexus

Conus arteriosus

Atrium cordis dextrum

A. coronaria sinistra, R. interventricularis anterior

V. interventricularis anterior

V. cardiaca [cordis] parva

Ventriculus cordis sinister

A. coronaria dextra

Ventriculus cordis dexter

Pericardium serosum, Lamina visceralis [Epicardium]

Apex cordis

Pericardium serosum, Lamina parietalis

Abb. 872   Heart, Cor.

Pericardium fibrosum

Pericardium serosum ⎫
Lamina parietalis ⎬ Pericardium
Lamina visceralis = Epicardium

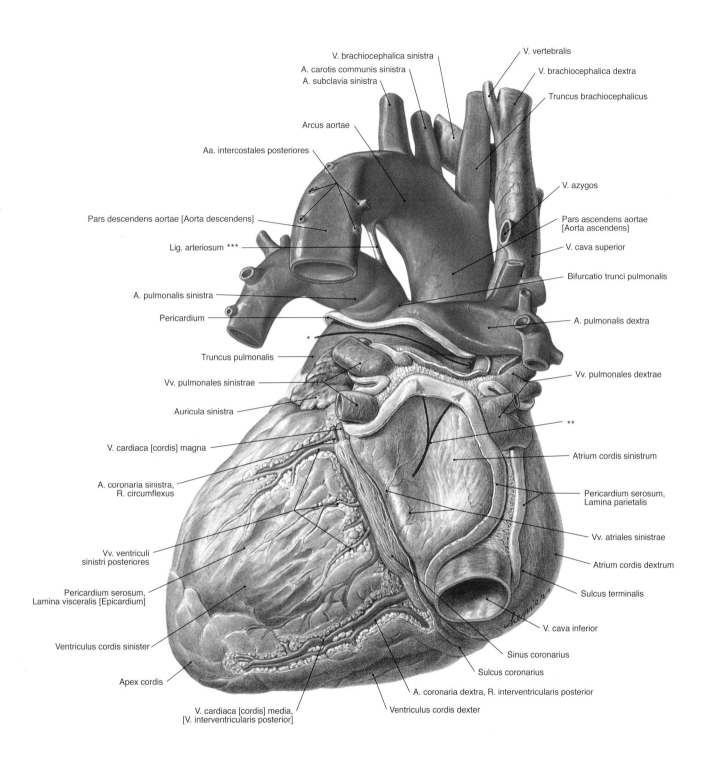

V. brachiocephalica sinistra
A. carotis communis sinistra
A. subclavia sinistra
V. vertebralis
V. brachiocephalica dextra
Truncus brachiocephalicus
Arcus aortae
Aa. intercostales posteriores
Pars descendens aortae [Aorta descendens]
V. azygos
Lig. arteriosum ***
Pars ascendens aortae [Aorta ascendens]
V. cava superior
A. pulmonalis sinistra
Bifurcatio trunci pulmonalis
Pericardium
A. pulmonalis dextra
Truncus pulmonalis
Vv. pulmonales sinistrae
Vv. pulmonales dextrae
Auricula sinistra
V. cardiaca [cordis] magna
Atrium cordis sinistrum
A. coronaria sinistra, R. circumflexus
Pericardium serosum, Lamina parietalis
Vv. ventriculi sinistri posteriores
Vv. atriales sinistrae
Atrium cordis dextrum
Pericardium serosum, Lamina visceralis [Epicardium]
Sulcus terminalis
Ventriculus cordis sinister
V. cava inferior
Apex cordis
Sinus coronarius
Sulcus coronarius
A. coronaria dextra, R. interventricularis posterior
V. cardiaca [cordis] media, [V. interventricularis posterior]
Ventriculus cordis dexter

Fig. 873 Heart, Cor, and great vessels; dorsal view.

*   Arrow in the transverse pericardial sinus
**   Double arrows in the oblique pericardial sinus
*** Remnants of the foetal ductus arteriosus (BOTALLO's ligament)

Myocardium

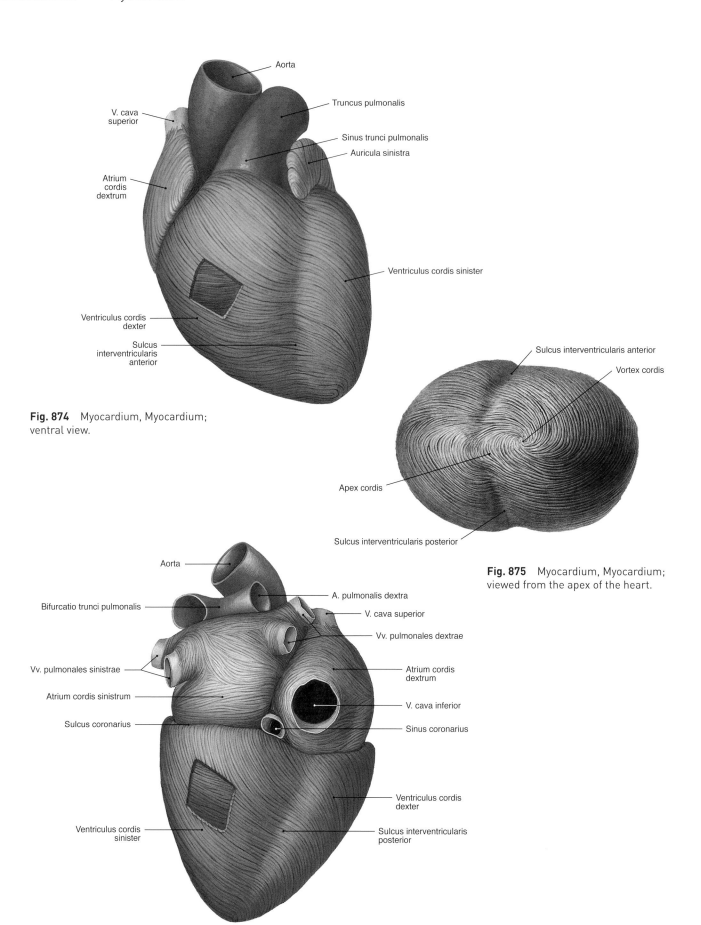

Fig. 874 Myocardium, Myocardium;
ventral view.

Fig. 875 Myocardium, Myocardium;
viewed from the apex of the heart.

Fig. 876 Myocardium, Myocardium;
dorsoinferior view.

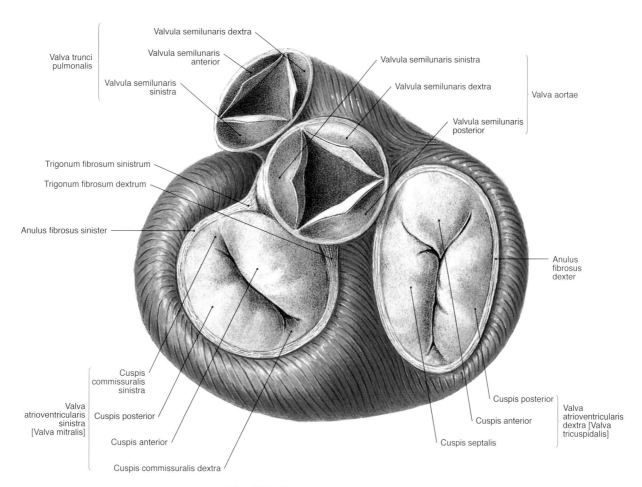

Valva trunci pulmonalis

Valvula semilunaris dextra
Valvula semilunaris anterior
Valvula semilunaris sinistra

Valvula semilunaris sinistra
Valvula semilunaris dextra
Valvula semilunaris posterior

Valva aortae

Trigonum fibrosum sinistrum
Trigonum fibrosum dextrum

Anulus fibrosus sinister

Anulus fibrosus dexter

Valva atrioventricularis sinistra [Valva mitralis]

Cuspis commissuralis sinistra
Cuspis posterior
Cuspis anterior
Cuspis commissuralis dextra

Cuspis posterior
Cuspis anterior
Cuspis septalis

Valva atrioventricularis dextra [Valva tricuspidalis]

Fig. 877 Valves of the heart, Valvae cordis; superior view.

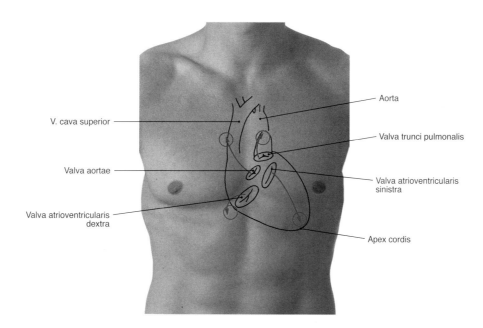

V. cava superior

Aorta

Valva trunci pulmonalis

Valva aortae

Valva atrioventricularis sinistra

Valva atrioventricularis dextra

Apex cordis

Fig. 878 Contour of the heart, valves of the heart, and points of auscultation projected onto the anterior thoracic wall (circles). The heart sounds and (where applicable) the heart murmurs are spreading in the direction of the arrows.

Internal spaces of the heart

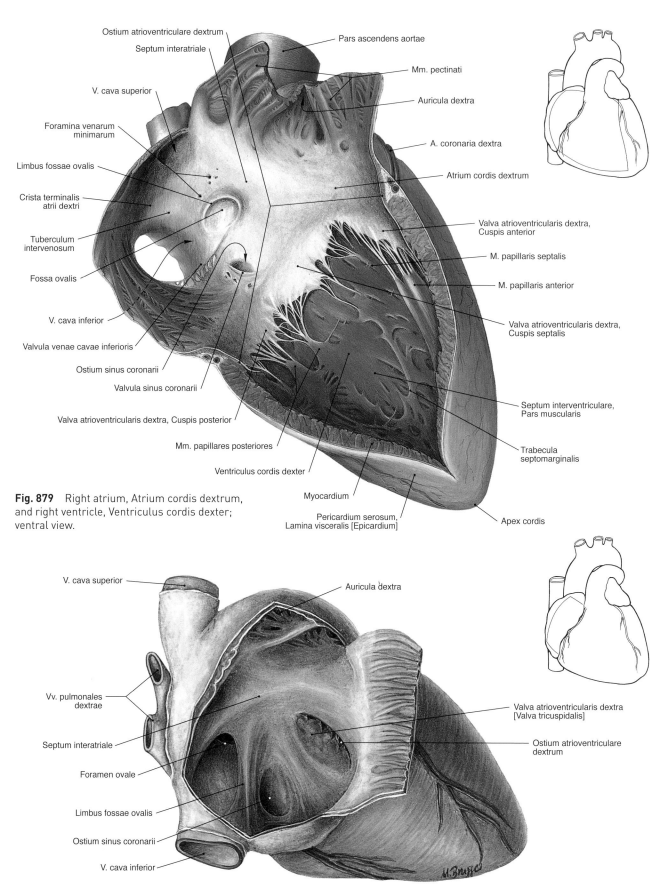

Ostium atrioventriculare dextrum

Septum interatriale

V. cava superior

Foramina venarum minimarum

Limbus fossae ovalis

Crista terminalis atrii dextri

Tuberculum intervenosum

Fossa ovalis

V. cava inferior

Valvula venae cavae inferioris

Ostium sinus coronarii

Valvula sinus coronarii

Valva atrioventricularis dextra, Cuspis posterior

Mm. papillares posteriores

Ventriculus cordis dexter

Myocardium

Pericardium serosum, Lamina visceralis [Epicardium]

Pars ascendens aortae

Mm. pectinati

Auricula dextra

A. coronaria dextra

Atrium cordis dextrum

Valva atrioventricularis dextra, Cuspis anterior

M. papillaris septalis

M. papillaris anterior

Valva atrioventricularis dextra, Cuspis septalis

Septum interventriculare, Pars muscularis

Trabecula septomarginalis

Apex cordis

Fig. 879   Right atrium, Atrium cordis dextrum, and right ventricle, Ventriculus cordis dexter; ventral view.

V. cava superior

Auricula dextra

Vv. pulmonales dextrae

Septum interatriale

Foramen ovale

Limbus fossae ovalis

Ostium sinus coronarii

V. cava inferior

Valva atrioventricularis dextra [Valva tricuspidalis]

Ostium atrioventriculare dextrum

Fig. 880   Right atrium, Atrium cordis dextrum, of a neonate; ventral view from the right.

Internal spaces of the heart

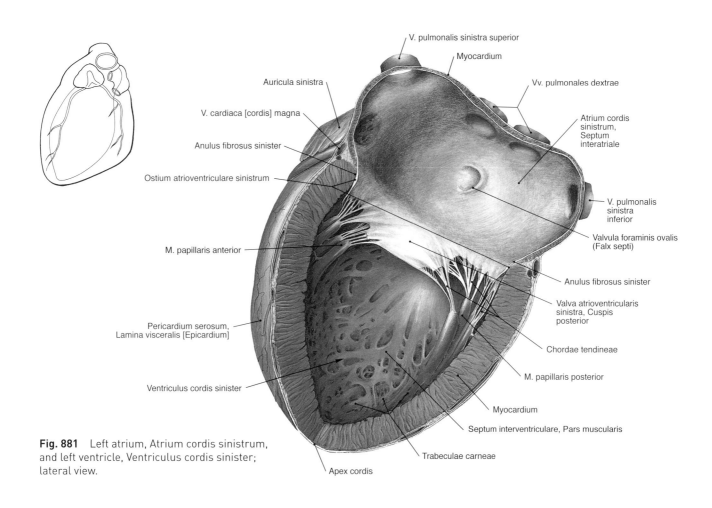

V. pulmonalis sinistra superior
Myocardium
Auricula sinistra
Vv. pulmonales dextrae
V. cardiaca [cordis] magna
Atrium cordis sinistrum, Septum interatriale
Anulus fibrosus sinister
Ostium atrioventriculare sinistrum
V. pulmonalis sinistra inferior
Valvula foraminis ovalis (Falx septi)
M. papillaris anterior
Anulus fibrosus sinister
Valva atrioventricularis sinistra, Cuspis posterior
Pericardium serosum, Lamina visceralis [Epicardium]
Chordae tendineae
M. papillaris posterior
Ventriculus cordis sinister
Myocardium
Septum interventriculare, Pars muscularis
Trabeculae carneae
Apex cordis

Fig. 881 Left atrium, Atrium cordis sinistrum, and left ventricle, Ventriculus cordis sinister; lateral view.

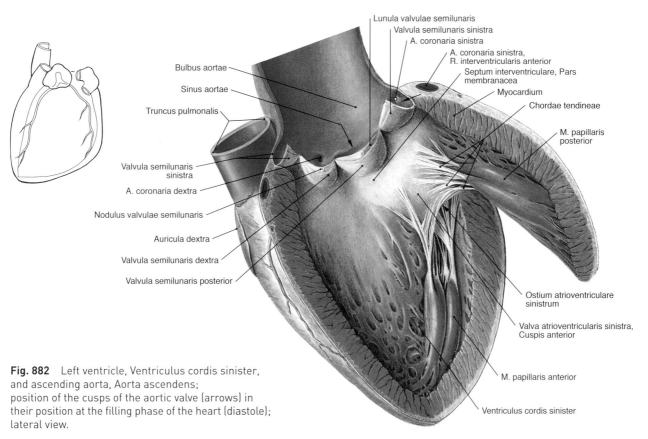

Lunula valvulae semilunaris
Valvula semilunaris sinistra
A. coronaria sinistra
A. coronaria sinistra, R. interventricularis anterior
Bulbus aortae
Septum interventriculare, Pars membranacea
Sinus aortae
Myocardium
Truncus pulmonalis
Chordae tendineae
M. papillaris posterior
Valvula semilunaris sinistra
A. coronaria dextra
Nodulus valvulae semilunaris
Auricula dextra
Valvula semilunaris dextra
Valvula semilunaris posterior
Ostium atrioventriculare sinistrum
Valva atrioventricularis sinistra, Cuspis anterior
M. papillaris anterior
Ventriculus cordis sinister

Fig. 882 Left ventricle, Ventriculus cordis sinister, and ascending aorta, Aorta ascendens; position of the cusps of the aortic valve (arrows) in their position at the filling phase of the heart (diastole); lateral view.

Internal spaces of the heart

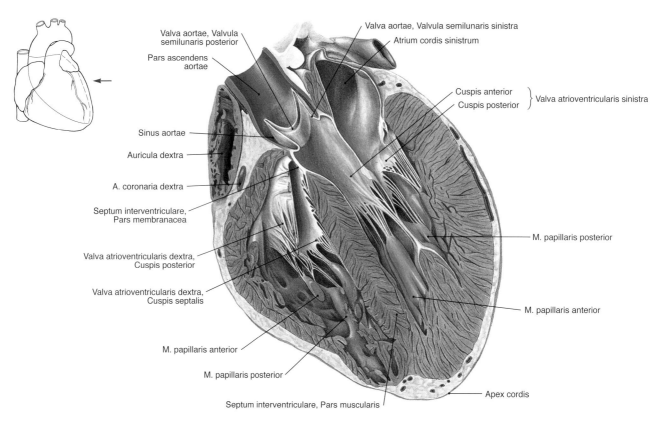

Valva aortae, Valvula
semilunaris posterior

Pars ascendens
aortae

Valva aortae, Valvula semilunaris sinistra

Atrium cordis sinistrum

Cuspis anterior ⎫
Cuspis posterior ⎭ Valva atrioventricularis sinistra

Sinus aortae

Auricula dextra

A. coronaria dextra

Septum interventriculare,
Pars membranacea

Valva atrioventricularis dextra,
Cuspis posterior

Valva atrioventricularis dextra,
Cuspis septalis

M. papillaris anterior

M. papillaris posterior

Septum interventriculare, Pars muscularis

M. papillaris posterior

M. papillaris anterior

Apex cordis

Fig. 883   Left and right ventricle, Ventriculus cordis
sinister et dexter.

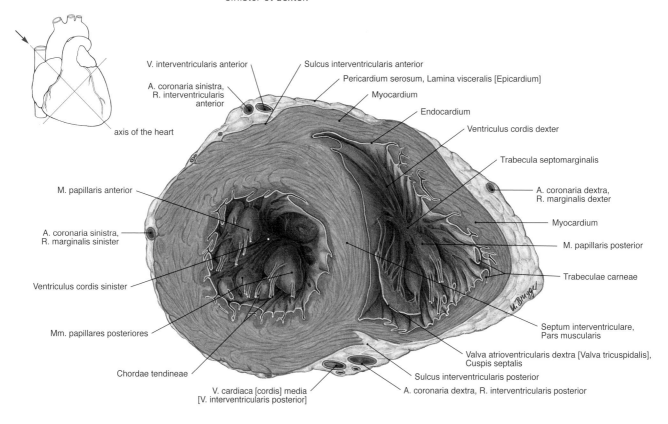

V. interventricularis anterior

A. coronaria sinistra,
R. interventricularis
anterior

axis of the heart

Sulcus interventricularis anterior

Pericardium serosum, Lamina visceralis [Epicardium]

Myocardium

Endocardium

Ventriculus cordis dexter

Trabecula septomarginalis

A. coronaria dextra,
R. marginalis dexter

Myocardium

M. papillaris posterior

Trabeculae carneae

Septum interventriculare,
Pars muscularis

Valva atrioventricularis dextra [Valva tricuspidalis],
Cuspis septalis

Sulcus interventricularis posterior

A. coronaria dextra, R. interventricularis posterior

M. papillaris anterior

A. coronaria sinistra,
R. marginalis sinister

Ventriculus cordis sinister

Mm. papillares posteriores

Chordae tendineae

V. cardiaca [cordis] media
[V. interventricularis posterior]

Fig. 884   Left and right ventricle, Ventriculus cordis
sinister et dexter;
superior view.

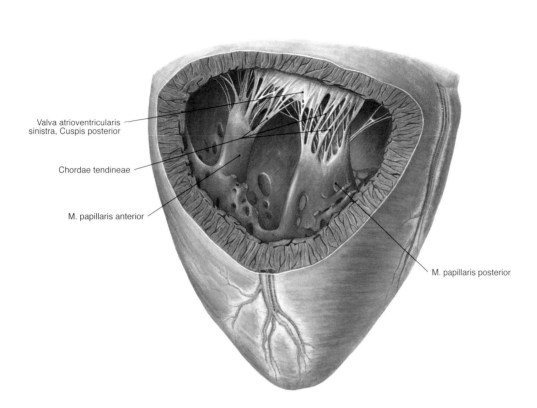
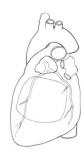

Valva atrioventricularis
sinistra, Cuspis posterior

Chordae tendineae

M. papillaris anterior

M. papillaris posterior

Fig. 885   Left ventricle, Ventriculus cordis sinister;
ventrosuperior view from the left.

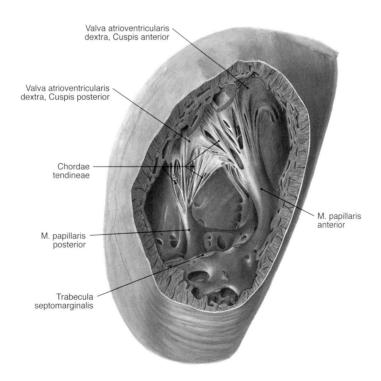
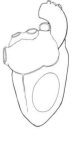

Valva atrioventricularis
dextra, Cuspis anterior

Valva atrioventricularis
dextra, Cuspis posterior

Chordae
tendineae

M. papillaris
anterior

M. papillaris
posterior

Trabecula
septomarginalis

Fig. 886   Right ventricle, Ventriculus cordis dexter;
dorsal view.

Conducting system

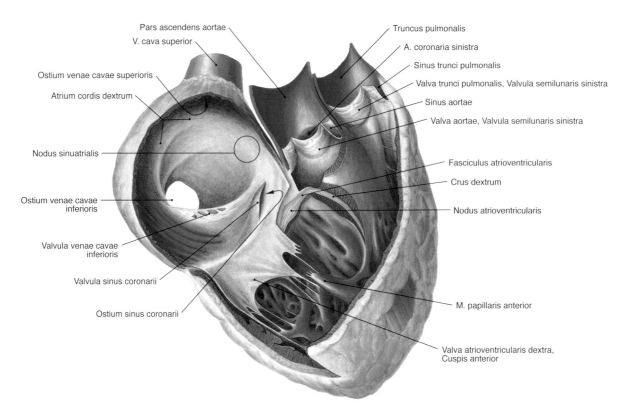

Fig. 887   Right atrium, Atrium cordis dextrum, and right ventricle, Ventriculus cordis dexter; conducting system, Complexus stimulans cordis [Systema conducente cordis], highlighted in yellow; ventral view.

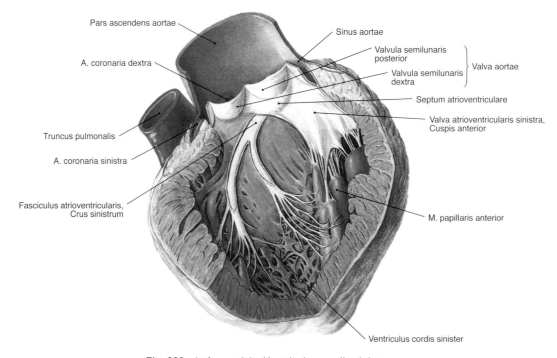

Fig. 888   Left ventricle, Ventriculus cordis sinister; conducting system, Complexus stimulans cordis [Systema conducente cordis], highlighted in yellow; ventral view from the left.

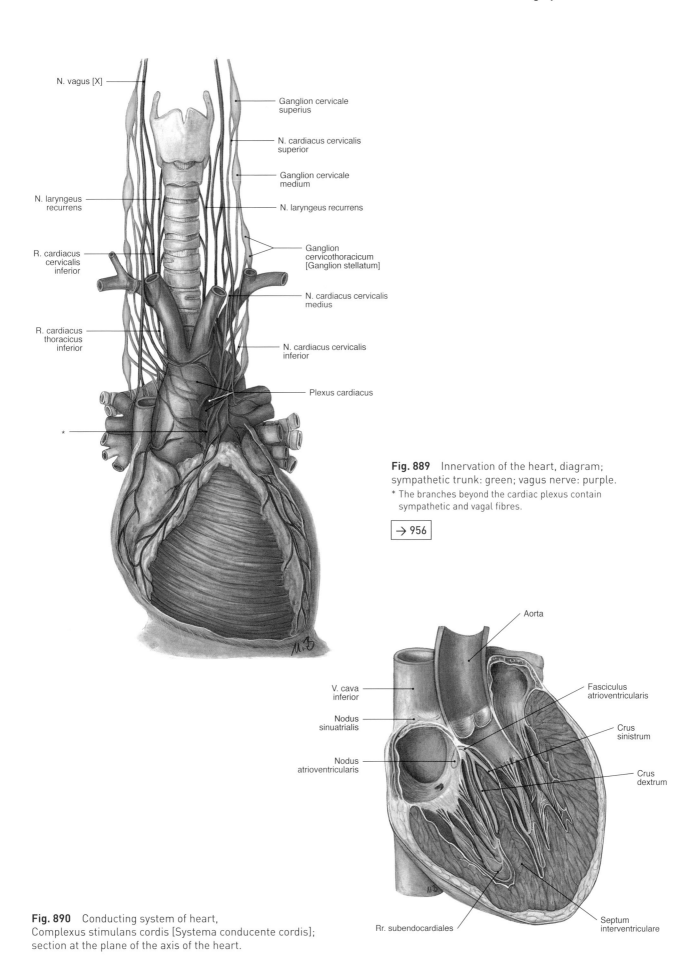

N. vagus [X]

Ganglion cervicale
superius

N. cardiacus cervicalis
superior

Ganglion cervicale
medium

N. laryngeus
recurrens

N. laryngeus recurrens

Ganglion
cervicothoracicum
[Ganglion stellatum]

R. cardiacus
cervicalis
inferior

N. cardiacus cervicalis
medius

R. cardiacus
thoracicus
inferior

N. cardiacus cervicalis
inferior

Plexus cardiacus

*

Fig. 889 Innervation of the heart, diagram;
sympathetic trunk: green; vagus nerve: purple.
* The branches beyond the cardiac plexus contain
sympathetic and vagal fibres.

→ 956

Aorta

V. cava
inferior

Fasciculus
atrioventricularis

Nodus
sinuatrialis

Crus
sinistrum

Nodus
atrioventricularis

Crus
dextrum

Rr. subendocardiales

Septum
interventriculare

Fig. 890 Conducting system of heart,
Complexus stimulans cordis [Systema conducente cordis];
section at the plane of the axis of the heart.

Coronary arteries

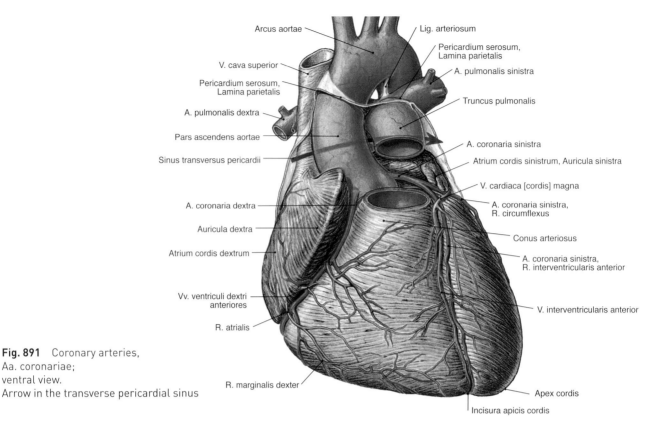

Arcus aortae
Lig. arteriosum
V. cava superior
Pericardium serosum, Lamina parietalis
A. pulmonalis sinistra
Pericardium serosum, Lamina parietalis
Truncus pulmonalis
A. pulmonalis dextra
Pars ascendens aortae
A. coronaria sinistra
Sinus transversus pericardii
Atrium cordis sinistrum, Auricula sinistra
V. cardiaca [cordis] magna
A. coronaria dextra
A. coronaria sinistra, R. circumflexus
Auricula dextra
Conus arteriosus
Atrium cordis dextrum
A. coronaria sinistra, R. interventricularis anterior
Vv. ventriculi dextri anteriores
V. interventricularis anterior
R. atrialis
R. marginalis dexter
Apex cordis
Incisura apicis cordis

Fig. 891 Coronary arteries, Aa. coronariae; ventral view. Arrow in the transverse pericardial sinus

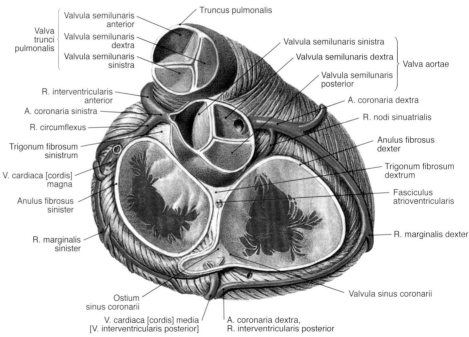

Valva trunci pulmonalis
Valvula semilunaris anterior
Truncus pulmonalis
Valvula semilunaris dextra
Valvula semilunaris sinistra
Valvula semilunaris sinistra
Valvula semilunaris dextra
Valva aortae
Valvula semilunaris posterior
R. interventricularis anterior
A. coronaria dextra
A. coronaria sinistra
R. nodi sinuatrialis
R. circumflexus
Trigonum fibrosum sinistrum
Anulus fibrosus dexter
V. cardiaca [cordis] magna
Trigonum fibrosum dextrum
Anulus fibrosus sinister
Fasciculus atrioventricularis
R. marginalis sinister
R. marginalis dexter
Valvula sinus coronarii
Ostium sinus coronarii
V. cardiaca [cordis] media [V. interventricularis posterior]
A. coronaria dextra, R. interventricularis posterior

Fig. 892 Coronary arteries, Aa. coronariae; superior view.

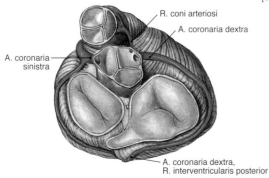

R. coni arteriosi
A. coronaria dextra
A. coronaria sinistra
A. coronaria dextra, R. interventricularis posterior

Fig. 893 Variability of the coronary arteries. The conus arteriosus branch arises from the aorta as an independent artery (~37%).

Vessels of the heart

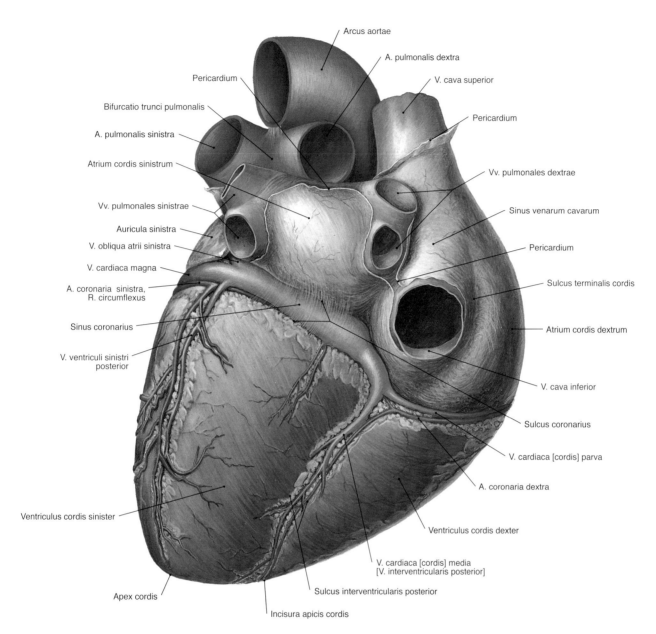

Arcus aortae

A. pulmonalis dextra

Pericardium

V. cava superior

Bifurcatio trunci pulmonalis

A. pulmonalis sinistra

Pericardium

Atrium cordis sinistrum

Vv. pulmonales dextrae

Vv. pulmonales sinistrae

Auricula sinistra

V. obliqua atrii sinistra

Sinus venarum cavarum

V. cardiaca magna

Pericardium

A. coronaria sinistra, R. circumflexus

Sulcus terminalis cordis

Sinus coronarius

V. ventriculi sinistri posterior

Atrium cordis dextrum

V. cava inferior

Sulcus coronarius

V. cardiaca [cordis] parva

A. coronaria dextra

Ventriculus cordis sinister

Ventriculus cordis dexter

V. cardiaca [cordis] media [V. interventricularis posterior]

Apex cordis

Sulcus interventricularis posterior

Incisura apicis cordis

Fig. 894 Veins of the heart, Vv. cordis.

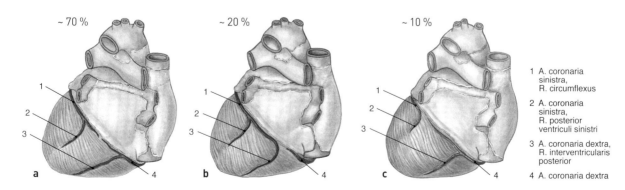

~ 70 %

~ 20 %

~ 10 %

a

b

c

1 A. coronaria sinistra, R. circumflexus

2 A. coronaria sinistra, R. posterior ventriculi sinistri

3 A. coronaria dextra, R. interventricularis posterior

4 A. coronaria dextra

Fig. 895 a–c Variations in the arterial supply of the posterior aspect of the heart; dorsal view.

a Balanced coronary artery supply
b Dominant left coronary artery supply
c Dominant right coronary artery supply

Coronary arteries, variability of supply

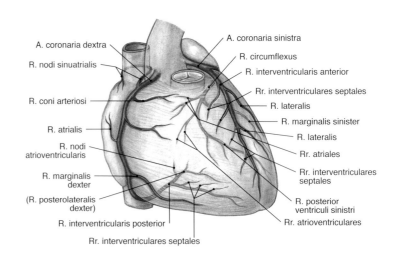

Fig. 896 Coronary arteries, Aa. coronariae;
posterior arterial branches are shown in a
lighter colour;
the posterior interventricular branch arises
from the right coronary artery (balanced coronary
artery supply);
ventral view.

A. coronaria dextra
R. nodi sinuatrialis
R. coni arteriosi
R. atrialis
R. nodi atrioventricularis
R. marginalis dexter
(R. posterolateralis dexter)
R. interventricularis posterior
Rr. interventriculares septales

A. coronaria sinistra
R. circumflexus
R. interventricularis anterior
Rr. interventriculares septales
R. lateralis
R. marginalis sinister
R. lateralis
Rr. atriales
Rr. interventriculares septales
R. posterior ventriculi sinistri
Rr. atrioventriculares

Fig. 897 Coronary arteries, Aa. coronariae;
the posterior interventricular branch arises from
the left coronary artery (dominant left coronary
artery supply);
ventral view.

A. coronaria dextra
R. nodi sinuatrialis
R. coni arteriosi
R. atrialis
R. marginalis dexter
R. interventricularis posterior

A. coronaria sinistra
R. circumflexus
R. interventricularis anterior
R. atrialis
R. lateralis
R. marginalis sinister
Rr. interventriculares septales
Rr. posteriores ventriculi sinistri
Rr. interventriculares septales

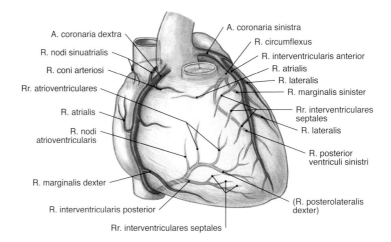

Fig. 898 Coronary arteries, Aa. coronariae;
the posterior wall of the ventricles is
mainly supplied by branches of the
right coronary artery (dominant right coronary
artery supply);
ventral view.

A. coronaria dextra
R. nodi sinuatrialis
R. coni arteriosi
Rr. atrioventriculares
R. atrialis
R. nodi atrioventricularis
R. marginalis dexter
R. interventricularis posterior
Rr. interventriculares septales

A. coronaria sinistra
R. circumflexus
R. interventricularis anterior
R. atrialis
R. lateralis
R. marginalis sinister
Rr. interventriculares septales
R. lateralis
R. posterior ventriculi sinistri
(R. posterolateralis dexter)

Coronary arteries, radiography

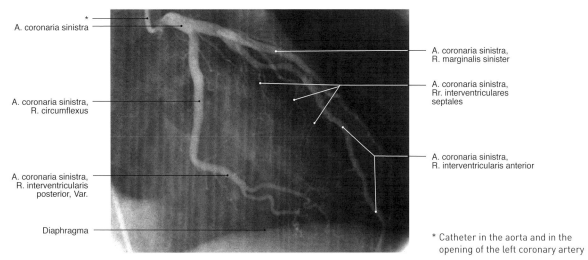

A. coronaria sinistra *

A. coronaria sinistra, R. marginalis sinister

A. coronaria sinistra, Rr. interventriculares septales

A. coronaria sinistra, R. circumflexus

A. coronaria sinistra, R. interventricularis anterior

A. coronaria sinistra, R. interventricularis posterior, Var.

Diaphragma

* Catheter in the aorta and in the opening of the left coronary artery

Fig. 899 Left coronary artery, A. coronaria sinistra; coronary angiography; the beam is directed obliquely from right anterior to left posterior (RAO).

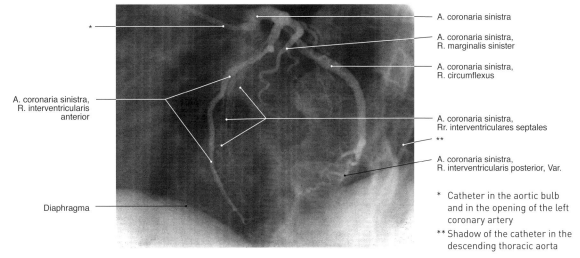

A. coronaria sinistra

A. coronaria sinistra, R. marginalis sinister

A. coronaria sinistra, R. circumflexus

A. coronaria sinistra, R. interventricularis anterior

A. coronaria sinistra, Rr. interventriculares septales

**

A. coronaria sinistra, R. interventricularis posterior, Var.

Diaphragma

* Catheter in the aortic bulb and in the opening of the left coronary artery
** Shadow of the catheter in the descending thoracic aorta

Fig. 900 Left coronary artery, A. coronaria sinistra; coronary angiography; the beam is directed obliquely from left anterior to right posterior (LAO).

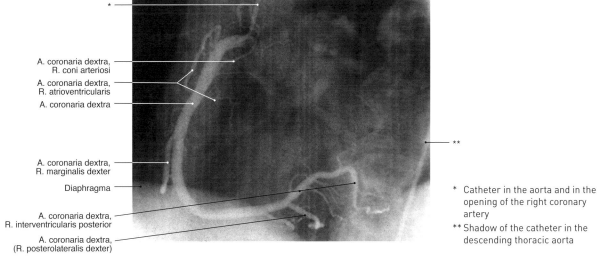

*

A. coronaria dextra, R. coni arteriosi

A. coronaria dextra, R. atrioventricularis

A. coronaria dextra

**

A. coronaria dextra, R. marginalis dexter

Diaphragma

A. coronaria dextra, R. interventricularis posterior

A. coronaria dextra, (R. posterolateralis dexter)

* Catheter in the aorta and in the opening of the right coronary artery
** Shadow of the catheter in the descending thoracic aorta

Fig. 901 Right coronary artery, A. coronaria dextra; coronary angiography; the beam is directed obliquely from left anterior to right posterior (LAO).

Heart situs

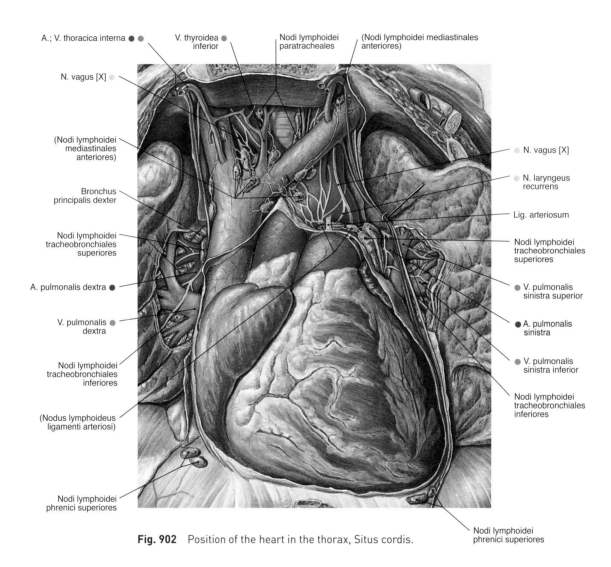

A.; V. thoracica interna ● ●

V. thyroidea ●
inferior

Nodi lymphoidei
paratracheales

(Nodi lymphoidei mediastinales
anteriores)

N. vagus [X] ●

(Nodi lymphoidei
mediastinales
anteriores)

Bronchus
principalis dexter

Nodi lymphoidei
tracheobronchiales
superiores

A. pulmonalis dextra ●

V. pulmonalis ●
dextra

Nodi lymphoidei
tracheobronchiales
inferiores

(Nodus lymphoideus
ligamenti arteriosi)

Nodi lymphoidei
phrenici superiores

N. vagus [X]

N. laryngeus
recurrens

Lig. arteriosum

Nodi lymphoidei
tracheobronchiales
superiores

● V. pulmonalis
sinistra superior

● A. pulmonalis
sinistra

● V. pulmonalis
sinistra inferior

Nodi lymphoidei
tracheobronchiales
inferiores

Nodi lymphoidei
phrenici superiores

Fig. 902   Position of the heart in the thorax, Situs cordis.

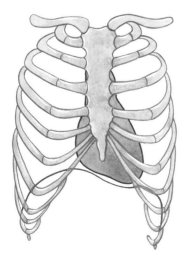

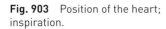

Fig. 903   Position of the heart;
inspiration.

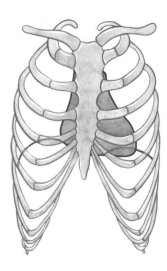

Fig. 904   Position of the heart;
expiration.

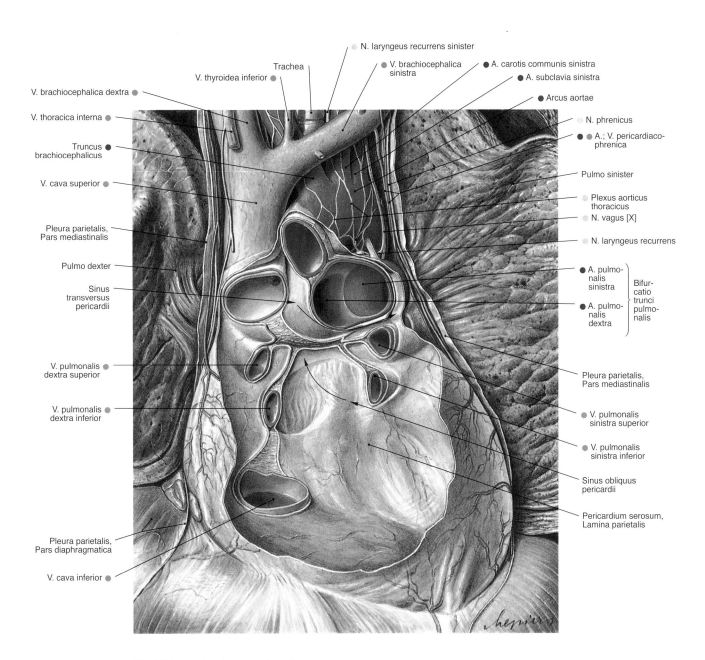

N. laryngeus recurrens sinister

Trachea

V. thyroidea inferior

V. brachiocephalica sinistra

A. carotis communis sinistra

A. subclavia sinistra

Arcus aortae

V. brachiocephalica dextra

V. thoracica interna

Truncus brachiocephalicus

V. cava superior

Pleura parietalis, Pars mediastinalis

Pulmo dexter

Sinus transversus pericardii

V. pulmonalis dextra superior

V. pulmonalis dextra inferior

Pleura parietalis, Pars diaphragmatica

V. cava inferior

N. phrenicus

A.; V. pericardiacophrenica

Pulmo sinister

Plexus aorticus thoracicus

N. vagus [X]

N. laryngeus recurrens

A. pulmonalis sinistra

A. pulmonalis dextra

} Bifurcatio trunci pulmonalis

Pleura parietalis, Pars mediastinalis

V. pulmonalis sinistra superior

V. pulmonalis sinistra inferior

Sinus obliquus pericardii

Pericardium serosum, Lamina parietalis

Fig. 905   Pericardium, Pericardium.

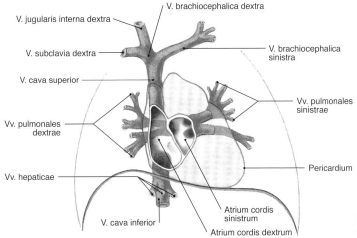

V. jugularis interna dextra

V. subclavia dextra

V. cava superior

Vv. pulmonales dextrae

Vv. hepaticae

V. cava inferior

V. brachiocephalica dextra

V. brachiocephalica sinistra

Vv. pulmonales sinistrae

Pericardium

Atrium cordis sinistrum

Atrium cordis dextrum

Fig. 906   Openings of the large veins into the heart; ventral view.

Trachea and bronchi

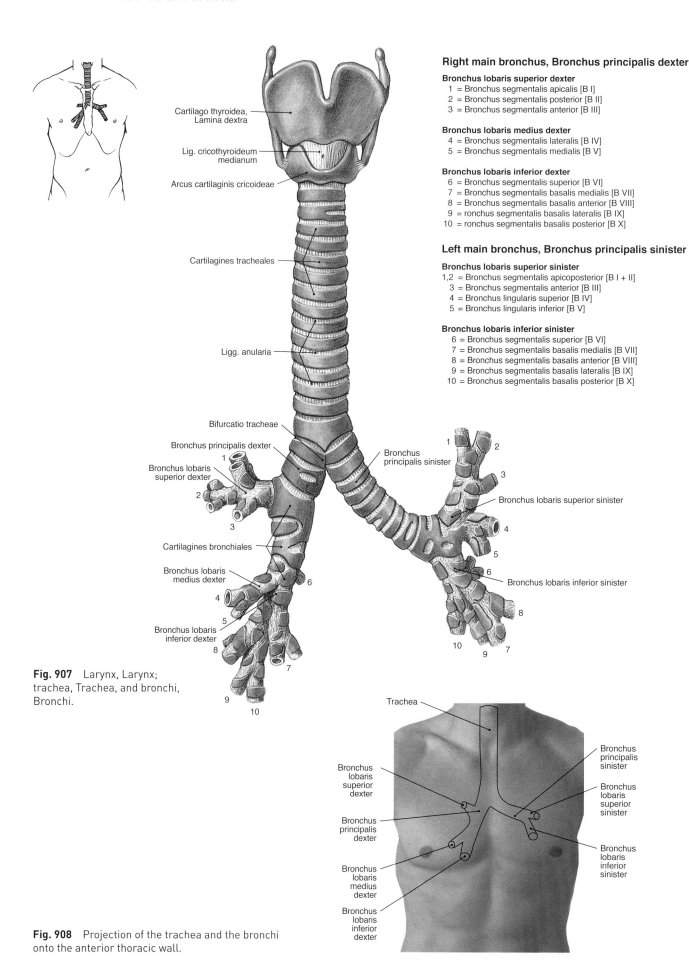

Cartilago thyroidea,
Lamina dextra

Lig. cricothyroideum
medianum

Arcus cartilaginis cricoideae

Cartilagines tracheales

Ligg. anularia

Bifurcatio tracheae

Bronchus principalis dexter

Bronchus lobaris
superior dexter

Cartilagines bronchiales

Bronchus lobaris
medius dexter

Bronchus lobaris
inferior dexter

Bronchus
principalis sinister

Bronchus lobaris superior sinister

Bronchus lobaris inferior sinister

Right main bronchus, Bronchus principalis dexter

Bronchus lobaris superior dexter
1 = Bronchus segmentalis apicalis [B I]
2 = Bronchus segmentalis posterior [B II]
3 = Bronchus segmentalis anterior [B III]

Bronchus lobaris medius dexter
4 = Bronchus segmentalis lateralis [B IV]
5 = Bronchus segmentalis medialis [B V]

Bronchus lobaris inferior dexter
6 = Bronchus segmentalis superior [B VI]
7 = Bronchus segmentalis basalis medialis [B VII]
8 = Bronchus segmentalis basalis anterior [B VIII]
9 = ronchus segmentalis basalis lateralis [B IX]
10 = ronchus segmentalis basalis posterior [B X]

Left main bronchus, Bronchus principalis sinister

Bronchus lobaris superior sinister
1,2 = Bronchus segmentalis apicoposterior [B I + II]
3 = Bronchus segmentalis anterior [B III]
4 = Bronchus lingularis superior [B IV]
5 = Bronchus lingularis inferior [B V]

Bronchus lobaris inferior sinister
6 = Bronchus segmentalis superior [B VI]
7 = Bronchus segmentalis basalis medialis [B VII]
8 = Bronchus segmentalis basalis anterior [B VIII]
9 = Bronchus segmentalis basalis lateralis [B IX]
10 = Bronchus segmentalis basalis posterior [B X]

Fig. 907 Larynx, Larynx;
trachea, Trachea, and bronchi,
Bronchi.

Trachea

Bronchus
lobaris
superior
dexter

Bronchus
principalis
dexter

Bronchus
lobaris
medius
dexter

Bronchus
lobaris
inferior
dexter

Bronchus
principalis
sinister

Bronchus
lobaris
superior
sinister

Bronchus
lobaris
inferior
sinister

Fig. 908 Projection of the trachea and the bronchi
onto the anterior thoracic wall.

Trachea, structure

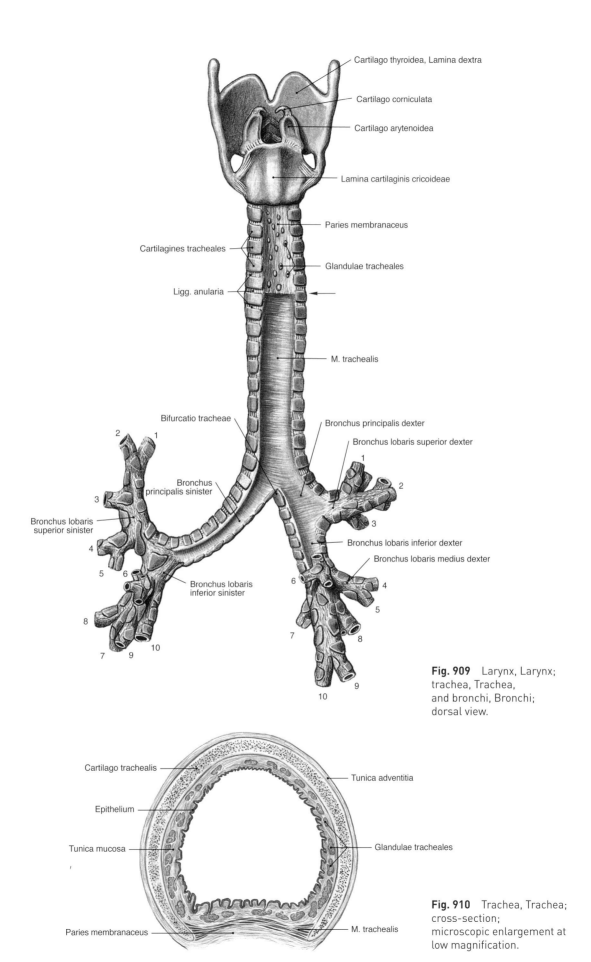

Cartilago thyroidea, Lamina dextra

Cartilago corniculata

Cartilago arytenoidea

Lamina cartilaginis cricoideae

Paries membranaceus

Cartilagines tracheales

Glandulae tracheales

Ligg. anularia

M. trachealis

Bifurcatio tracheae

Bronchus principalis dexter

Bronchus lobaris superior dexter

Bronchus principalis sinister

Bronchus lobaris superior sinister

Bronchus lobaris inferior sinister

Bronchus lobaris inferior dexter

Bronchus lobaris medius dexter

Fig. 909 Larynx, Larynx; trachea, Trachea, and bronchi, Bronchi; dorsal view.

Cartilago trachealis

Tunica adventitia

Epithelium

Tunica mucosa

Glandulae tracheales

Paries membranaceus

M. trachealis

Fig. 910 Trachea, Trachea; cross-section; microscopic enlargement at low magnification.

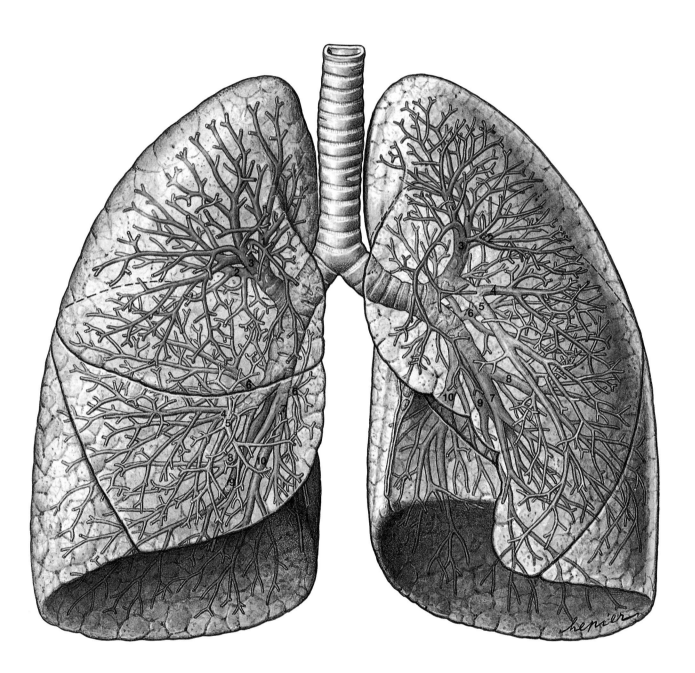

Fig. 911 Bronchi, Bronchi;
the lobar and the segmental bronchi have been projected
onto the lungs and are illustrated with different colours;
ventral view.
Numbers indicate the segmental bronchi (see p. 90).

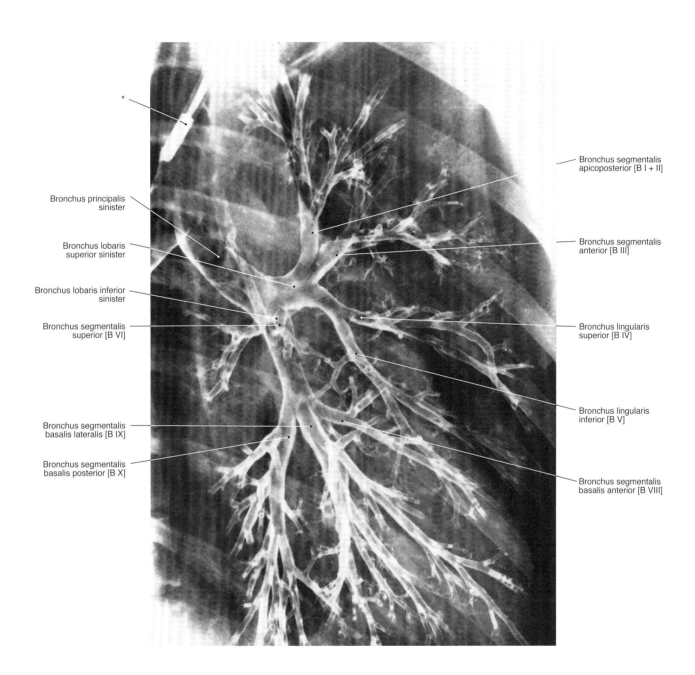

Bronchus segmentalis
apicoposterior [B I + II]

Bronchus principalis
sinister

Bronchus lobaris
superior sinister

Bronchus segmentalis
anterior [B III]

Bronchus lobaris inferior
sinister

Bronchus segmentalis
superior [B VI]

Bronchus lingularis
superior [B IV]

Bronchus lingularis
inferior [B V]

Bronchus segmentalis
basalis lateralis [B IX]

Bronchus segmentalis
basalis posterior [B X]

Bronchus segmentalis
basalis anterior [B VIII]

Fig. 912 Bronchi, Bronchi;
AP-radiograph; bronchography of the left lung.
* Bronchography catheter in the trachea

Lungs

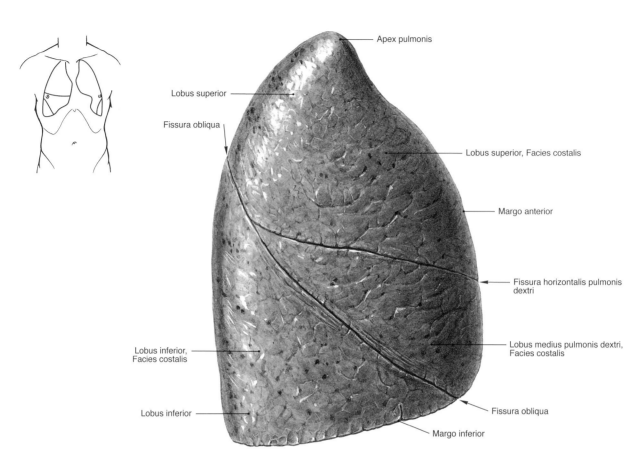

Fig. 913 Right lung, Pulmo dexter; lateral view.

Labels (Fig. 913):
- Apex pulmonis
- Lobus superior
- Fissura obliqua
- Lobus superior, Facies costalis
- Margo anterior
- Fissura horizontalis pulmonis dextri
- Lobus inferior, Facies costalis
- Lobus medius pulmonis dextri, Facies costalis
- Lobus inferior
- Fissura obliqua
- Margo inferior

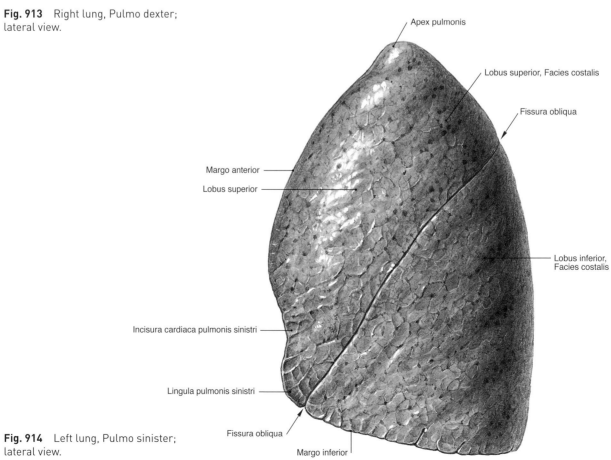

Fig. 914 Left lung, Pulmo sinister; lateral view.

Labels (Fig. 914):
- Apex pulmonis
- Lobus superior, Facies costalis
- Fissura obliqua
- Margo anterior
- Lobus superior
- Lobus inferior, Facies costalis
- Incisura cardiaca pulmonis sinistri
- Lingula pulmonis sinistri
- Fissura obliqua
- Margo inferior

Lungs

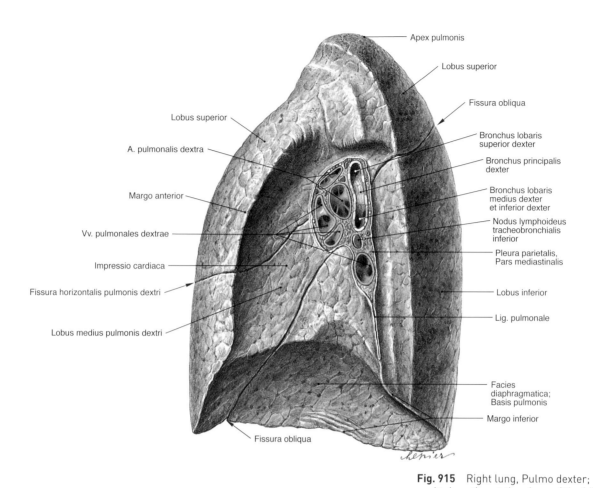

Apex pulmonis

Lobus superior

Fissura obliqua

Bronchus lobaris superior dexter

Bronchus principalis dexter

Bronchus lobaris medius dexter et inferior dexter

Nodus lymphoideus tracheobronchialis inferior

Pleura parietalis, Pars mediastinalis

Lobus inferior

Lig. pulmonale

Facies diaphragmatica; Basis pulmonis

Margo inferior

Lobus superior

A. pulmonalis dextra

Margo anterior

Vv. pulmonales dextrae

Impressio cardiaca

Fissura horizontalis pulmonis dextri

Lobus medius pulmonis dextri

Fissura obliqua

Fig. 915 Right lung, Pulmo dexter; sagittal section at the plane of the hilum of the lung; medial view.

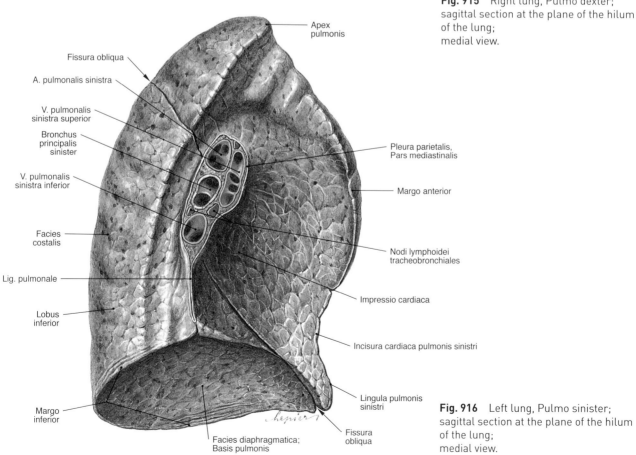

Apex pulmonis

Fissura obliqua

A. pulmonalis sinistra

V. pulmonalis sinistra superior

Bronchus principalis sinister

V. pulmonalis sinistra inferior

Facies costalis

Lig. pulmonale

Lobus inferior

Margo inferior

Facies diaphragmatica; Basis pulmonis

Pleura parietalis, Pars mediastinalis

Margo anterior

Nodi lymphoidei tracheobronchiales

Impressio cardiaca

Incisura cardiaca pulmonis sinistri

Lingula pulmonis sinistri

Fissura obliqua

Fig. 916 Left lung, Pulmo sinister; sagittal section at the plane of the hilum of the lung; medial view.

Bronchopulmonary segments

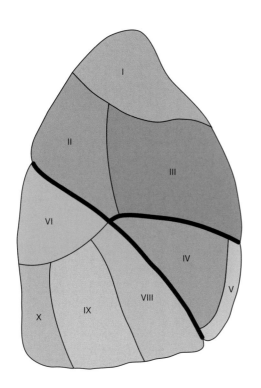

Pulmo dexter

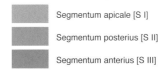

Pulmo dexter, Lobus superior

Segmentum apicale [S I]

Segmentum posterius [S II]

Segmentum anterius [S III]

Pulmo dexter, Lobus medius

Segmentum laterale [S IV]

Segmentum mediale [S V]

Pulmo dexter, Lobus inferior

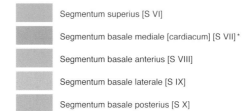

Segmentum superius [S VI]

Segmentum basale mediale [cardiacum] [S VII] *

Segmentum basale anterius [S VIII]

Segmentum basale laterale [S IX]

Segmentum basale posterius [S X]

* This segment is generally not an independent segment, but rather fused with the anterior basal segment [S VIII].

Fig. 917 Right lung, Pulmo dexter; bronchopulmonary segments, Segmenta bronchopulmonalia; lateral view.

Pulmo sinister

Pulmo sinister, Lobus superior

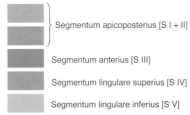

Segmentum apicoposterius [S I + II]

Segmentum anterius [S III]

Segmentum lingulare superius [S IV]

Segmentum lingulare inferius [S V]

Pulmo sinister, Lobus inferior

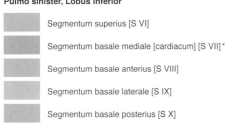

Segmentum superius [S VI]

Segmentum basale mediale [cardiacum] [S VII] *

Segmentum basale anterius [S VIII]

Segmentum basale laterale [S IX]

Segmentum basale posterius [S X]

* This segment is generally not an independent segment, but rather fused with the anterior basal segment [S VIII].

Fig. 918 Left lung, Pulmo sinister; bronchopulmonary segments, Segmenta bronchopulmonalia; lateral view.

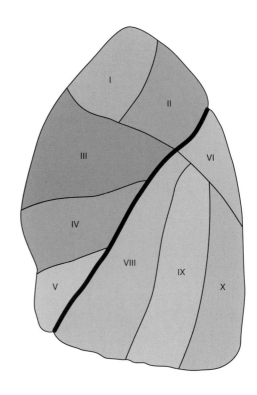

Bronchopulmonary segments

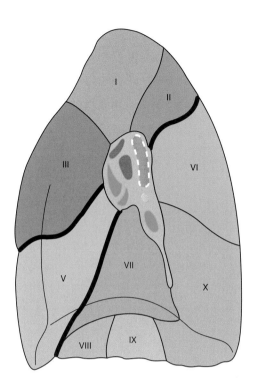

Fig. 919   Right lung, Pulmo dexter;
bronchopulmonary segments,
Segmenta bronchopulmonalia;
medial view.

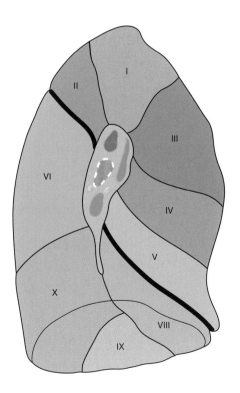

Fig. 920   Left lung, Pulmo sinister;
bronchopulmonary segments,
Segmenta bronchopulmonalia;
medial view.

Lungs, structure

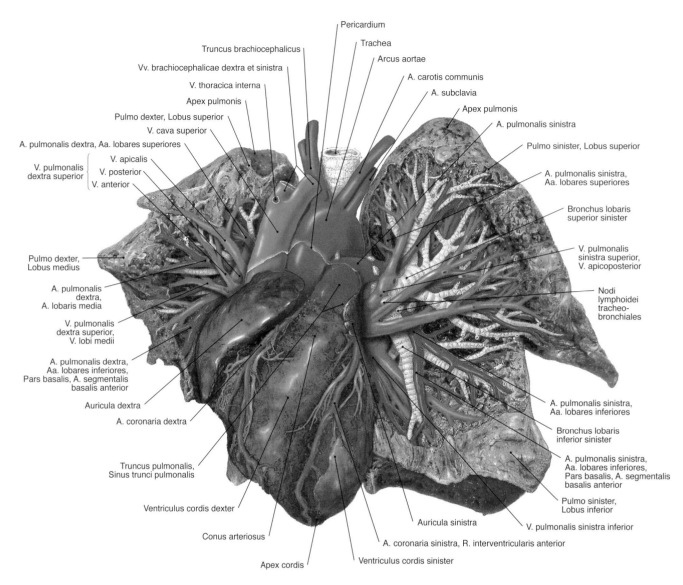

Pericardium
Trachea
Truncus brachiocephalicus
Arcus aortae
Vv. brachiocephalicae dextra et sinistra
A. carotis communis
V. thoracica interna
A. subclavia
Apex pulmonis
Apex pulmonis
Pulmo dexter, Lobus superior
A. pulmonalis sinistra
V. cava superior
A. pulmonalis dextra, Aa. lobares superiores
Pulmo sinister, Lobus superior
V. apicalis
A. pulmonalis sinistra,
V. pulmonalis
Aa. lobares superiores
dextra superior
V. posterior
V. anterior
Bronchus lobaris
superior sinister
Pulmo dexter,
V. pulmonalis
Lobus medius
sinistra superior,
V. apicoposterior
A. pulmonalis
dextra,
Nodi
A. lobaris media
lymphoidei
tracheo-
V. pulmonalis
bronchiales
dextra superior,
V. lobi medii
A. pulmonalis dextra,
Aa. lobares inferiores,
A. pulmonalis sinistra,
Pars basalis, A. segmentalis
Aa. lobares inferiores
basalis anterior
Bronchus lobaris
Auricula dextra
inferior sinister
A. coronaria dextra
A. pulmonalis sinistra,
Aa. lobares inferiores,
Pars basalis, A. segmentalis
basalis anterior
Truncus pulmonalis,
Pulmo sinister,
Sinus trunci pulmonalis
Lobus inferior
Ventriculus cordis dexter
Auricula sinistra
V. pulmonalis sinistra inferior
Conus arteriosus
A. coronaria sinistra, R. interventricularis anterior
Apex cordis
Ventriculus cordis sinister

Fig. 921 Lungs, Pulmones, and heart, Cor;
the arteries, the veins and the bronchi have been
dissected up to the external surface of the lungs.

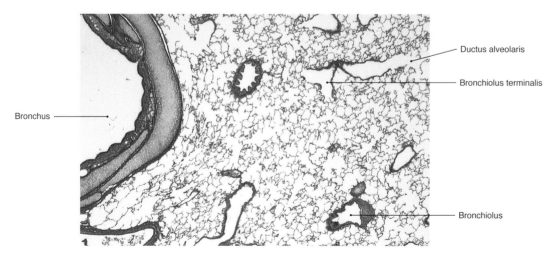

Ductus alveolaris
Bronchiolus terminalis
Bronchus
Bronchiolus

Fig. 922 Lung, Pulmo;
overview of the lung structure;
microscopic enlargement at low magnification.

Vessels of the lungs and bronchi

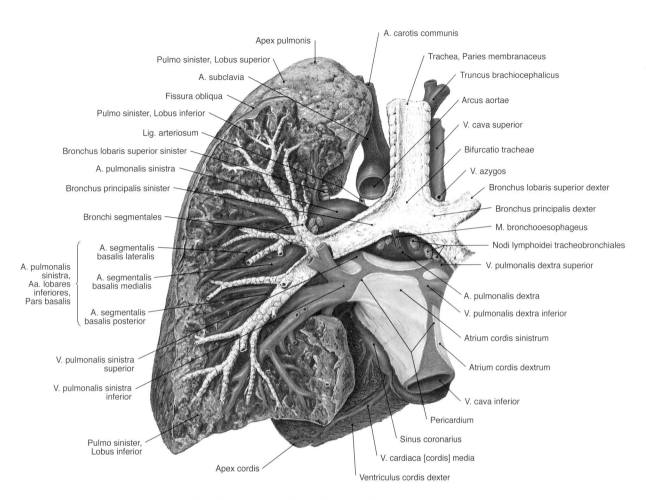

Apex pulmonis
A. carotis communis
Pulmo sinister, Lobus superior
Trachea, Paries membranaceus
A. subclavia
Truncus brachiocephalicus
Fissura obliqua
Arcus aortae
Pulmo sinister, Lobus inferior
V. cava superior
Lig. arteriosum
Bifurcatio tracheae
Bronchus lobaris superior sinister
V. azygos
A. pulmonalis sinistra
Bronchus lobaris superior dexter
Bronchus principalis sinister
Bronchus principalis dexter
M. bronchooesophageus
Bronchi segmentales
Nodi lymphoidei tracheobronchiales
A. segmentalis basalis lateralis
V. pulmonalis dextra superior
A. pulmonalis sinistra, Aa. lobares inferiores, Pars basalis
A. segmentalis basalis medialis
A. pulmonalis dextra
V. pulmonalis dextra inferior
A. segmentalis basalis posterior
Atrium cordis sinistrum
V. pulmonalis sinistra superior
Atrium cordis dextrum
V. pulmonalis sinistra inferior
V. cava inferior
Pulmo sinister, Lobus inferior
Pericardium
Sinus coronarius
Apex cordis
V. cardiaca [cordis] media
Ventriculus cordis dexter

Fig. 923   Vessels of the left lung, Pulmo sinister; dorsal view.

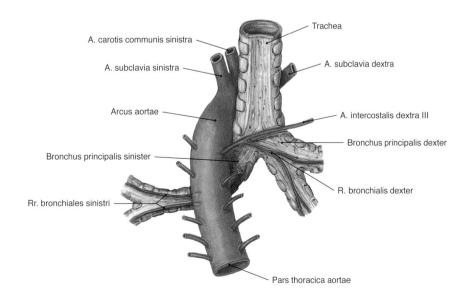

A. carotis communis sinistra
Trachea
A. subclavia sinistra
A. subclavia dextra
Arcus aortae
A. intercostalis dextra III
Bronchus principalis sinister
Bronchus principalis dexter
R. bronchialis dexter
Rr. bronchiales sinistri
Pars thoracica aortae

Fig. 924   Bronchi, Bronchi; arterial supply.

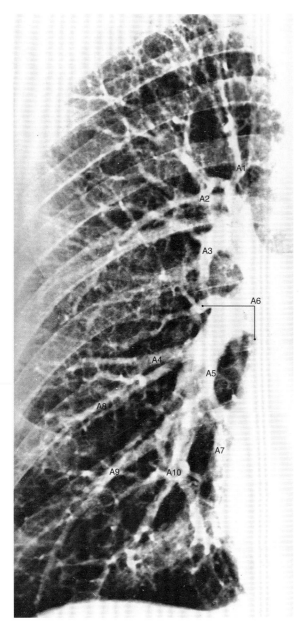

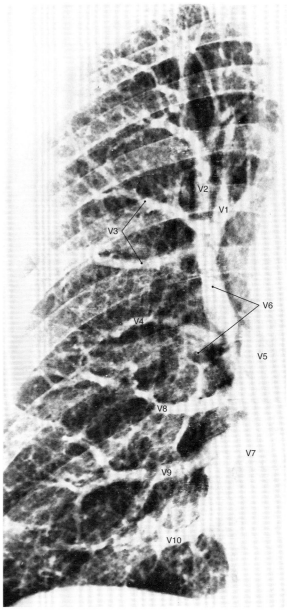

Fig. 925 Arteries of the right lung,
Aa. pulmonales dextrae;
AP-radiograph (pulmonary angiography); after
injection of a contrast medium into the right ventricle;
ventral view.
The numbers designate the segmental arteries
(compare p. 96).

Fig. 926 Veins of the right lung,
Vv. pulmonales dextrae;
AP-radiograph (return via pulmonary veins of the contrast
medium injected into the right ventricle);
ventral view.
Numbers indicate the segmental veins (compare p. 96).

Thoracic viscera, radiography

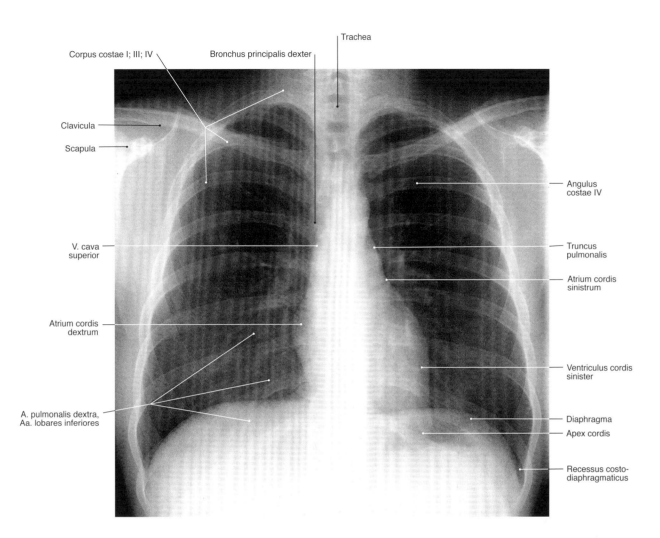

Trachea

Corpus costae I; III; IV

Bronchus principalis dexter

Clavicula

Scapula

V. cava superior

Atrium cordis dextrum

A. pulmonalis dextra, Aa. lobares inferiores

Angulus costae IV

Truncus pulmonalis

Atrium cordis sinistrum

Ventriculus cordis sinister

Diaphragma

Apex cordis

Recessus costo-diaphragmaticus

Fig. 927 Thoracic cage, Cavea thoracis, and thoracic viscera; PA-radiograph of a 27-year-old male (thorax radiograph).

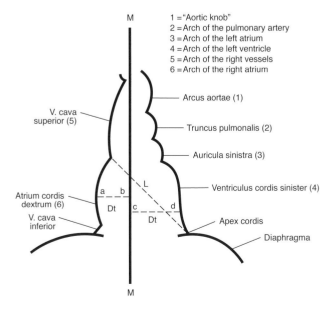

M

1 = "Aortic knob"
2 = Arch of the pulmonary artery
3 = Arch of the left atrium
4 = Arch of the left ventricle
5 = Arch of the right vessels
6 = Arch of the right atrium

Arcus aortae (1)

V. cava superior (5)

Truncus pulmonalis (2)

Auricula sinistra (3)

Ventriculus cordis sinister (4)

Atrium cordis dextrum (6)

V. cava inferior

Apex cordis

Diaphragma

M

Fig. 928 Outline of the heart shadow in the radiograph;
Dt = Transverse diameter,
      ab + cd = 13–14 cm
L = Longitudinal axis of the heart (from the superior border of the right atrial contour to the apex of the heart) = 15–16 cm
M = Median plane of the body

Bronchoscopy

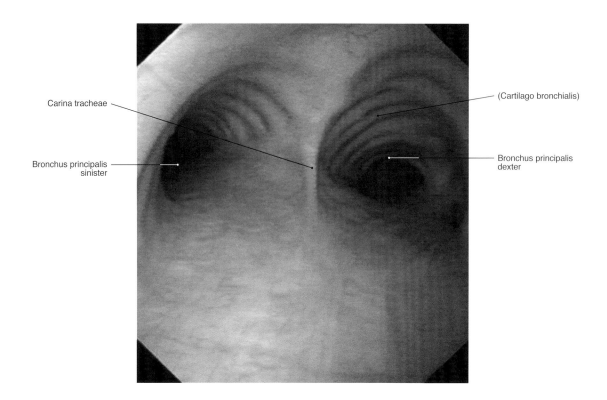

Carina tracheae

Bronchus principalis sinister

(Cartilago bronchialis)

Bronchus principalis dexter

Fig. 929 Bronchi, Bronchi;
bronchoscopy of a healthy individual displaying the tracheal bifurcation and the carina of trachea.

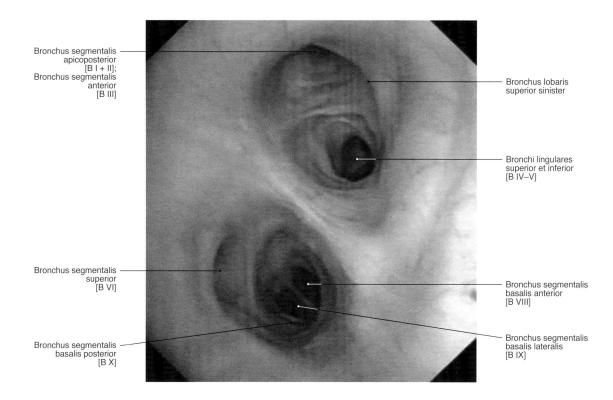

Bronchus segmentalis apicoposterior [B I + II]; Bronchus segmentalis anterior [B III]

Bronchus segmentalis superior [B VI]

Bronchus segmentalis basalis posterior [B X]

Bronchus lobaris superior sinister

Bronchi lingulares superior et inferior [B IV–V]

Bronchus segmentalis basalis anterior [B VIII]

Bronchus segmentalis basalis lateralis [B IX]

Fig. 930 Bronchi, Bronchi;
bronchoscopic view of the left segmental bronchi.

Lungs, surface projections

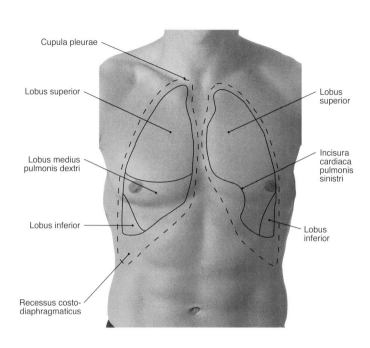

Cupula pleurae

Lobus superior

Lobus medius pulmonis dextri

Lobus inferior

Recessus costo-diaphragmaticus

Lobus superior

Incisura cardiaca pulmonis sinistri

Lobus inferior

Vertebra cervicalis VII [prominens]

Lobus superior

Spina scapulae

Lobus inferior

Recessus costodiaphragmaticus

Costa XII

Crista iliaca

Fig. 931 Projection of the pulmonary and the pleural borders onto the anterior thoracic wall.

Fig. 932 Projection of the pulmonary and the pleural borders onto the posterior thoracic wall.

Borders of the lungs – line
Borders of the pleura – dashed line

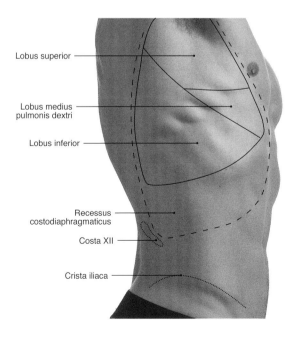

Lobus superior

Lobus medius pulmonis dextri

Lobus inferior

Recessus costodiaphragmaticus

Costa XII

Crista iliaca

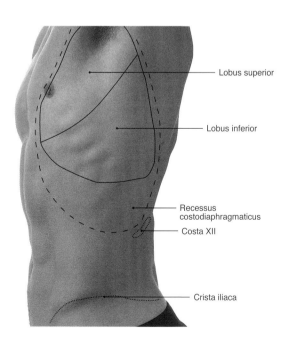

Lobus superior

Lobus inferior

Recessus costodiaphragmaticus

Costa XII

Crista iliaca

Fig. 933 Projection of the pulmonary and the pleural borders onto the lateral thoracic wall.

Fig. 934 Projection of the pulmonary and the pleural borders onto the lateral thoracic wall.

Oesophagus

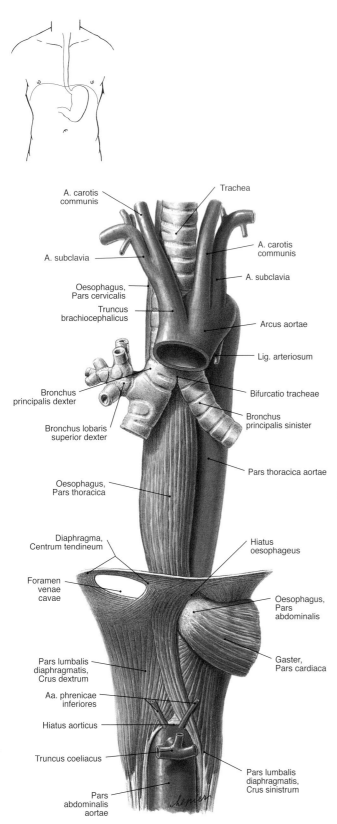

A. carotis communis

Trachea

A. subclavia

A. carotis communis

Oesophagus, Pars cervicalis

A. subclavia

Truncus brachiocephalicus

Arcus aortae

Lig. arteriosum

Bronchus principalis dexter

Bifurcatio tracheae

Bronchus lobaris superior dexter

Bronchus principalis sinister

Oesophagus, Pars thoracica

Pars thoracica aortae

Diaphragma, Centrum tendineum

Hiatus oesophageus

Foramen venae cavae

Oesophagus, Pars abdominalis

Pars lumbalis diaphragmatis, Crus dextrum

Gaster, Pars cardiaca

Aa. phrenicae inferiores

Hiatus aorticus

Truncus coeliacus

Pars lumbalis diaphragmatis, Crus sinistrum

Pars abdominalis aortae

Fig. 935 Oesophagus, Oesophagus; trachea, Trachea, and the thoracic aorta, Pars thoracica aortae; ventral view.

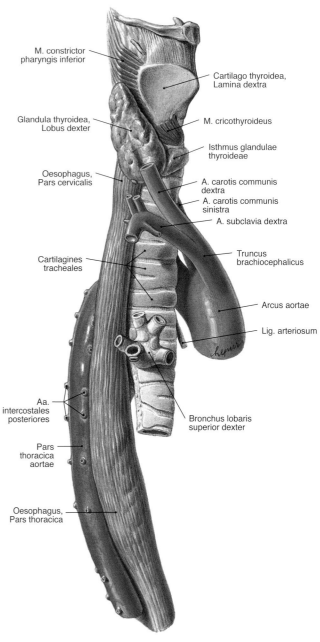

M. constrictor pharyngis inferior

Cartilago thyroidea, Lamina dextra

Glandula thyroidea, Lobus dexter

M. cricothyroideus

Isthmus glandulae thyroideae

Oesophagus, Pars cervicalis

A. carotis communis dextra

A. carotis communis sinistra

A. subclavia dextra

Cartilagines tracheales

Truncus brachiocephalicus

Arcus aortae

Lig. arteriosum

Aa. intercostales posteriores

Pars thoracica aortae

Bronchus lobaris superior dexter

Oesophagus, Pars thoracica

Fig. 936 Oesophagus, Oesophagus; trachea, Trachea, and the thoracic aorta, Pars thoracica aortae; viewed from the right.

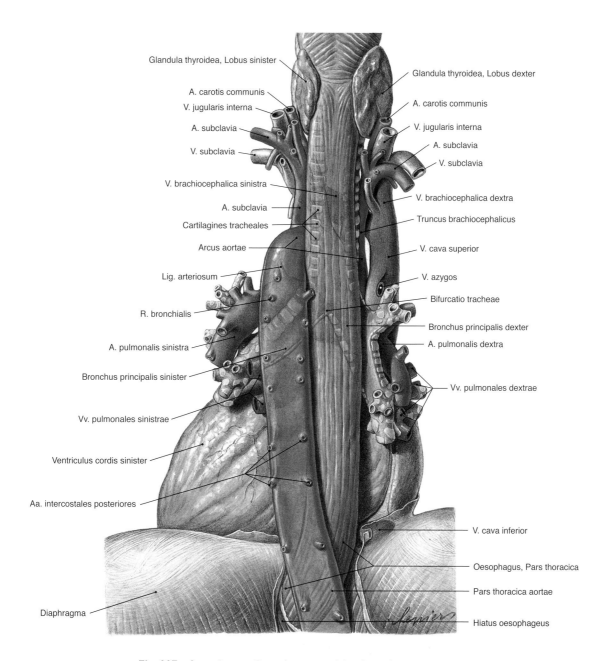

Glandula thyroidea, Lobus sinister
A. carotis communis
V. jugularis interna
A. subclavia
V. subclavia
V. brachiocephalica sinistra
A. subclavia
Cartilagines tracheales
Arcus aortae
Lig. arteriosum
R. bronchialis
A. pulmonalis sinistra
Bronchus principalis sinister
Vv. pulmonales sinistrae
Ventriculus cordis sinister
Aa. intercostales posteriores
Diaphragma

Glandula thyroidea, Lobus dexter
A. carotis communis
V. jugularis interna
A. subclavia
V. subclavia
V. brachiocephalica dextra
Truncus brachiocephalicus
V. cava superior
V. azygos
Bifurcatio tracheae
Bronchus principalis dexter
A. pulmonalis dextra
Vv. pulmonales dextrae
V. cava inferior
Oesophagus, Pars thoracica
Pars thoracica aortae
Hiatus oesophageus

Fig. 937 Oesophagus, Oesophagus, and the thoracic aorta,
Pars thoracica aortae;
dorsal view.

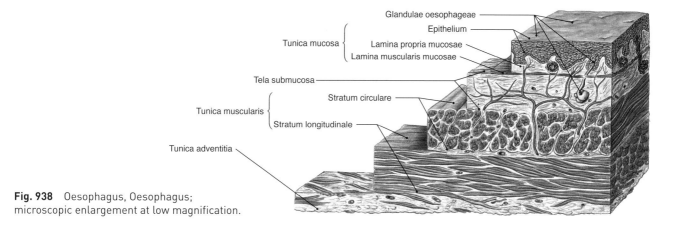

Glandulae oesophageae
Epithelium
Tunica mucosa
Lamina propria mucosae
Lamina muscularis mucosae
Tela submucosa
Stratum circulare
Tunica muscularis
Stratum longitudinale
Tunica adventitia

Fig. 938 Oesophagus, Oesophagus;
microscopic enlargement at low magnification.

Vessels of the oesophagus

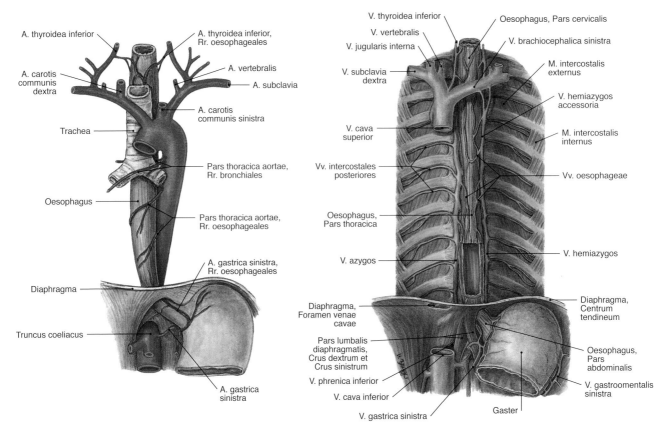

A. thyroidea inferior

A. thyroidea inferior, Rr. oesophageales

A. carotis communis dextra

A. vertebralis

A. subclavia

A. carotis communis sinistra

Trachea

Pars thoracica aortae, Rr. bronchiales

Oesophagus

Pars thoracica aortae, Rr. oesophageales

A. gastrica sinistra, Rr. oesophageales

Diaphragma

Truncus coeliacus

A. gastrica sinistra

V. thyroidea inferior

V. vertebralis

V. jugularis interna

V. subclavia dextra

Oesophagus, Pars cervicalis

V. brachiocephalica sinistra

M. intercostalis externus

V. hemiazygos accessoria

M. intercostalis internus

V. cava superior

Vv. intercostales posteriores

Vv. oesophageae

Oesophagus, Pars thoracica

V. azygos

V. hemiazygos

Diaphragma, Foramen venae cavae

Diaphragma, Centrum tendineum

Pars lumbalis diaphragmatis, Crus dextrum et Crus sinistrum

Oesophagus, Pars abdominalis

V. phrenica inferior

V. gastroomentalis sinistra

V. cava inferior

V. gastrica sinistra

Gaster

Fig. 939 Oesophagus, Oesophagus; supplying arteries; ventral view.

Fig. 940 Veins of the oesophagus, Vv. oesophageae.

→ 1077, 1078

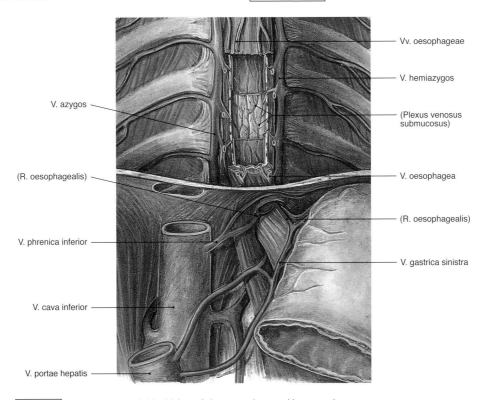

Vv. oesophageae

V. hemiazygos

V. azygos

(Plexus venosus submucosus)

(R. oesophagealis)

V. oesophagea

V. phrenica inferior

(R. oesophagealis)

V. gastrica sinistra

V. cava inferior

V. portae hepatis

→ 1078

Fig. 941 Veins of the oesophagus, Vv. oesophageae; magnification of Fig. 940; demonstration of anastomoses between branches of the hepatic portal vein and the superior vena cava.

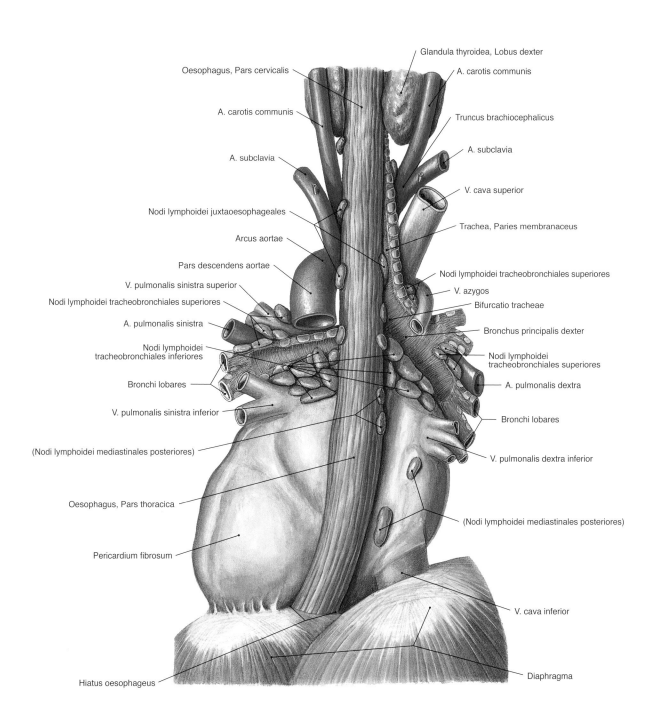

Glandula thyroidea, Lobus dexter

A. carotis communis

Oesophagus, Pars cervicalis

A. carotis communis

Truncus brachiocephalicus

A. subclavia

A. subclavia

V. cava superior

Nodi lymphoidei juxtaoesophageales

Trachea, Paries membranaceus

Arcus aortae

Nodi lymphoidei tracheobronchiales superiores

Pars descendens aortae

V. azygos

V. pulmonalis sinistra superior

Bifurcatio tracheae

Nodi lymphoidei tracheobronchiales superiores

Bronchus principalis dexter

A. pulmonalis sinistra

Nodi lymphoidei
tracheobronchiales inferiores

Nodi lymphoidei
tracheobronchiales superiores

Bronchi lobares

A. pulmonalis dextra

V. pulmonalis sinistra inferior

Bronchi lobares

(Nodi lymphoidei mediastinales posteriores)

V. pulmonalis dextra inferior

Oesophagus, Pars thoracica

(Nodi lymphoidei mediastinales posteriores)

Pericardium fibrosum

V. cava inferior

Hiatus oesophageus

Diaphragma

Fig. 942 Thoracic lymph nodes;
Nodi lymphoidei thoracis;
dorsal view.

Oesophagus, radiography and oesophagoscopy

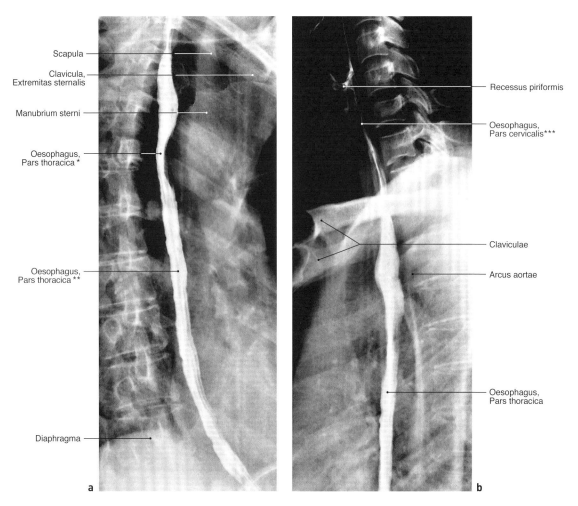

Scapula
Clavicula, Extremitas sternalis
Manubrium sterni
Oesophagus, Pars thoracica *
Oesophagus, Pars thoracica **
Diaphragma

a

Recessus piriformis
Oesophagus, Pars cervicalis***
Claviculae
Arcus aortae
Oesophagus, Pars thoracica

b

Fig. 943 a, b Oesophagus, Oesophagus;
radiograph after swallowing of a contrast medium.
a Right anterior oblique position, oblique diameter I (beam directed from left anterior to right posterior)
b Left anterior oblique position, oblique diameter II (beam directed from right anterior to left posterior)

*   Oesophageal constriction caused by the aortic arch
** Retrocardial portion of the oesophagus
***Oesophageal constriction at the junction of the pharynx with the oesophagus

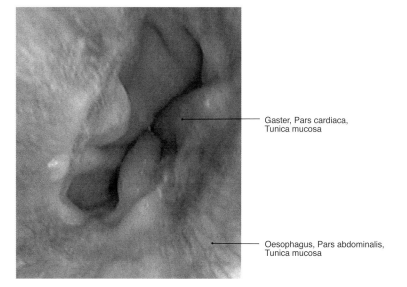

Gaster, Pars cardiaca, Tunica mucosa

Oesophagus, Pars abdominalis, Tunica mucosa

Fig. 944 Oesophagus, Oesophagus;
oesophagoscopy (technical details see Fig. 986);
superior view.

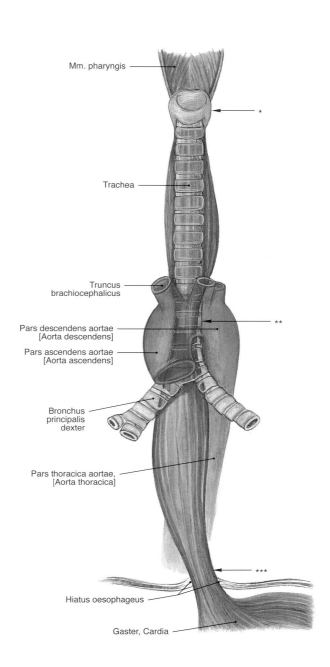

Mm. pharyngis

Trachea

Truncus
brachiocephalicus

Pars descendens aortae
[Aorta descendens]

Pars ascendens aortae
[Aorta ascendens]

Bronchus
principalis
dexter

Pars thoracica aortae,
[Aorta thoracica]

Hiatus oesophageus

Gaster, Cardia

*

**

***

Fig. 945 Oesophagus, Oesophagus;
constrictions.

* Upper oesophageal sphincter
** Narrowing caused by the aortic arch
***Diaphragmatic constriction

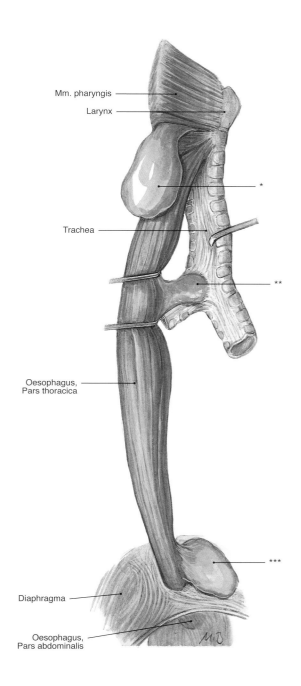

Mm. pharyngis
Larynx

Trachea

Oesophagus,
Pars thoracica

Diaphragma

Oesophagus,
Pars abdominalis

*

**

***

Fig. 946 Oesophagus, Oesophagus;
typical location and frequency of diverticula.

* Cervical diverticulum
  (ZENKER's diverticulum), (~70%)
** Mid-oesophageal diverticulum (~22%)
***Epiphrenic diverticulum (~8%)

Thymus

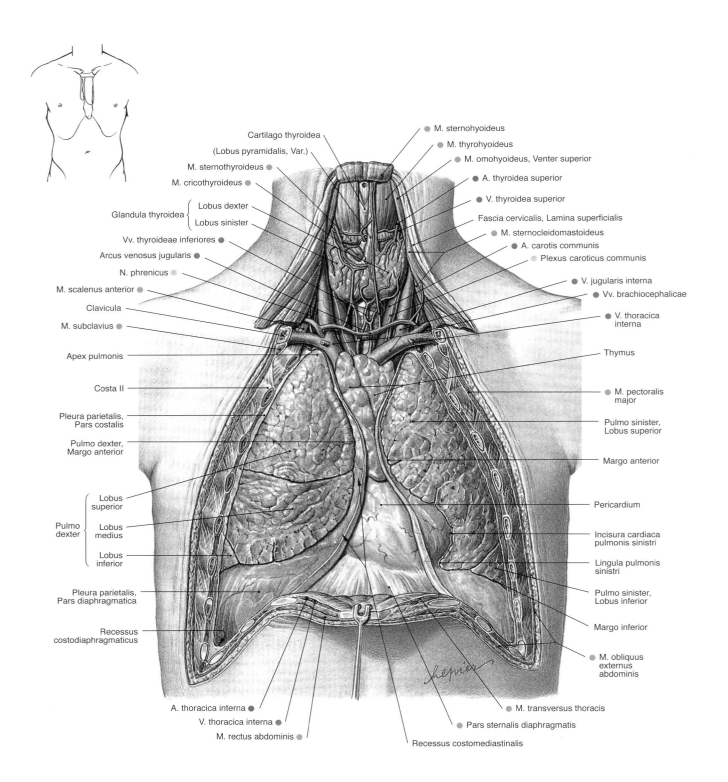

Cartilago thyroidea

(Lobus pyramidalis, Var.)

M. sternothyroideus

M. cricothyroideus

Glandula thyroidea { Lobus dexter
Lobus sinister }

Vv. thyroideae inferiores

Arcus venosus jugularis

N. phrenicus

M. scalenus anterior

Clavicula

M. subclavius

Apex pulmonis

Costa II

Pleura parietalis, Pars costalis

Pulmo dexter, Margo anterior

Pulmo dexter { Lobus superior
Lobus medius
Lobus inferior }

Pleura parietalis, Pars diaphragmatica

Recessus costodiaphragmaticus

A. thoracica interna

V. thoracica interna

M. rectus abdominis

M. sternohyoideus

M. thyrohyoideus

M. omohyoideus, Venter superior

A. thyroidea superior

V. thyroidea superior

Fascia cervicalis, Lamina superficialis

M. sternocleidomastoideus

A. carotis communis

Plexus caroticus communis

V. jugularis interna

Vv. brachiocephalicae

V. thoracica interna

Thymus

M. pectoralis major

Pulmo sinister, Lobus superior

Margo anterior

Pericardium

Incisura cardiaca pulmonis sinistri

Lingula pulmonis sinistri

Pulmo sinister, Lobus inferior

Margo inferior

M. obliquus externus abdominis

M. transversus thoracis

Pars sternalis diaphragmatis

Recessus costomediastinalis

→ 1049

Fig. 947 Thymus, Thymus; pericardium, Pericardium, and lungs, Pulmones, of an adolescent.
Note the size of the adolescent thymus. In older individuals, the thymic tissue is almost entirely replaced by adipose tissue.

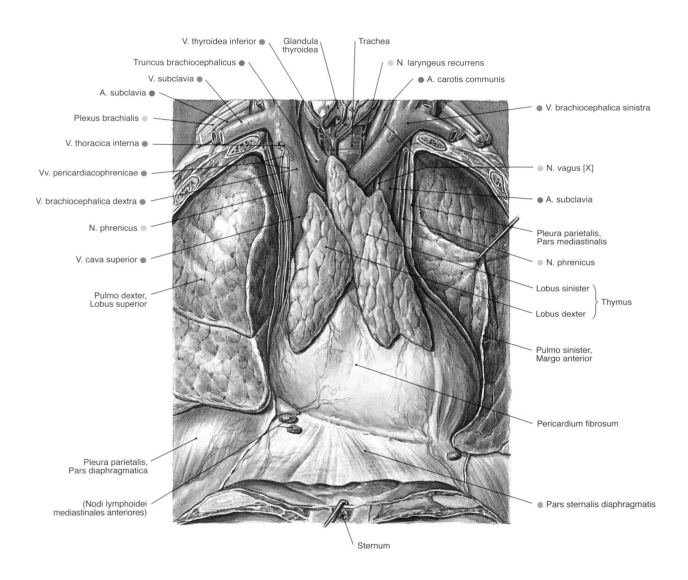

V. thyroidea inferior ●   Glandula thyroidea   Trachea

Truncus brachiocephalicus ●

V. subclavia ●

A. subclavia ●

Plexus brachialis ●

V. thoracica interna ●

Vv. pericardiacophrenicae ●

V. brachiocephalica dextra ●

N. phrenicus ●

V. cava superior ●

Pulmo dexter, Lobus superior

Pleura parietalis, Pars diaphragmatica

(Nodi lymphoidei mediastinales anteriores)

● N. laryngeus recurrens

● A. carotis communis

● V. brachiocephalica sinistra

● N. vagus [X]

● A. subclavia

Pleura parietalis, Pars mediastinalis

● N. phrenicus

Lobus sinister

Lobus dexter   } Thymus

Pulmo sinister, Margo anterior

Pericardium fibrosum

● Pars sternalis diaphragmatis

Sternum

Fig. 948   Thymus, Thymus, of an adolescent.

→ 1049

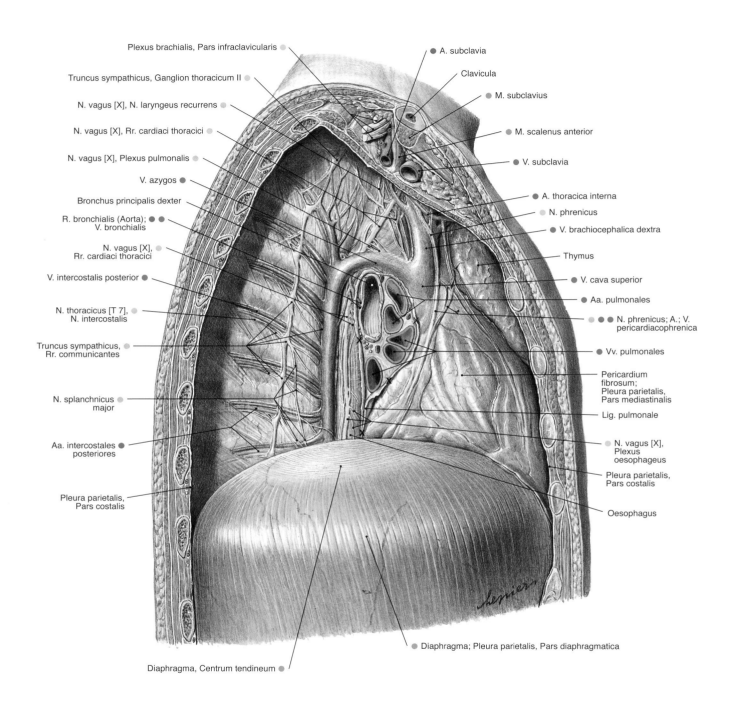

Plexus brachialis, Pars infraclavicularis ●

Truncus sympathicus, Ganglion thoracicum II ●

N. vagus [X], N. laryngeus recurrens ●

N. vagus [X], Rr. cardiaci thoracici ●

N. vagus [X], Plexus pulmonalis ●

V. azygos ●

Bronchus principalis dexter ●

R. bronchialis (Aorta); ● ●
V. bronchialis

N. vagus [X], ●
Rr. cardiaci thoracici

V. intercostalis posterior ●

N. thoracicus [T 7], ●
N. intercostalis

Truncus sympathicus, ●
Rr. communicantes

N. splanchnicus ●
major

Aa. intercostales ●
posteriores

Pleura parietalis,
Pars costalis

Diaphragma, Centrum tendineum ●

● A. subclavia

Clavicula

● M. subclavius

● M. scalenus anterior

● V. subclavia

● A. thoracica interna

● N. phrenicus

● V. brachiocephalica dextra

Thymus

● V. cava superior

● Aa. pulmonales

● ● ● N. phrenicus; A.; V.
pericardiacophrenica

● Vv. pulmonales

Pericardium
fibrosum;
Pleura parietalis,
Pars mediastinalis

Lig. pulmonale

● N. vagus [X],
Plexus
oesophageus

Pleura parietalis,
Pars costalis

Oesophagus

● Diaphragma; Pleura parietalis, Pars diaphragmatica

Fig. 949 Pleural cavity, Cavitas pleuralis, and mediastinum, Mediastinum, of an adolescent;
lateral thoracic wall and right lung have been removed; viewed from the right.
The x indicate the areas at the root of the lung and the pulmonary ligament, respectively, where the visceral pleura folds back into the parietal pleura.

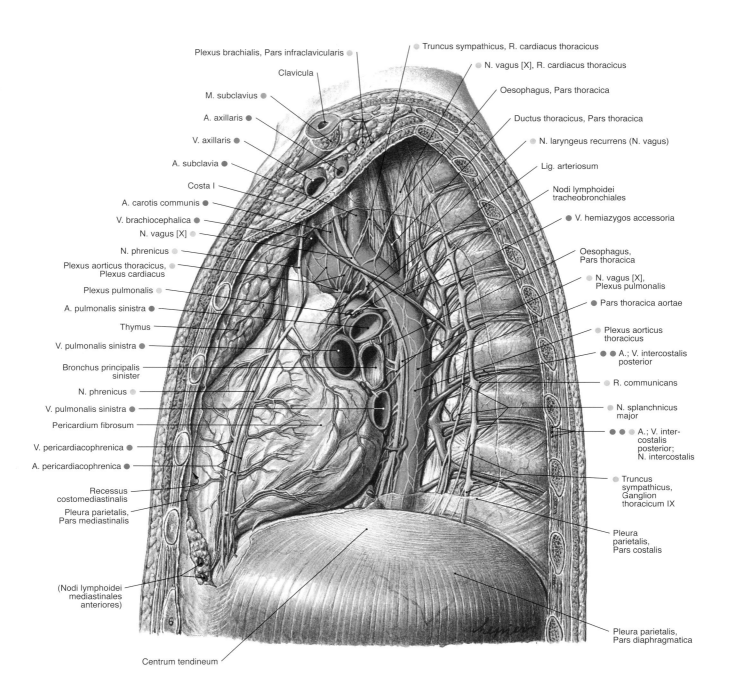

Plexus brachialis, Pars infraclavicularis ●

Clavicula

M. subclavius ●

A. axillaris ●

V. axillaris ●

A. subclavia ●

Costa I

A. carotis communis ●

V. brachiocephalica ●

N. vagus [X] ●

N. phrenicus ●

Plexus aorticus thoracicus, ●
Plexus cardiacus

Plexus pulmonalis ●

A. pulmonalis sinistra ●

Thymus

V. pulmonalis sinistra ●

Bronchus principalis
sinister

N. phrenicus ●

V. pulmonalis sinistra ●

Pericardium fibrosum

V. pericardiacophrenica ●

A. pericardiacophrenica ●

Recessus
costomediastinalis

Pleura parietalis,
Pars mediastinalis

(Nodi lymphoidei
mediastinales
anteriores)

Centrum tendineum

● Truncus sympathicus, R. cardiacus thoracicus

● N. vagus [X], R. cardiacus thoracicus

Oesophagus, Pars thoracica

Ductus thoracicus, Pars thoracica

● N. laryngeus recurrens (N. vagus)

Lig. arteriosum

Nodi lymphoidei
tracheobronchiales

● V. hemiazygos accessoria

Oesophagus,
Pars thoracica

● N. vagus [X],
Plexus pulmonalis

● Pars thoracica aortae

● Plexus aorticus
thoracicus

● ● A.; V. intercostalis
posterior

● R. communicans

● N. splanchnicus
major

● ● ● A.; V. inter-
costalis
posterior;
N. intercostalis

● Truncus
sympathicus,
Ganglion
thoracicum IX

Pleura
parietalis,
Pars costalis

Pleura parietalis,
Pars diaphragmatica

Fig. 950 Pleural cavity, Cavitas pleuralis, and mediastinum,
Mediastinum, of an adolescent;
viewed from the left.
In older individuals, the thymic tissue is almost entirely
replaced by adipose tissue.

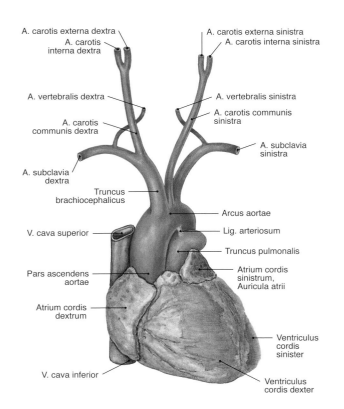

Fig. 951 Heart, Cor, and aortic arch, Arcus aortae,

with the origins of the major arteries;
ventral view.

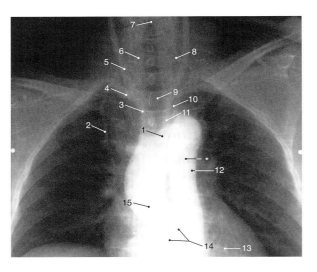

1 Arcus aortae
2 A. thoracica interna
3 Truncus brachiocephalicus
4 A. subclavia dextra
5 A. carotis communis dextra
6 A. vertebralis dextra
7 Rima glottidis
8 A. vertebralis sinistra

9 Trachea
10 A. subclavia sinistra
11 A. carotis communis sinistra
12 Pars descendens aortae
13 Cor
14 Valva aortae
15 Pars ascendens aortae

Fig. 952 Aortic arch, Arcus aortae, and branches;
AP-radiograph after injection of a contrast medium
into the aortic bulb;
ventral view.
* Catheter

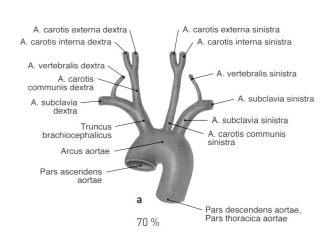

Fig. 953 a–e Variability of the origin of the major arteries
from the aortic arch, Arcus aortae.
a "Textbook case"
b Common origin of the brachiocephalic trunk and the left
common carotid artery
c Common trunk for the brachiocephalic trunk and the left
common carotid artery

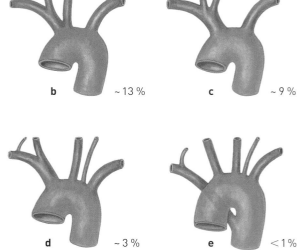

d Left vertebral artery branching off the aortic arch
independently
e Right subclavian artery as the ultimate branch of the
aortic arch
This abnormal artery frequently passes behind the
oesophagus to the right, which can result in swallowing
difficulties (Dysphagia lusoria).

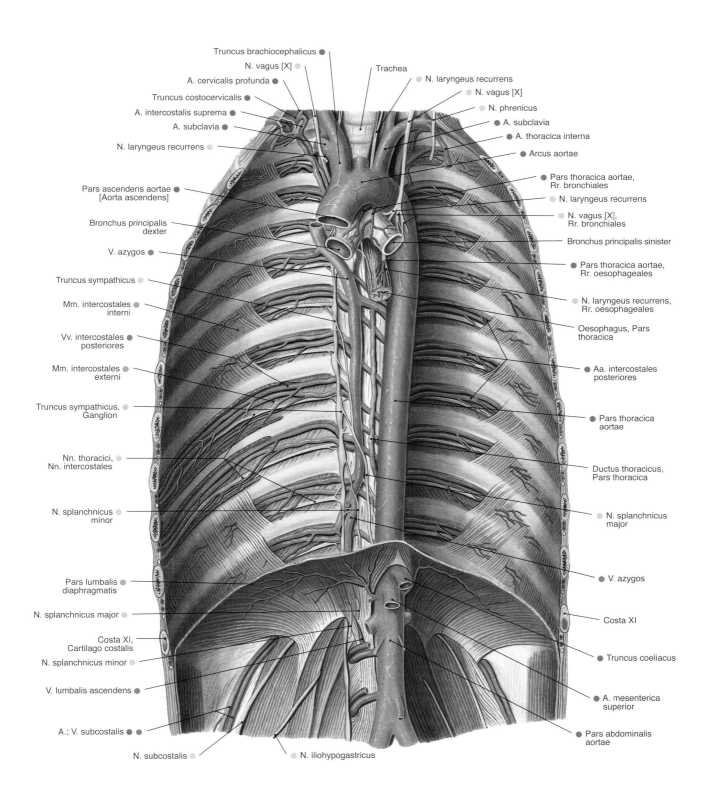

Truncus brachiocephalicus ●
N. vagus [X] ●
A. cervicalis profunda ●
Truncus costocervicalis ●
A. intercostalis suprema ●
A. subclavia ●
N. laryngeus recurrens ●

Trachea
N. laryngeus recurrens ●
N. vagus [X] ●
N. phrenicus ●
● A. subclavia
● A. thoracica interna
● Arcus aortae

Pars ascendens aortae ●
[Aorta ascendens]

● Pars thoracica aortae,
Rr. bronchiales
● N. laryngeus recurrens
● N. vagus [X],
Rr. bronchiales

Bronchus principalis
dexter

Bronchus principalis sinister

V. azygos ●

● Pars thoracica aortae,
Rr. oesophageales

Truncus sympathicus ●

● N. laryngeus recurrens,
Rr. oesophageales

Mm. intercostales ●
interni

Oesophagus, Pars
thoracica

Vv. intercostales ●
posteriores

● Aa. intercostales
posteriores

Mm. intercostales ●
externi

Truncus sympathicus, ●
Ganglion

● Pars thoracica
aortae

Nn. thoracici, ●
Nn. intercostales

Ductus thoracicus,
Pars thoracica

N. splanchnicus ●
minor

● N. splanchnicus
major

● V. azygos

Pars lumbalis ●
diaphragmatis

N. splanchnicus major ●

Costa XI

Costa XI, ●
Cartilago costalis

N. splanchnicus minor ●

● Truncus coeliacus

V. lumbalis ascendens ●

● A. mesenterica
superior

A.; V. subcostalis ● ●

● Pars abdominalis
aortae

N. subcostalis ●
N. iliohypogastricus ●

Fig. 954   Thoracic and abdominal aorta, Pars thoracica
aortae et Pars abdominalis aortae.

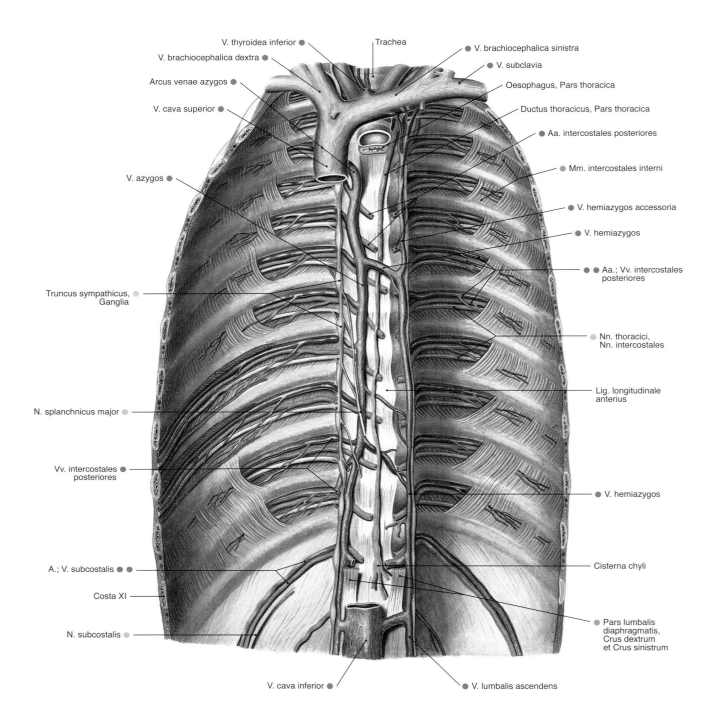

V. thyroidea inferior ●

Trachea

● V. brachiocephalica sinistra

V. brachiocephalica dextra ●

● V. subclavia

Arcus venae azygos ●

Oesophagus, Pars thoracica

V. cava superior ●

Ductus thoracicus, Pars thoracica

● Aa. intercostales posteriores

V. azygos ●

● Mm. intercostales interni

● V. hemiazygos accessoria

● V. hemiazygos

Truncus sympathicus, Ganglia ●

● ● Aa.; Vv. intercostales posteriores

● Nn. thoracici, Nn. intercostales

Lig. longitudinale anterius

N. splanchnicus major ●

Vv. intercostales posteriores ●

● V. hemiazygos

A.; V. subcostalis ● ●

Cisterna chyli

Costa XI

N. subcostalis ●

● Pars lumbalis diaphragmatis, Crus dextrum et Crus sinistrum

V. cava inferior ●

● V. lumbalis ascendens

Fig. 955 Vessels and nerves of the posterior mediastinum, Mediastinum posterius.

Posterior mediastinum

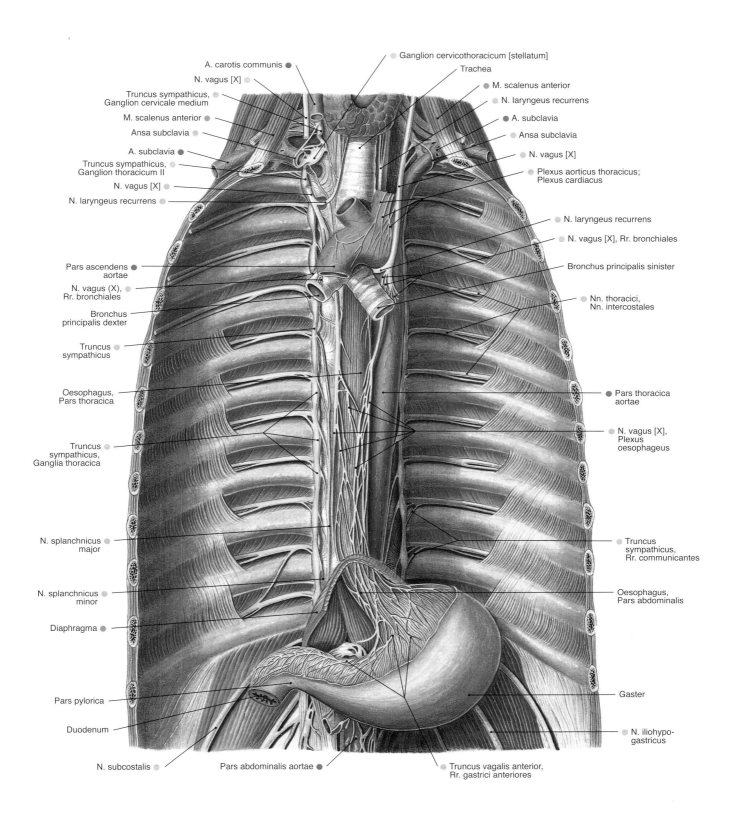

A. carotis communis ●
N. vagus [X] ●
Truncus sympathicus, ●
Ganglion cervicale medium
M. scalenus anterior ●
Ansa subclavia ●
A. subclavia ●
Truncus sympathicus, ●
Ganglion thoracicum II
N. vagus [X] ●
N. laryngeus recurrens ●

Pars ascendens ●
aortae
N. vagus (X), ●
Rr. bronchiales
Bronchus
principalis dexter
Truncus ●
sympathicus

Oesophagus,
Pars thoracica

Truncus ●
sympathicus,
Ganglia thoracica

N. splanchnicus ●
major

N. splanchnicus ●
minor

Diaphragma ●

Pars pylorica ●

Duodenum ●

N. subcostalis ●   Pars abdominalis aortae ●

● Ganglion cervicothoracicum [stellatum]
Trachea
● M. scalenus anterior
● N. laryngeus recurrens
● A. subclavia
● Ansa subclavia
● N. vagus [X]
● Plexus aorticus thoracicus;
Plexus cardiacus

● N. laryngeus recurrens
● N. vagus [X], Rr. bronchiales

Bronchus principalis sinister

● Nn. thoracici,
Nn. intercostales

● Pars thoracica
aortae

● N. vagus [X],
Plexus
oesophageus

● Truncus
sympathicus,
Rr. communicantes

Oesophagus,
Pars abdominalis

Gaster

● N. iliohypo-
gastricus

● Truncus vagalis anterior,
Rr. gastrici anteriores

Fig. 956   Autonomous nervous system of the thoracic cavity,
Pars thoracica autonomica.

→ 49, 50

Phrenic nerve

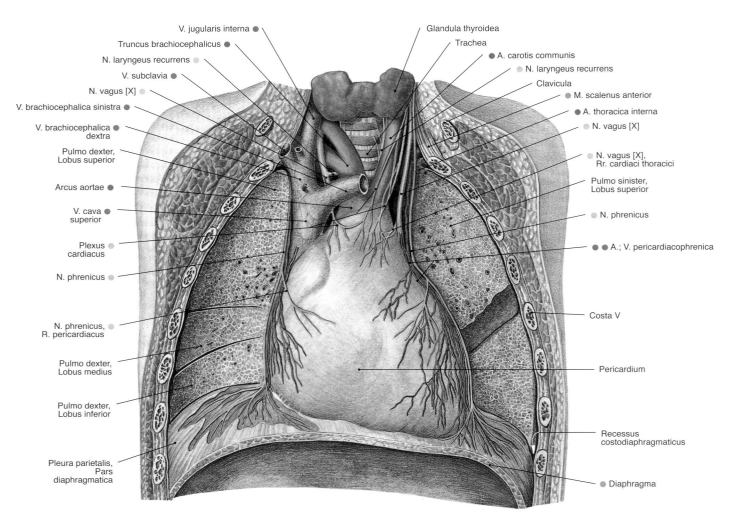

V. jugularis interna ●
Truncus brachiocephalicus ●
N. laryngeus recurrens ●
V. subclavia ●
N. vagus [X] ●
V. brachiocephalica sinistra ●
V. brachiocephalica ● dextra
Pulmo dexter, Lobus superior
Arcus aortae ●
V. cava ● superior
Plexus ● cardiacus
N. phrenicus ●
N. phrenicus, ● R. pericardiacus
Pulmo dexter, Lobus medius
Pulmo dexter, Lobus inferior
Pleura parietalis, Pars diaphragmatica

Glandula thyroidea
Trachea
● A. carotis communis
● N. laryngeus recurrens
Clavicula
● M. scalenus anterior
● A. thoracica interna
● N. vagus [X]
● N. vagus [X], Rr. cardiaci thoracici
Pulmo sinister, Lobus superior
● N. phrenicus
● ● A.; V. pericardiacophrenica
Costa V
Pericardium
Recessus costodiaphragmaticus
● Diaphragma

Fig. 957 Thoracic viscera of an adult; the anterior thoracic wall has been removed, and the right and the left lung have been sectioned in the frontal plane; ventral view.

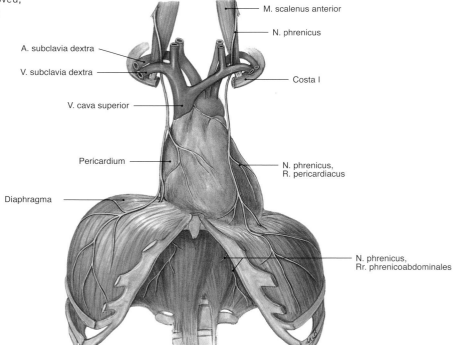

A. subclavia dextra
V. subclavia dextra
V. cava superior
Pericardium
Diaphragma

M. scalenus anterior
N. phrenicus
Costa I
N. phrenicus, R. pericardiacus
N. phrenicus, Rr. phrenicoabdominales

Fig. 958 Course of the phrenic nerve, N. phrenicus.

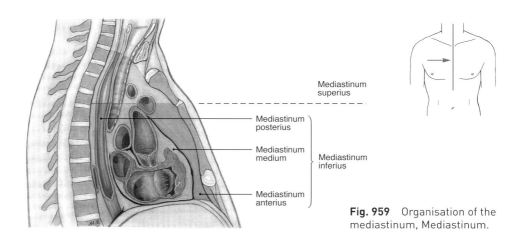

Mediastinum
superius

Mediastinum
posterius

Mediastinum
medium

Mediastinum
anterius

Mediastinum
inferius

Fig. 959 Organisation of the mediastinum, Mediastinum.

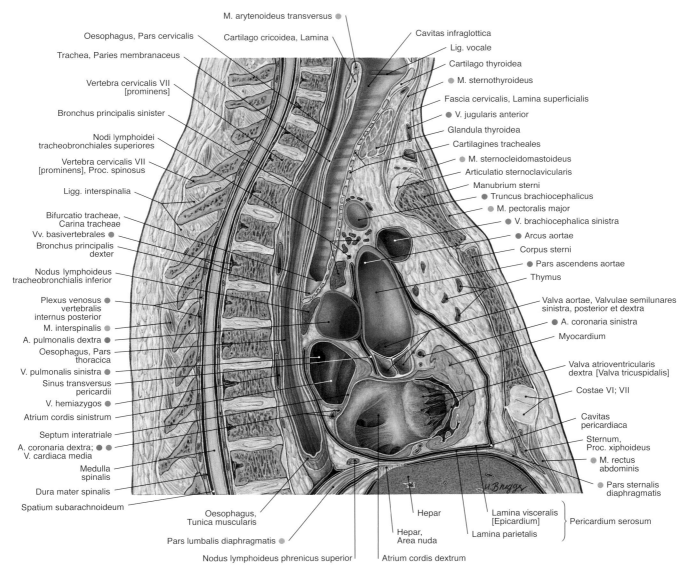

M. arytenoideus transversus ●
Oesophagus, Pars cervicalis
Cartilago cricoidea, Lamina
Trachea, Paries membranaceus
Vertebra cervicalis VII [prominens]
Bronchus principalis sinister
Nodi lymphoidei tracheobronchiales superiores
Vertebra cervicalis VII [prominens], Proc. spinosus
Ligg. interspinalia
Bifurcatio tracheae, Carina tracheae
Vv. basivertebrales ●
Bronchus principalis dexter
Nodus lymphoideus tracheobronchialis inferior
Plexus venosus ● vertebralis internus posterior
M. interspinalis ●
A. pulmonalis dextra ●
Oesophagus, Pars thoracica
V. pulmonalis sinistra ●
Sinus transversus pericardii
V. hemiazygos ●
Atrium cordis sinistrum
Septum interatriale
A. coronaria dextra; ● ● ● V. cardiaca media
Medulla spinalis
Dura mater spinalis
Spatium subarachnoideum

Cavitas infraglottica
Lig. vocale
Cartilago thyroidea
● M. sternothyroideus
Fascia cervicalis, Lamina superficialis
● V. jugularis anterior
Glandula thyroidea
Cartilagines tracheales
● M. sternocleidomastoideus
Articulatio sternoclavicularis
Manubrium sterni
● Truncus brachiocephalicus
● M. pectoralis major
● V. brachiocephalica sinistra
● Arcus aortae
Corpus sterni
● Pars ascendens aortae
Thymus
Valva aortae, Valvulae semilunares sinistra, posterior et dextra
● A. coronaria sinistra
Myocardium
Valva atrioventricularis dextra [Valva tricuspidalis]
Costae VI; VII
Cavitas pericardiaca
Sternum, Proc. xiphoideus
● M. rectus abdominis
● Pars sternalis diaphragmatis

Oesophagus, Tunica muscularis
Pars lumbalis diaphragmatis ●
Nodus lymphoideus phrenicus superior

Hepar
Hepar, Area nuda
Atrium cordis dextrum

Lamina visceralis [Epicardium]
Lamina parietalis
Pericardium serosum

Fig. 960 Thoracic cavity, Cavitas thoracis, and mediastinum, Mediastinum; median sagittal section through the neck and the thorax; lateral view from the right.

Thorax, frontal sections

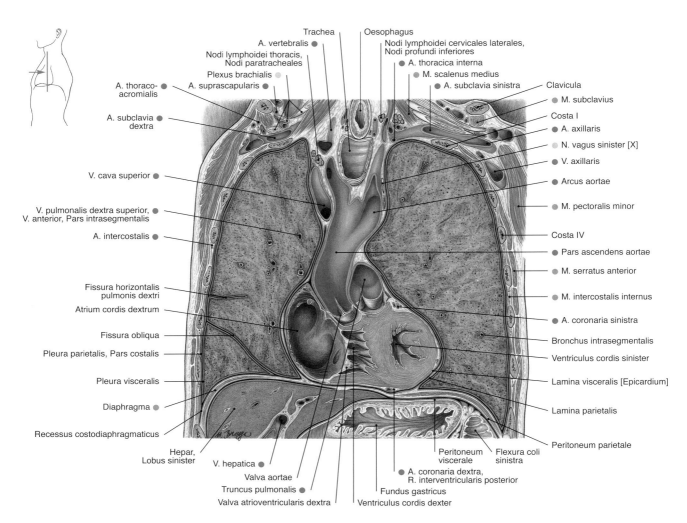

Fig. 961 Thoracic cavity, Cavitas thoracis.

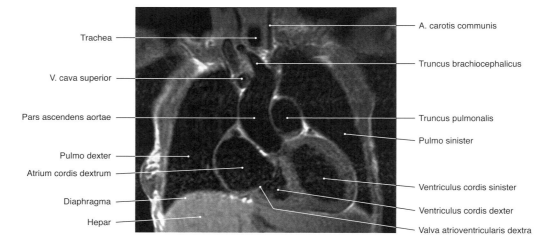

Fig. 962 Thoracic cavity, Cavitas thoracis; magnetic resonance tomographic image (MRI); frontal section at the level of the superior vena cava; ventral view.

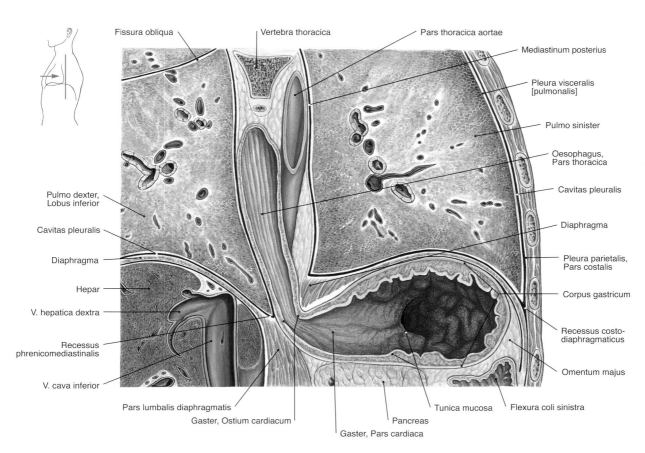

Fissura obliqua — Vertebra thoracica — Pars thoracica aortae

Mediastinum posterius

Pleura visceralis [pulmonalis]

Pulmo sinister

Oesophagus, Pars thoracica

Cavitas pleuralis

Diaphragma

Pleura parietalis, Pars costalis

Corpus gastricum

Recessus costo-diaphragmaticus

Omentum majus

Pulmo dexter, Lobus inferior

Cavitas pleuralis

Diaphragma

Hepar

V. hepatica dextra

Recessus phrenicomediastinalis

V. cava inferior

Pars lumbalis diaphragmatis

Gaster, Ostium cardiacum

Gaster, Pars cardiaca

Pancreas

Tunica mucosa

Flexura coli sinistra

Fig. 963 Diaphragm, Diaphragma, and oesophagus, Oesophagus, with its transition into the stomach, Gaster; frontal section through the lower part of the thoracic cavity and the upper part of the abdominal cavity.

→ 1187

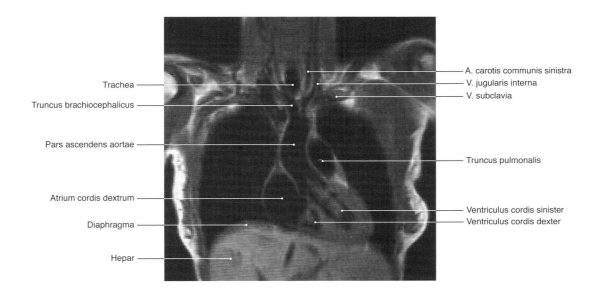

Trachea

Truncus brachiocephalicus

Pars ascendens aortae

Atrium cordis dextrum

Diaphragma

Hepar

A. carotis communis sinistra

V. jugularis interna

V. subclavia

Truncus pulmonalis

Ventriculus cordis sinister

Ventriculus cordis dexter

Fig. 964 Thoracic cavity, Cavitas thoracis; magnetic resonance tomographic image (MRI); frontal section at the level of the aortic valve; ventral view.

Thorax, frontal sections

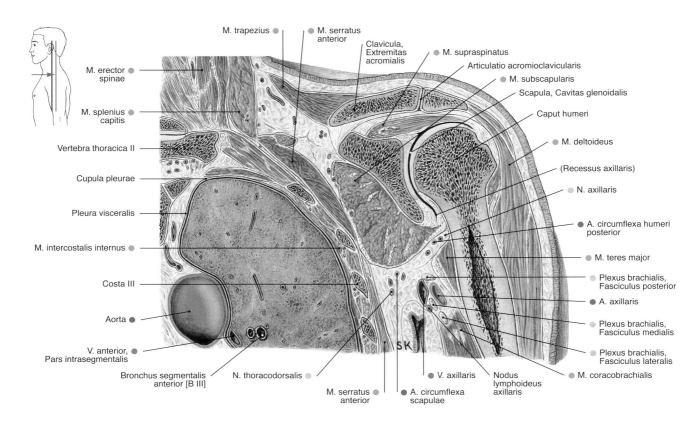

M. trapezius

M. serratus anterior

Clavicula, Extremitas acromialis

M. supraspinatus

Articulatio acromioclavicularis

M. subscapularis

Scapula, Cavitas glenoidalis

Caput humeri

M. deltoideus

(Recessus axillaris)

N. axillaris

A. circumflexa humeri posterior

M. teres major

Plexus brachialis, Fasciculus posterior

A. axillaris

Plexus brachialis, Fasciculus medialis

Plexus brachialis, Fasciculus lateralis

M. coracobrachialis

M. erector spinae

M. splenius capitis

Vertebra thoracica II

Cupula pleurae

Pleura visceralis

M. intercostalis internus

Costa III

Aorta

V. anterior, Pars intrasegmentalis

Bronchus segmentalis anterior [B III]

N. thoracodorsalis

M. serratus anterior

A. circumflexa scapulae

V. axillaris

Nodus lymphoideus axillaris

Fig. 965 Thoracic cavity, Cavitas thoracis; axilla, Axilla, and shoulder joint, Articulatio humeri.

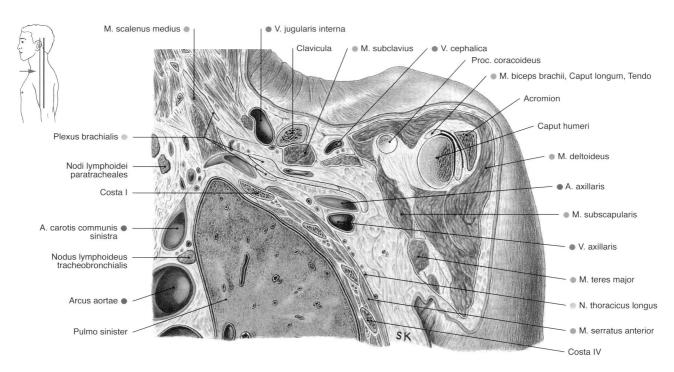

M. scalenus medius

V. jugularis interna

Clavicula

M. subclavius

V. cephalica

Proc. coracoideus

M. biceps brachii, Caput longum, Tendo

Acromion

Caput humeri

M. deltoideus

A. axillaris

M. subscapularis

V. axillaris

M. teres major

N. thoracicus longus

M. serratus anterior

Costa IV

Plexus brachialis

Nodi lymphoidei paratracheales

Costa I

A. carotis communis sinistra

Nodus lymphoideus tracheobronchialis

Arcus aortae

Pulmo sinister

Fig. 966 Thoracic cavity, Cavitas thoracis; axilla, Axilla, and shoulder joint, Articulatio humeri.

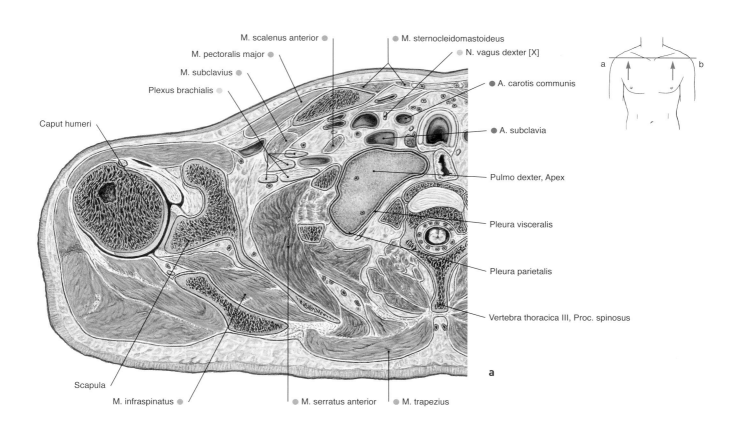

M. scalenus anterior ●
M. pectoralis major ●
M. subclavius ●
Plexus brachialis ●
Caput humeri
● M. sternocleidomastoideus
● N. vagus dexter [X]
● A. carotis communis
● A. subclavia
Pulmo dexter, Apex
Pleura visceralis
Pleura parietalis
Vertebra thoracica III, Proc. spinosus
Scapula
M. infraspinatus ●
● M. serratus anterior
● M. trapezius

a

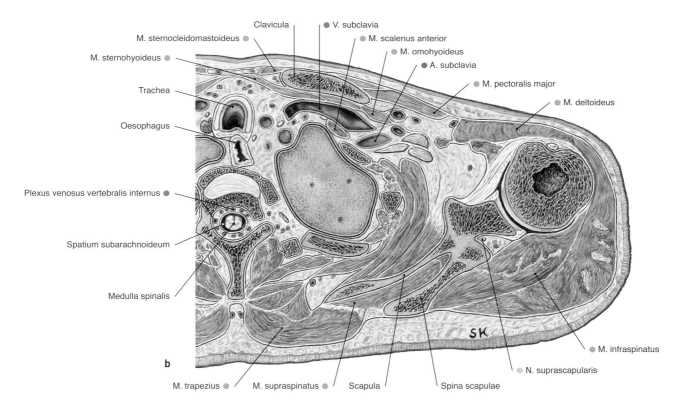

Clavicula
● V. subclavia
M. sternocleidomastoideus ●
M. sternohyoideus ●
Trachea
Oesophagus
● M. scalenus anterior
● M. omohyoideus
● A. subclavia
● M. pectoralis major
● M. deltoideus
Plexus venosus vertebralis internus ●
Spatium subarachnoideum
Medulla spinalis
SK
● M. infraspinatus
● N. suprascapularis
M. trapezius ●
M. supraspinatus ●
Scapula
Spina scapulae

b

Fig. 967 a, b   Thoracic cavity, Cavitas thoracis; axilla, Axilla, and shoulder joint, Articulatio humeri.

a Right part of the body
b Left part of the body

→ 294

Thorax, transverse sections

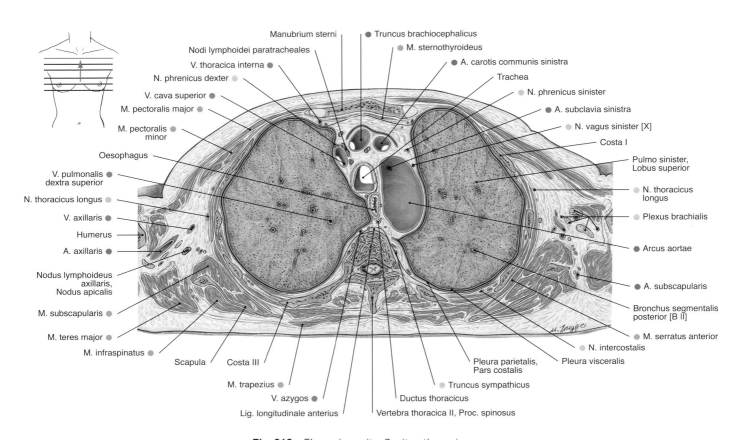

Manubrium sterni — Truncus brachiocephalicus
Nodi lymphoidei paratracheales — M. sternothyroideus
V. thoracica interna — A. carotis communis sinistra
N. phrenicus dexter — Trachea
V. cava superior — N. phrenicus sinister
M. pectoralis major — A. subclavia sinistra
M. pectoralis minor — N. vagus sinister [X]
Oesophagus — Costa I
V. pulmonalis dextra superior — Pulmo sinister, Lobus superior
N. thoracicus longus — N. thoracicus longus
V. axillaris — Plexus brachialis
Humerus — Arcus aortae
A. axillaris — A. subscapularis
Nodus lymphoideus axillaris, Nodus apicalis — Bronchus segmentalis posterior [B II]
M. subscapularis — M. serratus anterior
M. teres major — N. intercostalis
M. infraspinatus — Pleura visceralis
Scapula — Costa III — Pleura parietalis, Pars costalis
M. trapezius — Truncus sympathicus
V. azygos — Ductus thoracicus
Lig. longitudinale anterius — Vertebra thoracica II, Proc. spinosus

Fig. 968 Thoracic cavity, Cavitas thoracis.

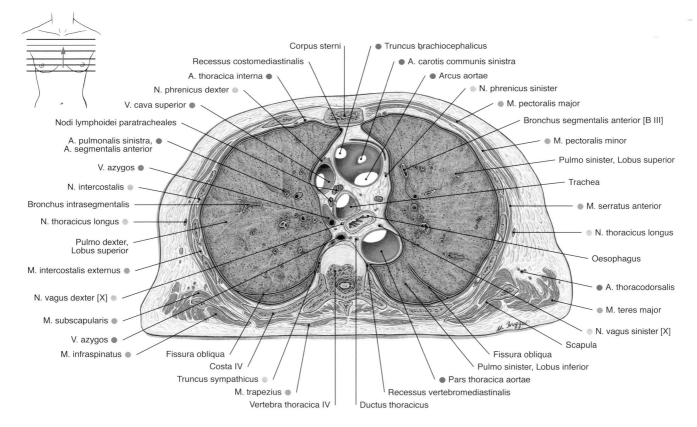

Corpus sterni — Truncus brachiocephalicus
Recessus costomediastinalis — A. carotis communis sinistra
A. thoracica interna — Arcus aortae
N. phrenicus dexter — N. phrenicus sinister
V. cava superior — M. pectoralis major
Nodi lymphoidei paratracheales — Bronchus segmentalis anterior [B III]
A. pulmonalis sinistra, A. segmentalis anterior — M. pectoralis minor
V. azygos — Pulmo sinister, Lobus superior
N. intercostalis — Trachea
Bronchus intrasegmentalis — M. serratus anterior
N. thoracicus longus — N. thoracicus longus
Pulmo dexter, Lobus superior — Oesophagus
M. intercostalis externus — A. thoracodorsalis
N. vagus dexter [X] — M. teres major
M. subscapularis — N. vagus sinister [X]
V. azygos — Scapula
M. infraspinatus — Fissura obliqua
Fissura obliqua — Pulmo sinister, Lobus inferior
Costa IV — Pars thoracica aortae
Truncus sympathicus — Recessus vertebromediastinalis
M. trapezius — Ductus thoracicus
Vertebra thoracica IV

Fig. 969 Thoracic cavity, Cavitas thoracis.

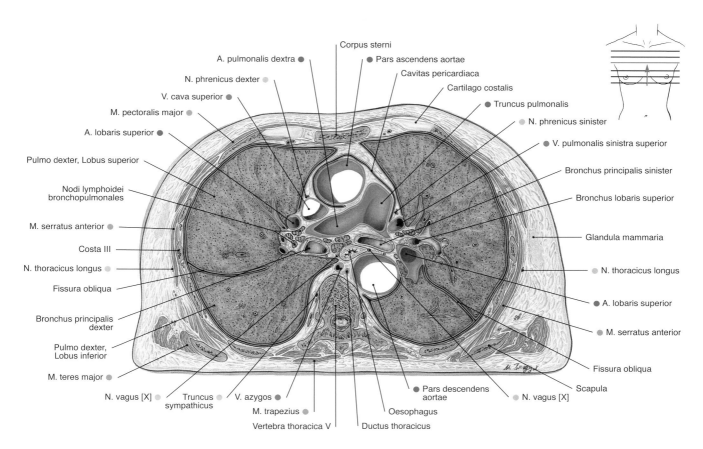

Corpus sterni
A. pulmonalis dextra ●
N. phrenicus dexter ●
V. cava superior ●
M. pectoralis major ●
A. lobaris superior ●
Pulmo dexter, Lobus superior
Nodi lymphoidei bronchopulmonales
M. serratus anterior ●
Costa III
N. thoracicus longus ●
Fissura obliqua
Bronchus principalis dexter
Pulmo dexter, Lobus inferior
M. teres major ●

● Pars ascendens aortae
Cavitas pericardiaca
Cartilago costalis
● Truncus pulmonalis
● N. phrenicus sinister
● V. pulmonalis sinistra superior
Bronchus principalis sinister
Bronchus lobaris superior
Glandula mammaria
● N. thoracicus longus
● A. lobaris superior
● M. serratus anterior
Fissura obliqua
Scapula

N. vagus [X] ●
Truncus sympathicus ●
V. azygos ●
M. trapezius ●
Vertebra thoracica V
Ductus thoracicus
● Pars descendens aortae
Oesophagus
● N. vagus [X]

Fig. 970 Thoracic cavity, Cavitas thoracis.

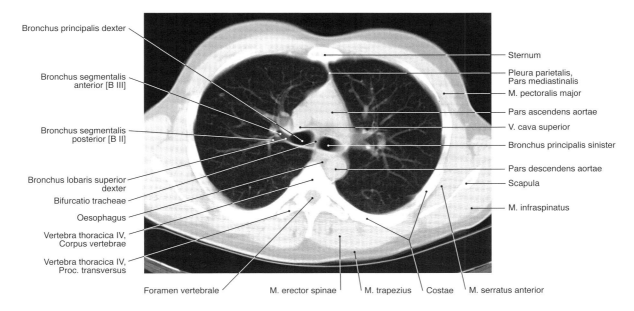

Bronchus principalis dexter
Bronchus segmentalis anterior [B III]
Bronchus segmentalis posterior [B II]
Bronchus lobaris superior dexter
Bifurcatio tracheae
Oesophagus
Vertebra thoracica IV, Corpus vertebrae
Vertebra thoracica IV, Proc. transversus

Sternum
Pleura parietalis, Pars mediastinalis
M. pectoralis major
Pars ascendens aortae
V. cava superior
Bronchus principalis sinister
Pars descendens aortae
Scapula
M. infraspinatus

Foramen vertebrale
M. erector spinae
M. trapezius
Costae
M. serratus anterior

Fig. 971 Thoracic cavity, Cavitas thoracis; computed tomographic cross-section (CT).

Thorax, transverse sections

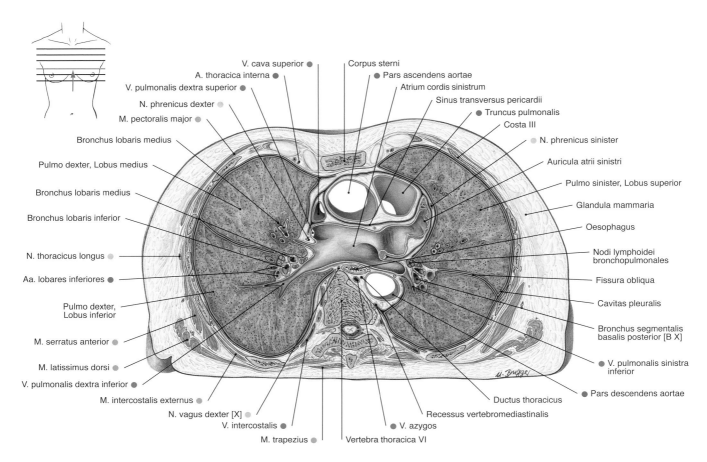

V. cava superior
A. thoracica interna
V. pulmonalis dextra superior
N. phrenicus dexter
M. pectoralis major
Bronchus lobaris medius
Pulmo dexter, Lobus medius
Bronchus lobaris medius
Bronchus lobaris inferior
N. thoracicus longus
Aa. lobares inferiores
Pulmo dexter, Lobus inferior
M. serratus anterior
M. latissimus dorsi
V. pulmonalis dextra inferior
M. intercostalis externus
N. vagus dexter [X]
V. intercostalis
M. trapezius

Corpus sterni
Pars ascendens aortae
Atrium cordis sinistrum
Sinus transversus pericardii
Truncus pulmonalis
Costa III
N. phrenicus sinister
Auricula atrii sinistri
Pulmo sinister, Lobus superior
Glandula mammaria
Oesophagus
Nodi lymphoidei bronchopulmonales
Fissura obliqua
Cavitas pleuralis
Bronchus segmentalis basalis posterior [B X]
V. pulmonalis sinistra inferior
Pars descendens aortae
Ductus thoracicus
Recessus vertebromediastinalis
V. azygos
Vertebra thoracica VI

Fig. 972   Thoracic cavity, Cavitas thoracis.

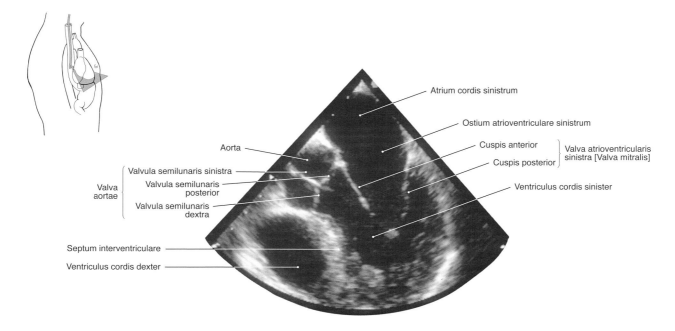

Aorta
Valvula semilunaris sinistra
Valva aortae {
Valvula semilunaris posterior
Valvula semilunaris dextra
Septum interventriculare
Ventriculus cordis dexter

Atrium cordis sinistrum
Ostium atrioventriculare sinistrum
Cuspis anterior
Cuspis posterior
} Valva atrioventricularis sinistra [Valva mitralis]
Ventriculus cordis sinister

Fig. 973   Heart, Cor;
ultrasound image viewed from the oesophagus
(transoesophageal echocardiography).

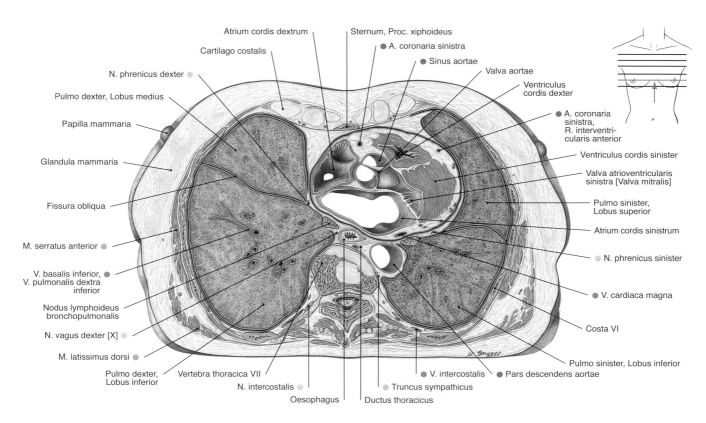

Atrium cordis dextrum
Cartilago costalis
N. phrenicus dexter
Pulmo dexter, Lobus medius
Papilla mammaria
Glandula mammaria
Fissura obliqua
M. serratus anterior
V. basalis inferior,
V. pulmonalis dextra
inferior
Nodus lymphoideus
bronchopulmonalis
N. vagus dexter [X]
M. latissimus dorsi
Pulmo dexter,
Lobus inferior
Vertebra thoracica VII
N. intercostalis
Oesophagus
Ductus thoracicus

Sternum, Proc. xiphoideus
A. coronaria sinistra
Sinus aortae
Valva aortae
Ventriculus
cordis dexter
A. coronaria
sinistra,
R. interventri-
cularis anterior
Ventriculus cordis sinister
Valva atrioventricularis
sinistra [Valva mitralis]
Pulmo sinister,
Lobus superior
Atrium cordis sinistrum
N. phrenicus sinister
V. cardiaca magna
Costa VI
Pulmo sinister, Lobus inferior
Pars descendens aortae
V. intercostalis
Truncus sympathicus

Fig. 974 Thoracic cavity, Cavitas thoracis.

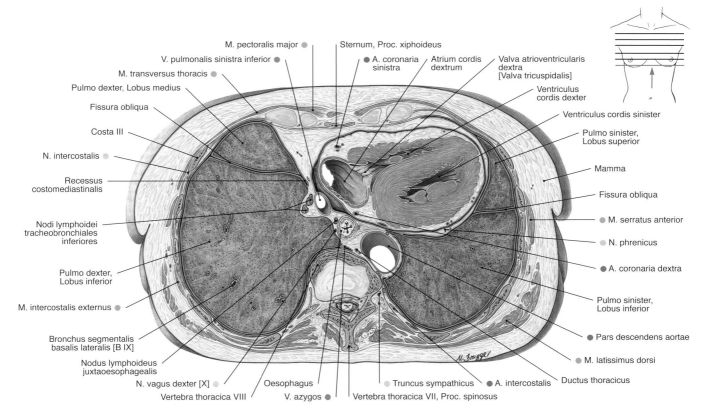

M. pectoralis major
V. pulmonalis sinistra inferior
M. transversus thoracis
Pulmo dexter, Lobus medius
Fissura obliqua
Costa III
N. intercostalis
Recessus
costomediastinalis
Nodi lymphoidei
tracheobronchiales
inferiores
Pulmo dexter,
Lobus inferior
M. intercostalis externus
Bronchus segmentalis
basalis lateralis [B IX]
Nodus lymphoideus
juxtaoesophagealis
N. vagus dexter [X]
Vertebra thoracica VIII
Oesophagus
V. azygos

Sternum, Proc. xiphoideus
A. coronaria
sinistra
Atrium cordis
dextrum
Valva atrioventricularis
dextra
[Valva tricuspidalis]
Ventriculus
cordis dexter
Ventriculus cordis sinister
Pulmo sinister,
Lobus superior
Mamma
Fissura obliqua
M. serratus anterior
N. phrenicus
A. coronaria dextra
Pulmo sinister,
Lobus inferior
Pars descendens aortae
M. latissimus dorsi
Ductus thoracicus
A. intercostalis
Truncus sympathicus
Vertebra thoracica VII, Proc. spinosus

Fig. 975 Thoracic cavity, Cavitas thoracis.

Stomach

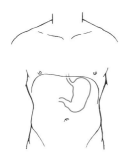

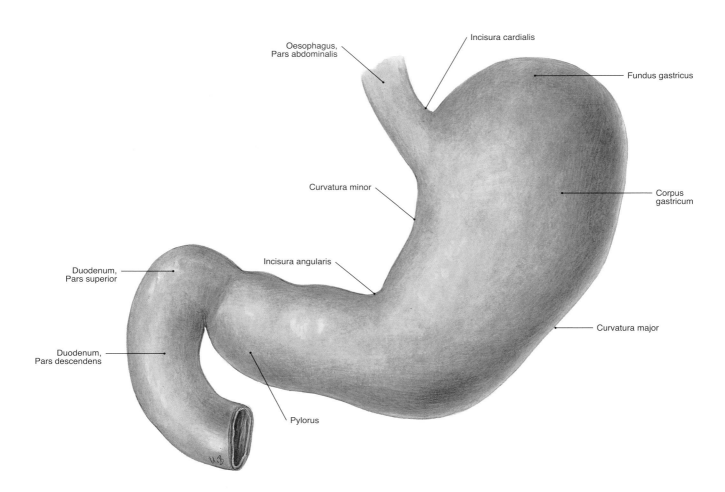

Oesophagus,
Pars abdominalis

Incisura cardialis

Fundus gastricus

Curvatura minor

Corpus
gastricum

Duodenum,
Pars superior

Incisura angularis

Curvatura major

Duodenum,
Pars descendens

Pylorus

Fig. 976   Stomach, Gaster;
ventral view.

Muscles of the stomach

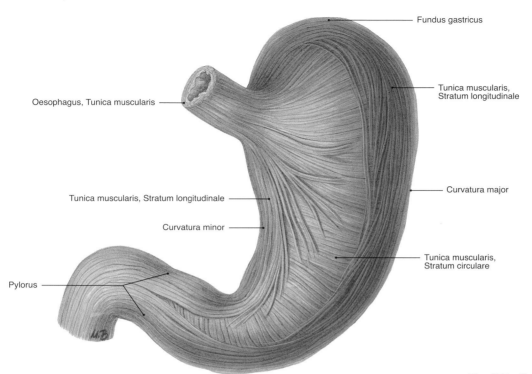

Fundus gastricus

Oesophagus, Tunica muscularis

Tunica muscularis, Stratum longitudinale

Tunica muscularis, Stratum longitudinale

Curvatura minor

Curvatura major

Pylorus

Tunica muscularis, Stratum circulare

Fig. 977 Stomach, Gaster; external muscle layers; ventral view.

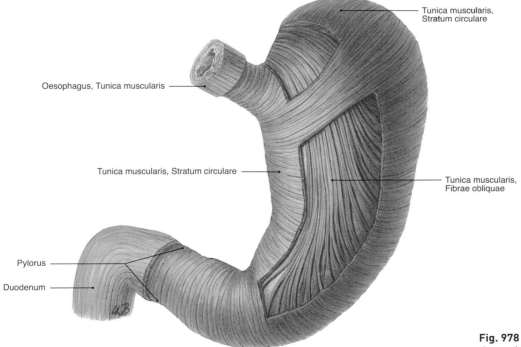

Tunica muscularis, Stratum circulare

Oesophagus, Tunica muscularis

Tunica muscularis, Stratum circulare

Tunica muscularis, Fibrae obliquae

Pylorus

Duodenum

Fig. 978 Stomach, Gaster; the peritoneum has been removed to demonstrate the internal muscle layers; ventral view.

Stomach, structure

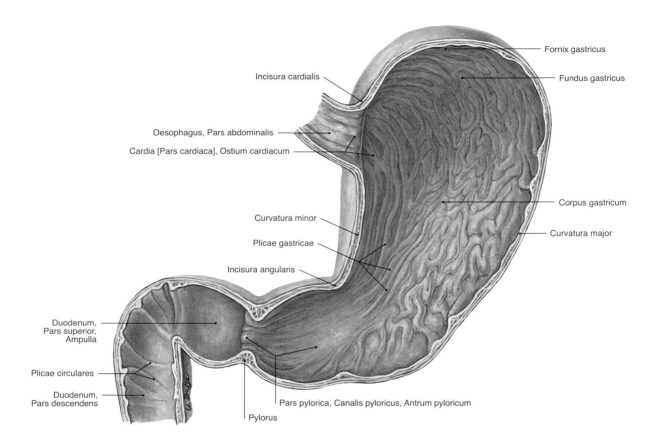

Incisura cardialis

Oesophagus, Pars abdominalis

Cardia [Pars cardiaca], Ostium cardiacum

Curvatura minor

Plicae gastricae

Incisura angularis

Duodenum, Pars superior, Ampulla

Plicae circulares

Duodenum, Pars descendens

Pars pylorica, Canalis pyloricus, Antrum pyloricum

Pylorus

Fornix gastricus

Fundus gastricus

Corpus gastricum

Curvatura major

Fig. 979 Stomach, Gaster, and duodenum, Duodenum; ventral view.

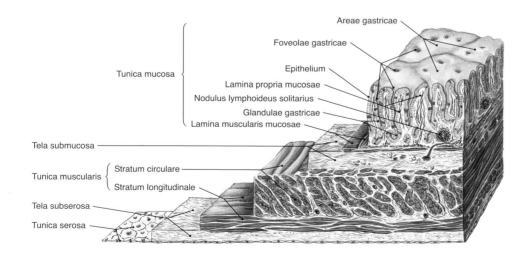

Areae gastricae

Foveolae gastricae

Epithelium

Lamina propria mucosae

Nodulus lymphoideus solitarius

Glandulae gastricae

Lamina muscularis mucosae

Tunica mucosa

Tela submucosa

Tunica muscularis

Stratum circulare

Stratum longitudinale

Tela subserosa

Tunica serosa

Fig. 980 Diagram of the stomach wall; the layers of the wall have been removed stepwise; microscopic enlargement at low magnification.

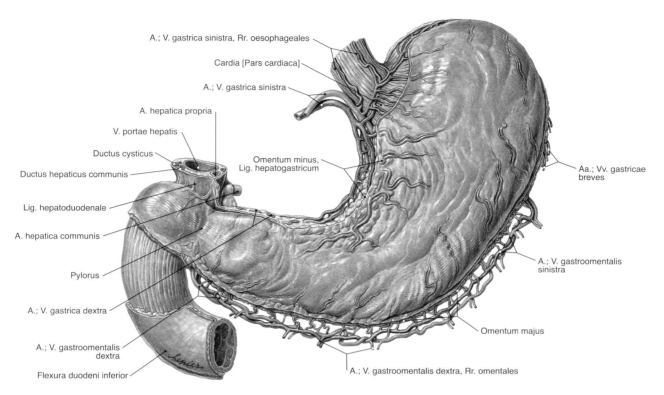

A.; V. gastrica sinistra, Rr. oesophageales

Cardia [Pars cardiaca]

A.; V. gastrica sinistra

A. hepatica propria

V. portae hepatis

Ductus cysticus

Ductus hepaticus communis

Omentum minus,
Lig. hepatogastricum

Lig. hepatoduodenale

A. hepatica communis

Pylorus

A.; V. gastrica dextra

A.; V. gastroomentalis
dextra

Flexura duodeni inferior

Aa.; Vv. gastricae
breves

A.; V. gastroomentalis
sinistra

Omentum majus

A.; V. gastroomentalis dextra, Rr. omentales

Fig. 981   Blood vessels of the stomach, Gaster;
ventral view.

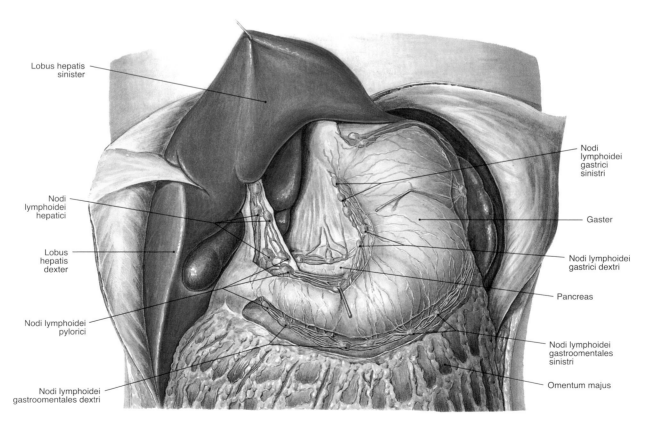

Lobus hepatis
sinister

Nodi
lymphoidei
hepatici

Lobus
hepatis
dexter

Nodi lymphoidei
pylorici

Nodi lymphoidei
gastroomentales dextri

Nodi
lymphoidei
gastrici
sinistri

Gaster

Nodi lymphoidei
gastrici dextri

Pancreas

Nodi lymphoidei
gastroomentales
sinistri

Omentum majus

Fig. 982   Stomach, Gaster, and liver, Hepar,
with lymph nodes, Nodi lymphoidei;
ventral view.

Stomach, radiography

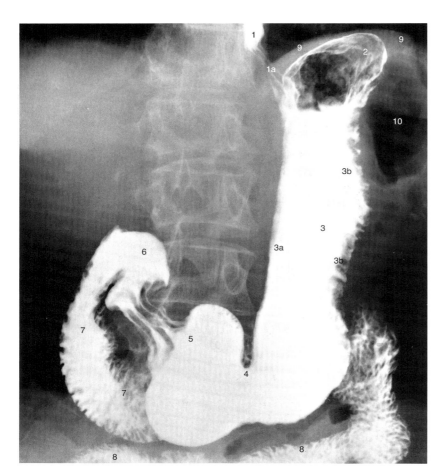

1 = Oesophagus with contrast medium. At the transition (1a) into the fundus of stomach, the grooves between the folds appear as dark striations.
2 = Fundus of stomach with air bubble
3 = Body of stomach
3a = Lesser curvature
3b = Greater curvature. In the linings of the latter, notches corresponding to the contour of the mucous are visible.
4 = Peristaltic constriction at the angular notch
5 = Pyloric part prior to the progression of a portion of the stomach's content
6 = Ampulla of duodenum
7 = Descending part of the duodenum with circular folds
8 = Jejunum
9 = Left "dome" of diaphragm
10 = Left colic flexure (filled with air)

Fig. 983 Stomach, Gaster, and duodenum, Duodenum; AP-radiograph after oral administration of a contrast medium; upright position; ventral view.

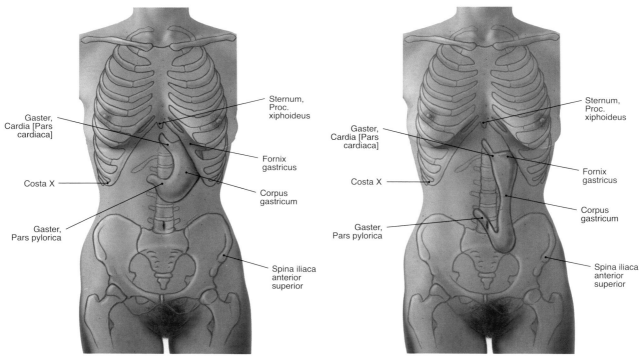

Fig. 984 Stomach, Gaster; projection of a "normal" stomach onto the anterior abdominal wall; upright position.

Fig. 985 Stomach, Gaster; projection of a "long" stomach onto the anterior abdominal wall; upright position.

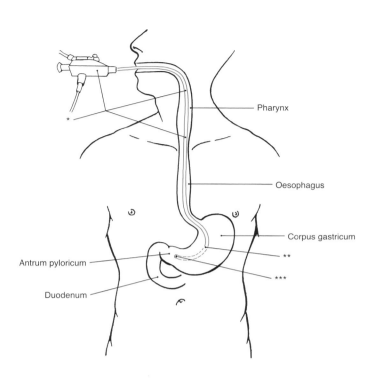

Fig. 986 Technical procedure of oesophagoscopy and gastroscopy.

* Gastroscope
** The gastroscope's tip located in the body of stomach (compare Fig. 987 a)
***The gastroscope's tip located in the pyloric antrum (compare Fig. 987 b)

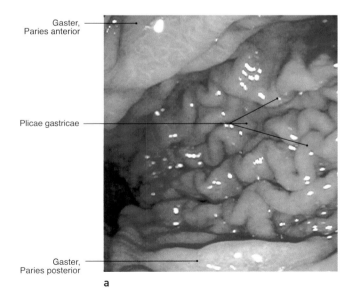

a

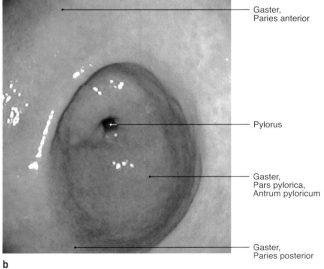

b

Fig. 987 a, b Stomach, Gaster; endoscopic image of the stomach (gastroscopy); superior view.

a View of the body of stomach, Corpus gastricum, with distinct longitudinal folds of the mucosa (Plica gastricae)
b View of the pyloric antrum, Antrum pyloricum, predominantly covered with smooth mucosa

Duodenum

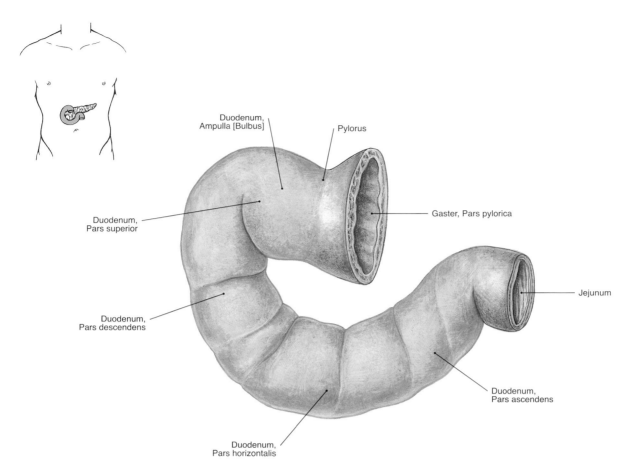

Duodenum,
Ampulla [Bulbus]

Pylorus

Duodenum,
Pars superior

Gaster, Pars pylorica

Jejunum

Duodenum,
Pars descendens

Duodenum,
Pars ascendens

Duodenum,
Pars horizontalis

Fig. 988 Duodenum, Duodenum.

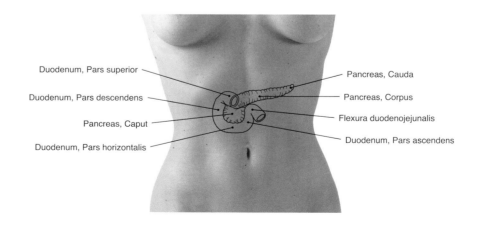

Duodenum, Pars superior

Pancreas, Cauda

Duodenum, Pars descendens

Pancreas, Corpus

Pancreas, Caput

Flexura duodenojejunalis

Duodenum, Pars horizontalis

Duodenum, Pars ascendens

Fig. 989 Duodenum, Duodenum, and
pancreas, Pancreas;
projected onto the anterior abdominal wall.

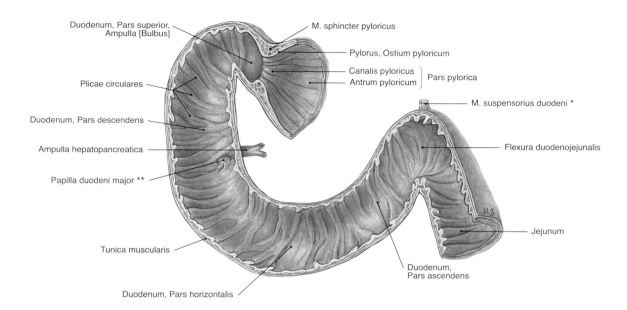

Duodenum, Pars superior, Ampulla [Bulbus]

M. sphincter pyloricus

Pylorus, Ostium pyloricum

Canalis pyloricus
Antrum pyloricum } Pars pylorica

Plicae circulares

M. suspensorius duodeni *

Duodenum, Pars descendens

Flexura duodenojejunalis

Ampulla hepatopancreatica

Papilla duodeni major **

Jejunum

Tunica muscularis

Duodenum, Pars ascendens

Duodenum, Pars horizontalis

Fig. 990 Duodenum, Duodenum;
ventral view.
* Clinical term: muscle of TREITZ
** Clinical term: papilla of VATER

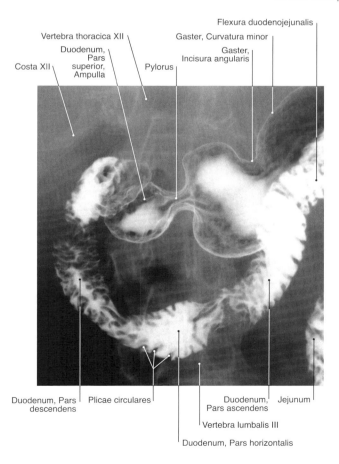

Vertebra thoracica XII

Flexura duodenojejunalis

Duodenum, Pars superior, Ampulla

Gaster, Curvatura minor

Gaster, Incisura angularis

Costa XII

Pylorus

Duodenum, Pars descendens

Plicae circulares

Duodenum, Pars ascendens

Jejunum

Vertebra lumbalis III

Duodenum, Pars horizontalis

Fig. 991 Duodenum, Duodenum;
AP-radiograph after oral administration of a contrast medium;
upright position;
ventral view.

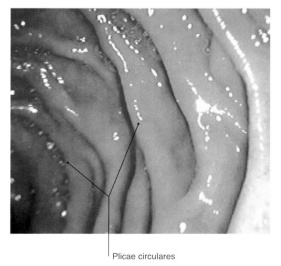

Plicae circulares

Fig. 992 Duodenum, Duodenum;
endoscopic image.

Small intestine, structure

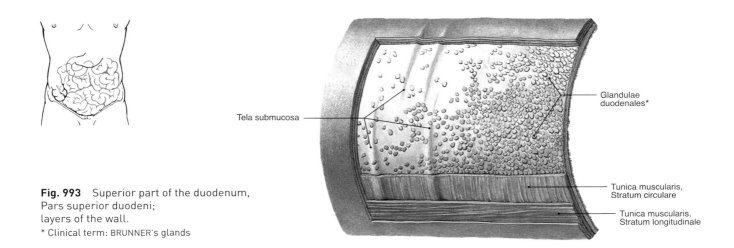

Fig. 993   Superior part of the duodenum,
Pars superior duodeni;
layers of the wall.
* Clinical term: BRUNNER's glands

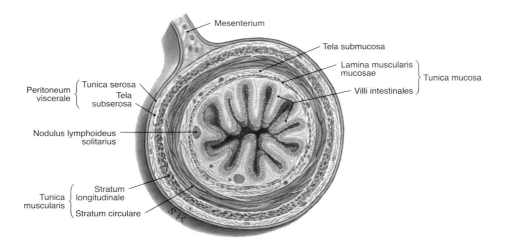

Fig. 994   Small intestine, Intestinum tenue;
cross-section through the upper small intestine.

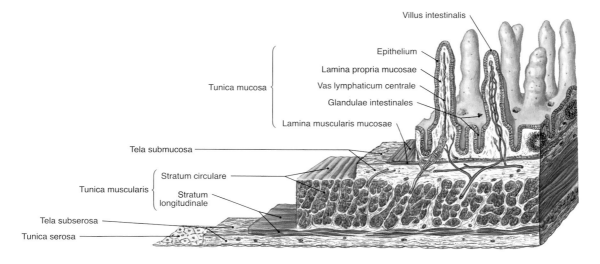

Fig. 995   Small intestine, Intestinum tenue;
layers of the wall;
microscopic enlargement at low magnification.

Mucosa of the small intestine

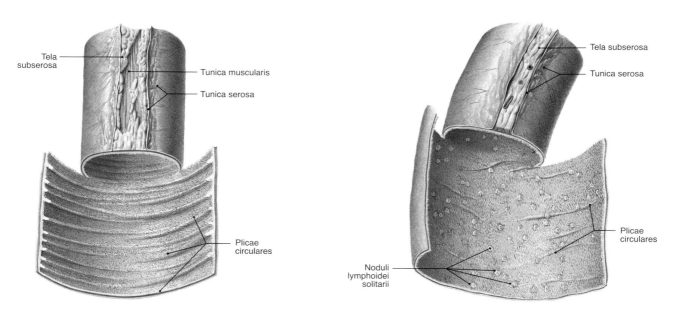

Fig. 996   Jejunum, Jejunum.

Fig. 997   Ileum, Ileum.

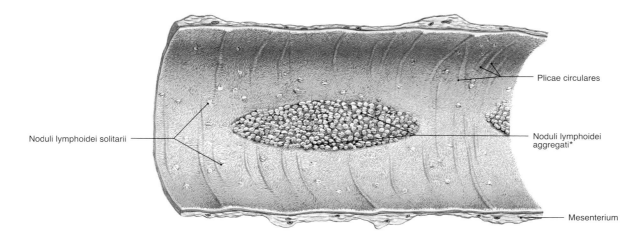

Fig. 998   Terminal ileum,
Pars terminalis ilei.
* Clinical term: PEYER's patches

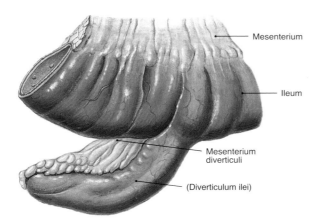

Fig. 999   MECKEL's diverticulum (Diverticulum ilei).
This vestige of the yolk stalk (Ductus omphaloentericus)
occurs in 1–3% of cases. It is located 30–70 cm oral to
the ileocaecal junction opposite to the attachment of the
mesentery.

Large intestine

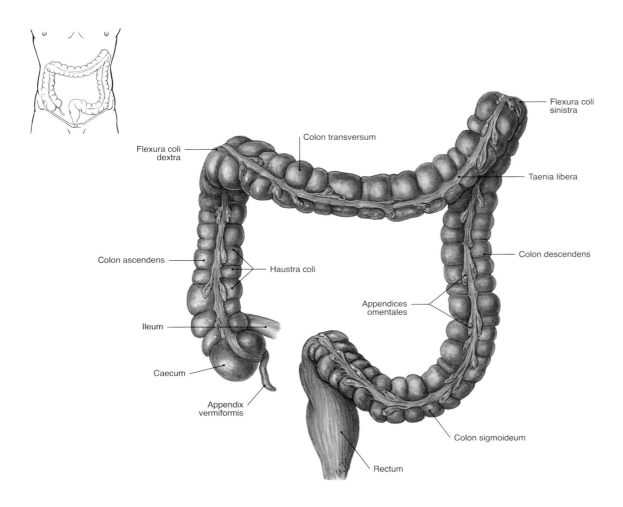

Flexura coli sinistra

Colon transversum

Flexura coli dextra

Taenia libera

Colon ascendens

Haustra coli

Colon descendens

Appendices omentales

Ileum

Caecum

Appendix vermiformis

Colon sigmoideum

Rectum

Fig. 1000 Large intestine, Intestinum crassum; ventral view.

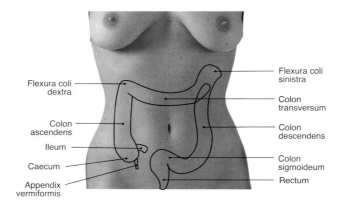

Flexura coli dextra

Flexura coli sinistra

Colon transversum

Colon ascendens

Ileum

Colon descendens

Caecum

Colon sigmoideum

Appendix vermiformis

Rectum

Fig. 1001 Large intestine, Intestinum crassum; projected onto the anterior abdominal wall.
The positions of the transverse colon and of the sigmoid colon are highly variable (compare Fig. 1010).

Large intestine, structure

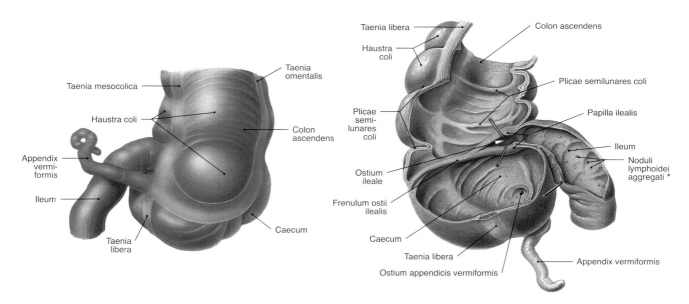

Fig. 1002   Caecum, Caecum; vermiform appendix,
Appendix vermiformis, and terminal ileum,
Pars terminalis ilei;
dorsal view.

Fig. 1003   Ascending colon, Colon ascendens;
caecum, Caecum, and vermiform appendix, Appendix vermiformis;
ventral view.
* Clinical term: PEYER's patches

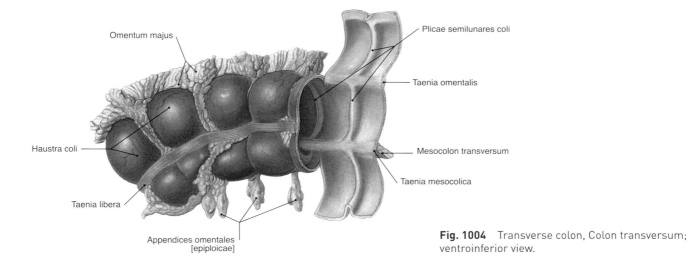

Fig. 1004   Transverse colon, Colon transversum;
ventroinferior view.

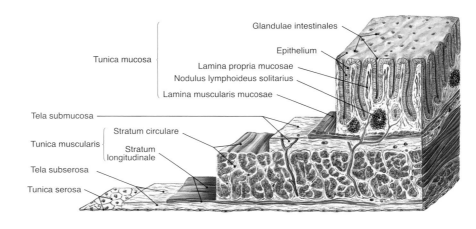

Fig. 1005   Colon, Colon;
layers of the wall;
microscopic enlargement
at low magnification.

Vermiform appendix

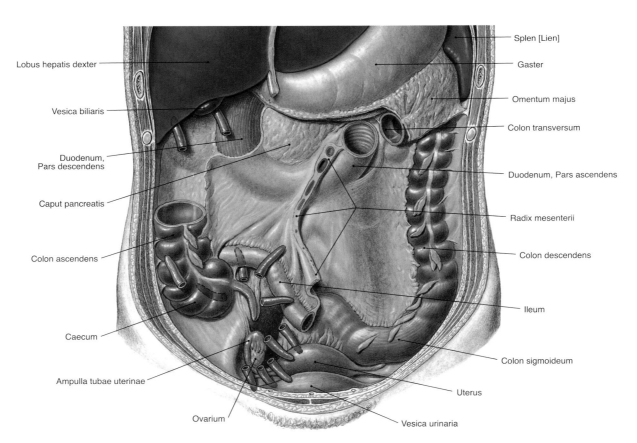

Fig. 1006 Vermiform appendix, Appendix vermiformis;
variations in its position;
ventral view.

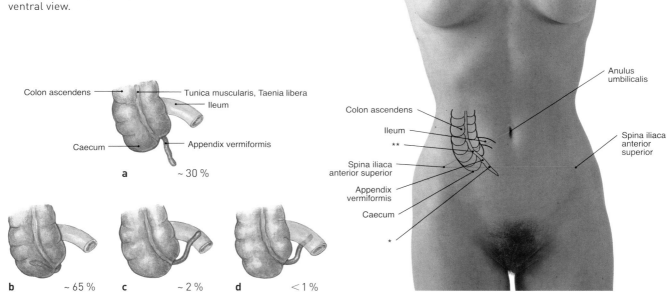

Fig. 1007 a–d Vermiform appendix, Appendix vermiformis;
variations in its position.
a Descending into the lesser pelvis
b Behind the caecum
c In front of the ileum
d Behind the ileum

Fig. 1008 Caecum, Caecum, and vermiform appendix,
Appendix vermiformis;
projection onto the anterior abdominal wall.

* Clinical term: v. LANZ's point, at the right third of a line
  connecting the anterior superior iliac spines, locates the tip
  of the vermiform appendix
** Clinical term: McBURNEY's point, at the outer third of a line
  connecting the right anterior superior iliac spine and the
  umbilicus, locates the base of the vermiform appendix

Large intestine, imaging

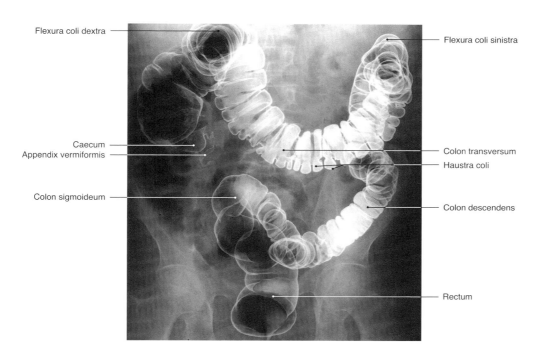

Flexura coli dextra
Flexura coli sinistra
Caecum
Appendix vermiformis
Colon transversum
Haustra coli
Colon sigmoideum
Colon descendens
Rectum

Fig. 1009 Colon, Colon, and rectum, Rectum; AP-radiograph after filling with a contrast medium and air (double contrast method).

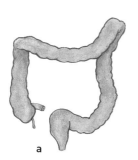 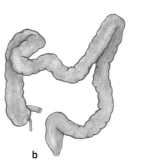 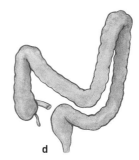

a b c d

Fig. 1010 a–d Transverse colon, Colon transversum; common variations in its position; ventral view.

a Normal position
b Twisted

c U-shaped
d V-shaped

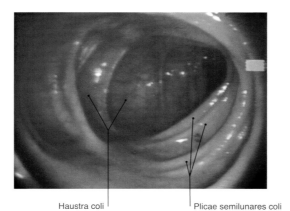

Haustra coli
Plicae semilunares coli

Fig. 1011 Ascending colon, Colon ascendens; endoscopic image after passage of the rectum, the sigmoid colon, the descending colon and the transverse colon (colonoscopy).

Liver

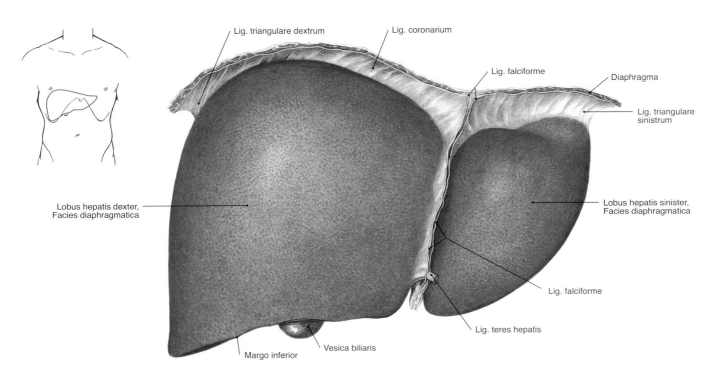

Fig. 1012 Liver, Hepar;
ventral view.

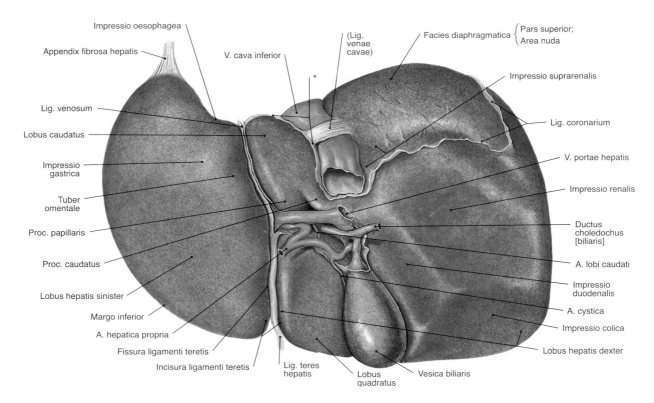

Fig. 1013 Liver, Hepar, and porta hepatis, Porta hepatis;
dorsal view.

* Borders of the superior recess of the omental bursa

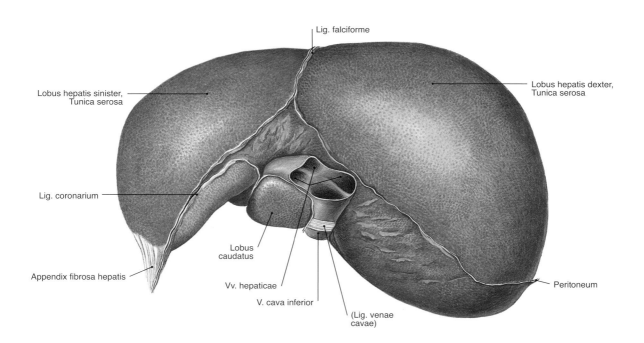

Lig. falciforme

Lobus hepatis sinister,
Tunica serosa

Lobus hepatis dexter,
Tunica serosa

Lig. coronarium

Lobus
caudatus

Appendix fibrosa hepatis

Vv. hepaticae

V. cava inferior

(Lig. venae
cavae)

Peritoneum

Fig. 1014 Liver, Hepar;
superior view.

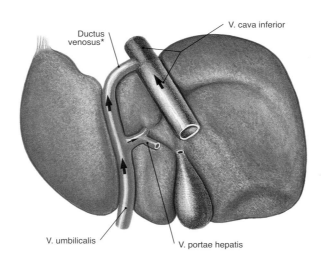

Ductus
venosus*

V. cava inferior

V. umbilicalis

V. portae hepatis

Fig. 1015 Liver, Hepar, of a foetus;
oxygen content of the blood is shown
by different colours and the direction
of flow by arrows;
dorsal view.
* Also: Ductus ARANTII

Liver puncture

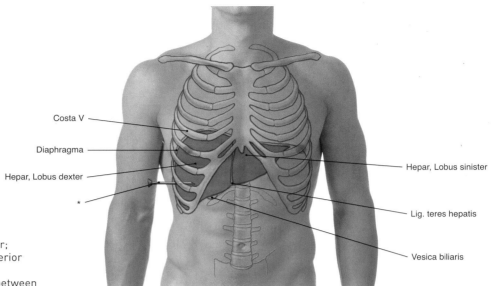

Fig. 1016 Liver, Hepar;
projection onto the anterior
abdominal wall;
intermediate position between
inspiration and expiration.
* Position of the needle for liver puncture

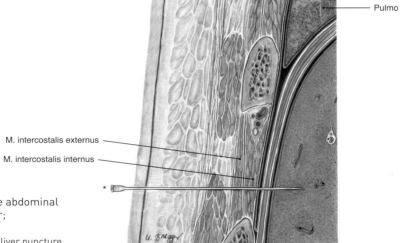

Fig. 1017 Layers of the abdominal
wall and the liver, Hepar;
frontal section.
* Position of the needle for liver puncture

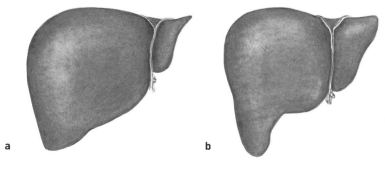

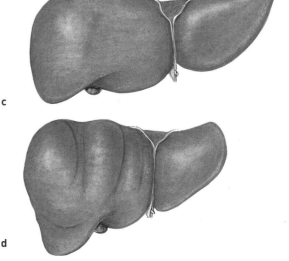

Fig. 1018 a–d Liver, Hepar;
variations in shape.
a Small left lobe of liver, Lobus hepatis sinister
b Tongue-shaped process of the right lobe of liver,
Lobus hepatis dexter
c Bridged flat shape
d Diaphragmatic furrows

Liver, structure

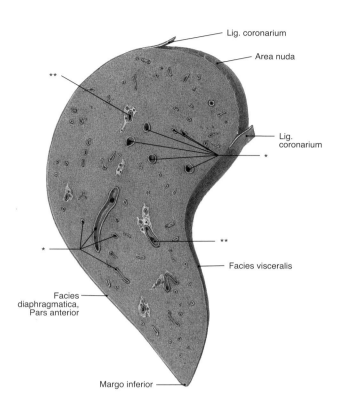

Lig. coronarium

Area nuda

Lig. coronarium

*

**

Facies visceralis

Facies
diaphragmatica,
Pars anterior

Margo inferior

Fig. 1019 Liver, Hepar;
sagittal section through the right lobe of liver to demonstrate
the branches of the hepatic veins and the hepatic portal vein.
* Intrahepatic branches of the hepatic veins
** Intrahepatic branches of the hepatic portal vein and the hepatic artery

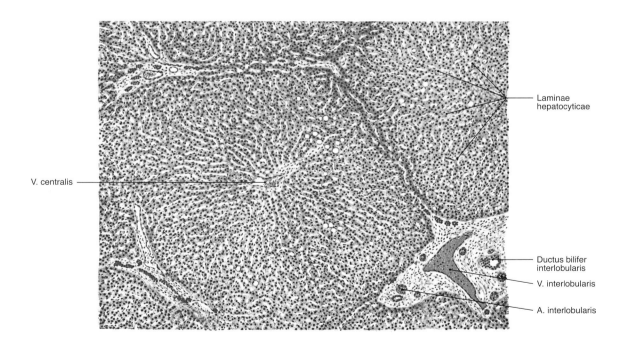

Laminae
hepatocyticae

V. centralis

Ductus bilifer
interlobularis

V. interlobularis

A. interlobularis

Fig. 1020 Liver, Hepar;
microscopic structure (microscopic enlargement at low
magnification);

trias of GLISSON (consists of a branch of the hepatic portal
vein, a branch of the hepatic artery proper and a small bile duct),
and a small liver lobule surrounding a central vein.

Blood vessels of the liver

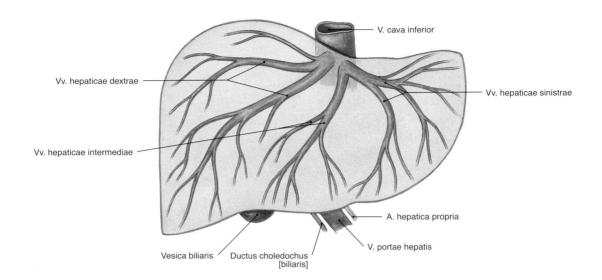

Fig. 1021 Liver, Hepar, and hepatic veins, Vv. hepaticae; ventral view.

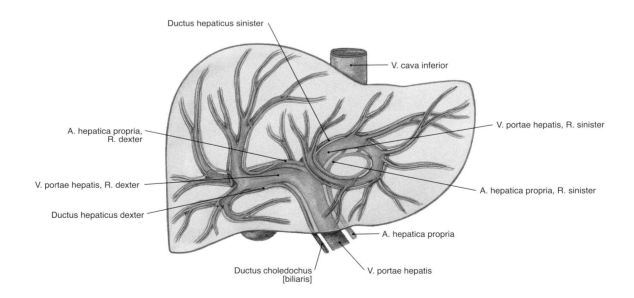

Fig. 1022 Liver, Hepar, and the hepatic portal vein, V. portae hepatis; ventral view.

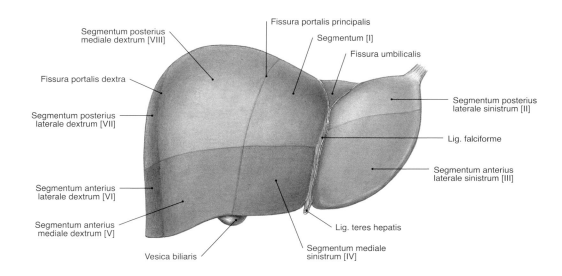

Fig. 1023 Liver, Hepar;
the segments of the lobes are shown in different colours;
ventral view.

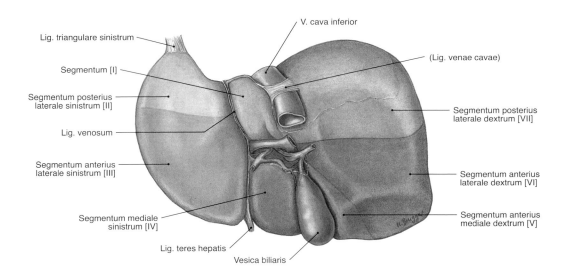

Fig. 1024 Liver, Hepar;
the segments of the lobes are shown in different colours;
dorsal view.

Liver, ultrasound

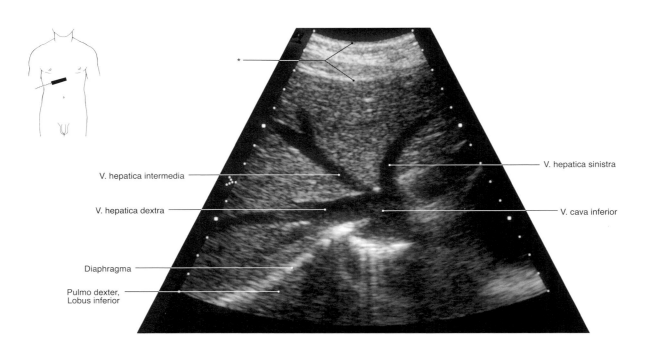

V. hepatica intermedia

V. hepatica dextra

V. hepatica sinistra

V. cava inferior

Diaphragma

Pulmo dexter,
Lobus inferior

→ 1021

Fig. 1025 Hepatic veins, Vv. hepaticae;
ultrasound image showing the opening of the hepatic veins
into the inferior vena cava;
inferior view.
* Abdominal wall

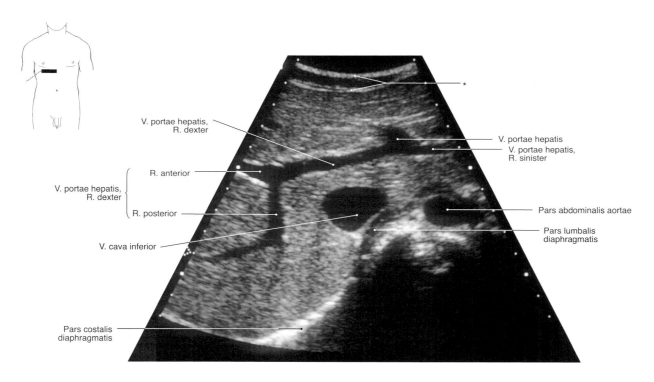

V. portae hepatis,
R. dexter

R. anterior

V. portae hepatis,
R. dexter

R. posterior

V. cava inferior

Pars costalis
diaphragmatis

V. portae hepatis

V. portae hepatis,
R. sinister

Pars abdominalis aortae

Pars lumbalis
diaphragmatis

→ 1022

Fig. 1026 Hepatic portal vein, V. portae hepatis;
ultrasound image showing the division of the hepatic portal vein
into the main branches;
inferior view.
* Abdominal wall

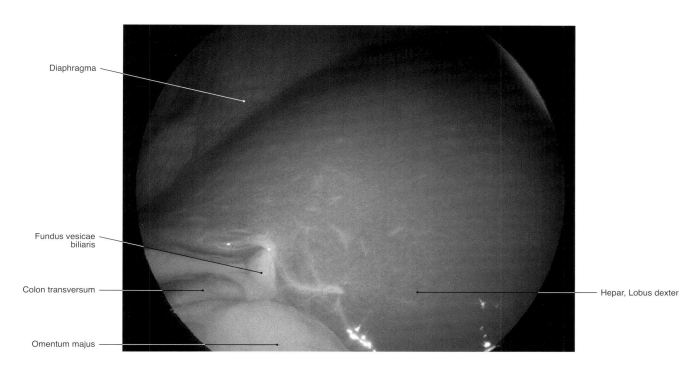

Diaphragma

Fundus vesicae biliaris

Colon transversum

Omentum majus

Hepar, Lobus dexter

Fig. 1027 Liver, Hepar, and gallbladder, Vesica biliaris [fellea];
laparoscopy;
oblique inferior view from the left.

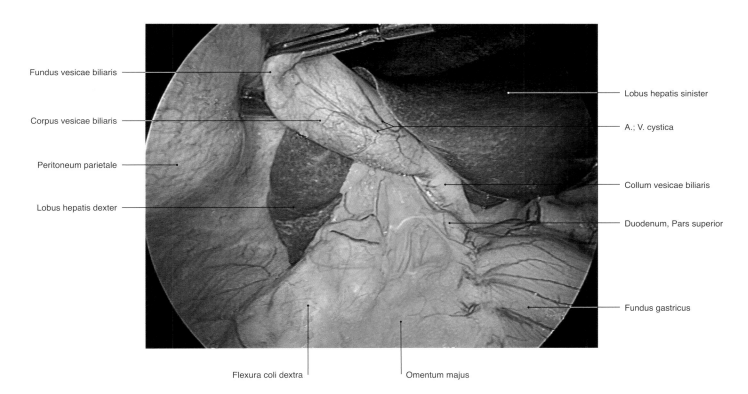

Fundus vesicae biliaris

Corpus vesicae biliaris

Peritoneum parietale

Lobus hepatis dexter

Lobus hepatis sinister

A.; V. cystica

Collum vesicae biliaris

Duodenum, Pars superior

Fundus gastricus

Flexura coli dextra

Omentum majus

Fig. 1028 Gallbladder, Vesica biliaris [fellea], and liver, Hepar;
laparoscopy;
ventral view.

Gallbladder and bile duct system

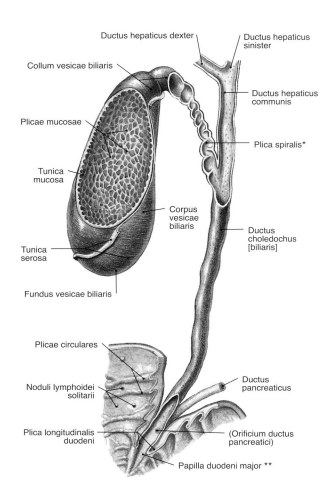

Ductus hepaticus dexter
Collum vesicae biliaris
Plicae mucosae
Tunica mucosa
Corpus vesicae biliaris
Tunica serosa
Fundus vesicae biliaris
Ductus hepaticus sinister
Ductus hepaticus communis
Plica spiralis*
Ductus choledochus [biliaris]
Plicae circulares
Noduli lymphoidei solitarii
Plica longitudinalis duodeni
Ductus pancreaticus
(Orificium ductus pancreatici)
Papilla duodeni major **

Fig. 1029 Gallbladder, Vesica biliaris [fellea], and bile duct system; ventral view.
* Clinical term: HEISTER's valve
** Clinical term: tubercle of VATER

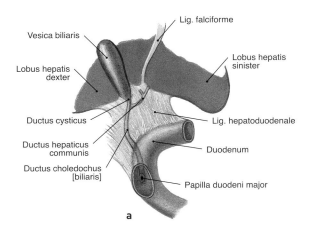

Vesica biliaris
Lobus hepatis dexter
Ductus cysticus
Ductus hepaticus communis
Ductus choledochus [biliaris]
Lig. falciforme
Lobus hepatis sinister
Lig. hepatoduodenale
Duodenum
Papilla duodeni major

a

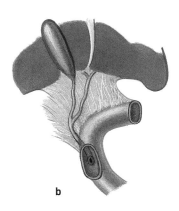

b

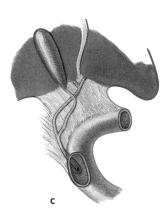

c

Fig. 1030 a–c Variations in the bile duct system: common hepatic duct, Ductus hepaticus communis, and bile duct, Ductus choledochus.
a High union of the common hepatic duct, Ductus hepaticus communis, and the cystic duct, Ductus cysticus
b Low union of the common hepatic duct, Ductus hepaticus communis, and the cystic duct, Ductus cysticus
c Low union after the cystic duct, Ductus cysticus, crosses over the common hepatic duct, Ductus hepaticus communis

Bile duct system, radiography

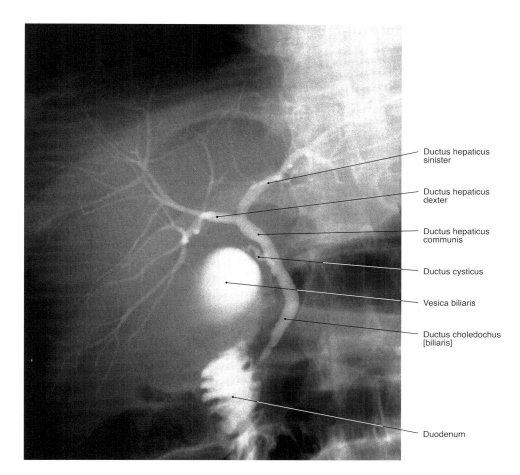

Ductus hepaticus sinister

Ductus hepaticus dexter

Ductus hepaticus communis

Ductus cysticus

Vesica biliaris

Ductus choledochus [biliaris]

Duodenum

Fig. 1031   Bile duct system;
AP-radiograph after administration of a contrast medium;
upright position;
ventral view.

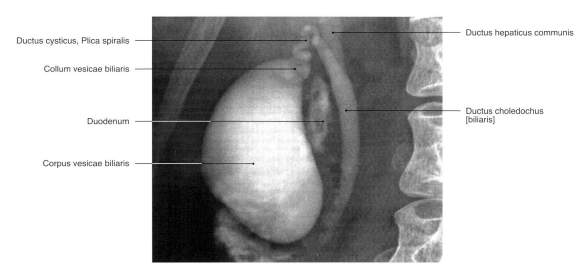

Ductus cysticus, Plica spiralis

Collum vesicae biliaris

Duodenum

Corpus vesicae biliaris

Ductus hepaticus communis

Ductus choledochus [biliaris]

Fig. 1032   Gallbladder, Vesica biliaris [fellea],
and bile duct system;
AP-radiograph after administration of a contrast medium;
upright position;
ventral view.

Pancreas

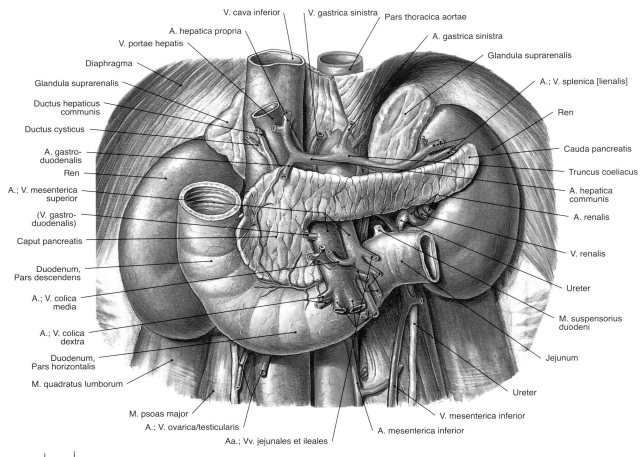

V. cava inferior
V. gastrica sinistra
Pars thoracica aortae
A. hepatica propria
V. portae hepatis
A. gastrica sinistra
Diaphragma
Glandula suprarenalis
Glandula suprarenalis
A.; V. splenica [lienalis]
Ductus hepaticus communis
Ren
Ductus cysticus
Cauda pancreatis
A. gastro-duodenalis
Truncus coeliacus
Ren
A. hepatica communis
A.; V. mesenterica superior
A. renalis
(V. gastro-duodenalis)
V. renalis
Caput pancreatis
Duodenum, Pars descendens
Ureter
A.; V. colica media
M. suspensorius duodeni
A.; V. colica dextra
Jejunum
Duodenum, Pars horizontalis
M. quadratus lumborum
Ureter
M. psoas major
V. mesenterica inferior
A.; V. ovarica/testicularis
A. mesenterica inferior
Aa.; Vv. jejunales et ileales

Fig. 1033 Retroperitoneal organs and vessels of the upper abdomen; ventral view.

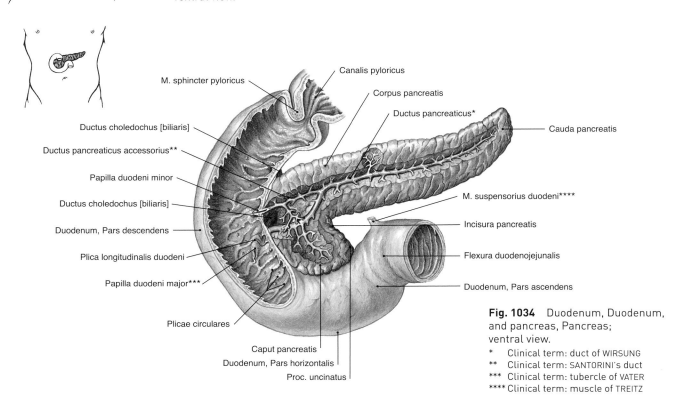

M. sphincter pyloricus
Canalis pyloricus
Corpus pancreatis
Ductus choledochus [biliaris]
Ductus pancreaticus*
Cauda pancreatis
Ductus pancreaticus accessorius**
Papilla duodeni minor
Ductus choledochus [biliaris]
M. suspensorius duodeni****
Duodenum, Pars descendens
Incisura pancreatis
Plica longitudinalis duodeni
Flexura duodenojejunalis
Papilla duodeni major***
Duodenum, Pars ascendens
Plicae circulares
Caput pancreatis
Duodenum, Pars horizontalis
Proc. uncinatus

Fig. 1034 Duodenum, Duodenum, and pancreas, Pancreas; ventral view.
* Clinical term: duct of WIRSUNG
** Clinical term: SANTORINI's duct
*** Clinical term: tubercle of VATER
**** Clinical term: muscle of TREITZ

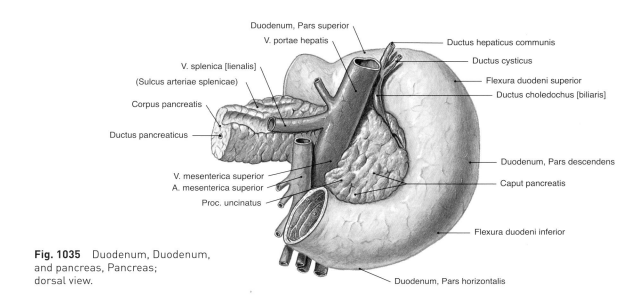

Duodenum, Pars superior
V. portae hepatis
Ductus hepaticus communis
Ductus cysticus
V. splenica [lienalis]
Flexura duodeni superior
(Sulcus arteriae splenicae)
Ductus choledochus [biliaris]
Corpus pancreatis
Ductus pancreaticus
Duodenum, Pars descendens
V. mesenterica superior
Caput pancreatis
A. mesenterica superior
Proc. uncinatus
Flexura duodeni inferior
Duodenum, Pars horizontalis

Fig. 1035 Duodenum, Duodenum, and pancreas, Pancreas; dorsal view.

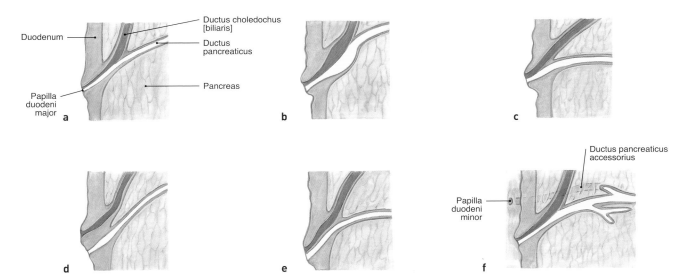

Ductus choledochus [biliaris]
Duodenum
Ductus pancreaticus
Pancreas
Papilla duodeni major

a   **b**   **c**

Ductus pancreaticus accessorius
Papilla duodeni minor

d   **e**   **f**

Fig. 1036 a–f   Variations in the opening of the bile duct, Ductus choledochus, and the pancreatic duct, Ductus pancreaticus.
a   Long common part
b   Ampullary enlargement at the terminal part

c   Short common part
d   Separate opening
e   Single opening with a septum dividing the common duct
f   Accessory duct, Ductus pancreaticus accessorius

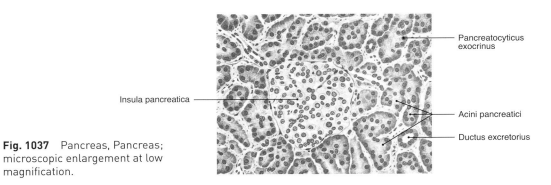

Pancreatocyticus exocrinus
Insula pancreatica
Acini pancreatici
Ductus excretorius

Fig. 1037   Pancreas, Pancreas; microscopic enlargement at low magnification.

Pancreas, imaging

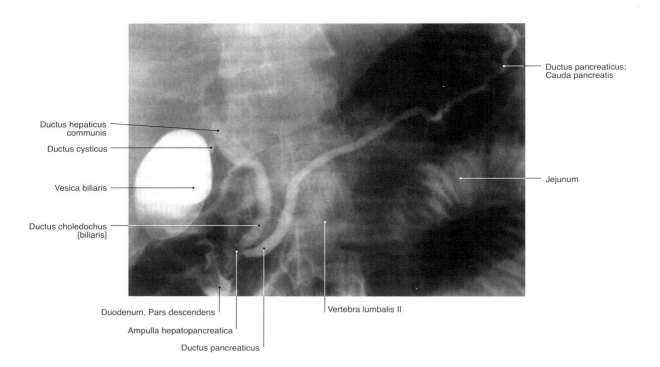

Ductus hepaticus communis

Ductus cysticus

Vesica biliaris

Ductus choledochus [biliaris]

Duodenum, Pars descendens

Ampulla hepatopancreatica

Ductus pancreaticus

Ductus pancreaticus; Cauda pancreatis

Jejunum

Vertebra lumbalis II

Fig. 1038 Pancreatic duct, Ductus pancreaticus; bile duct, Ductus choledochus, and gallbladder, Vesica biliaris [fellea]; AP-radiograph; supine position; after endoscopic intubation of the common excretory duct of the liver and the pancreas, as well as injection of a contrast medium; ventral view.
Clinical term: ERCP (endoscopic retrograde cholangio-pancreaticography).

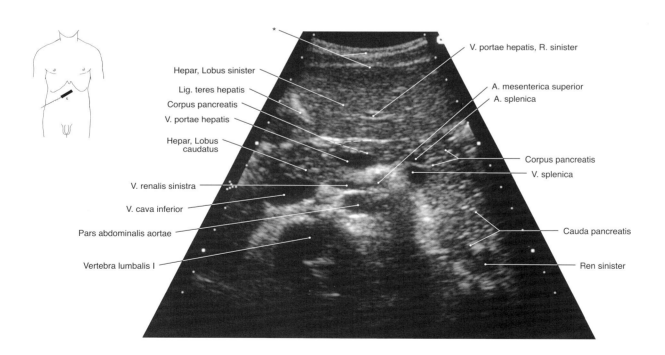

*

Hepar, Lobus sinister

Lig. teres hepatis

Corpus pancreatis

V. portae hepatis

Hepar, Lobus caudatus

V. renalis sinistra

V. cava inferior

Pars abdominalis aortae

Vertebra lumbalis I

V. portae hepatis, R. sinister

A. mesenterica superior

A. splenica

Corpus pancreatis

V. splenica

Cauda pancreatis

Ren sinister

Fig. 1039 Pancreas, Pancreas; ultrasound image showing the pancreas and adjacent large vessels in deep inspiration; oblique inferior view.
* Abdominal wall

Pancreas, imaging

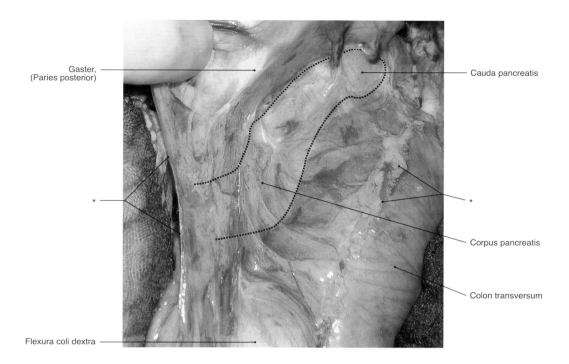

Gaster, (Paries posterior)

Cauda pancreatis

*

Corpus pancreatis

Colon transversum

*

Flexura coli dextra

Fig. 1040 Pancreas, Pancreas;
the gastrocolic ligament of the greater omentum has been
dissected to expose the omental bursa;
photograph taken during surgery.
* Dissection line at the greater omentum

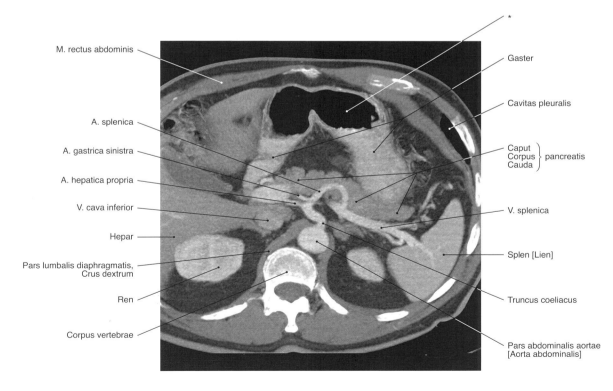

*

M. rectus abdominis

A. splenica

A. gastrica sinistra

A. hepatica propria

V. cava inferior

Hepar

Pars lumbalis diaphragmatis,
Crus dextrum

Ren

Corpus vertebrae

Gaster

Cavitas pleuralis

Caput
Corpus } pancreatis
Cauda

V. splenica

Splen [Lien]

Truncus coeliacus

Pars abdominalis aortae
[Aorta abdominalis]

Fig. 1041 Pancreas, Pancreas;
computed tomographic horizontal section (CT);
inferior view.
In this subject, the coeliac trunk is located remarkably low.
* Air bubble in the stomach

Spleen

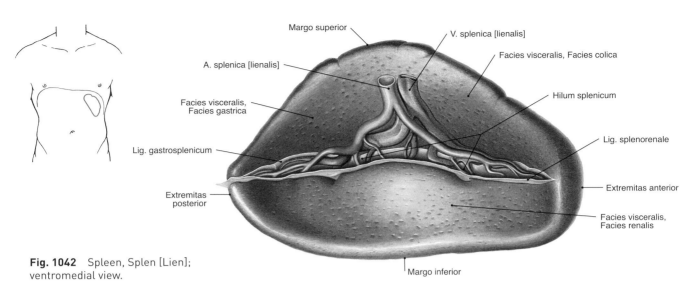

Fig. 1042 Spleen, Splen [Lien]; ventromedial view.

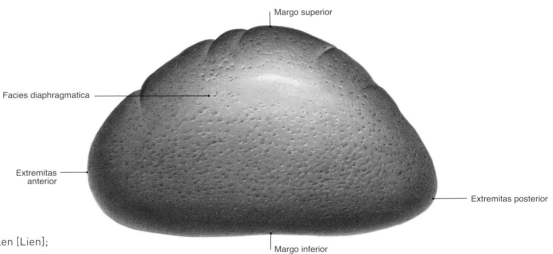

Fig. 1043 Spleen, Splen [Lien]; superolateral view.

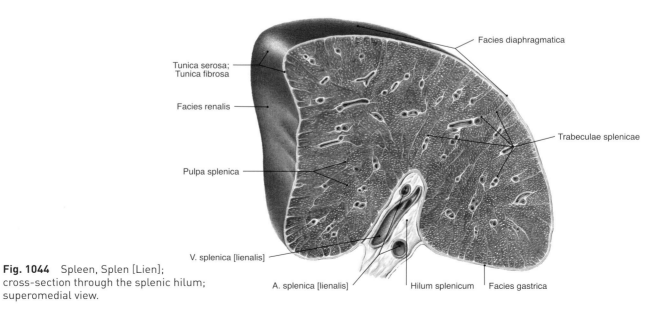

Fig. 1044 Spleen, Aplen [Lien]; cross-section through the splenic hilum; superomedial view.

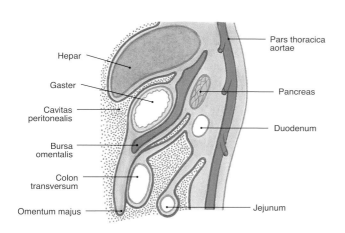

Fig. 1045 Development of the peritoneal cavity, Cavitas peritonealis, and the visceral relationships; schematic median section; lateral view.

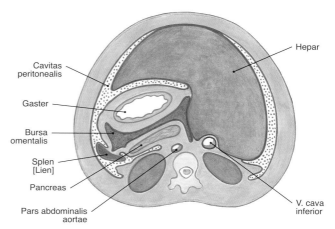

Fig. 1046 Development of the peritoneal cavity, Cavitas peritonealis; schematic horizontal section; superior view.

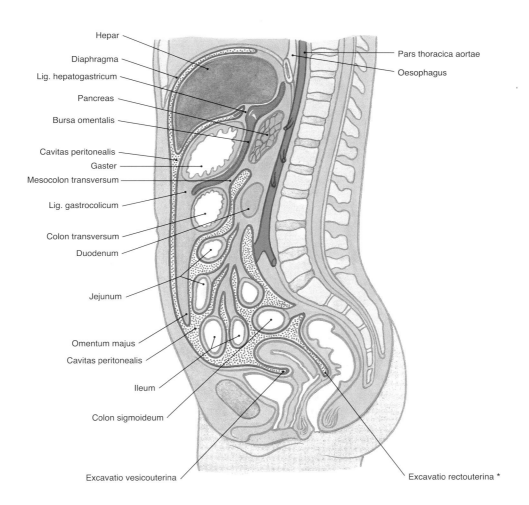

Fig. 1047 Development of the peritoneal cavity, Cavitas peritonealis, and the visceral relationships of the female; final state of the peritoneal cavity with adhesion of the greater omentum to the transverse colon;

schematic median section; lateral view.
The omental bursa corresponds with the peritoneal cavity via the omental foramen.
* Clinical term: pouch of DOUGLAS

Greater omentum

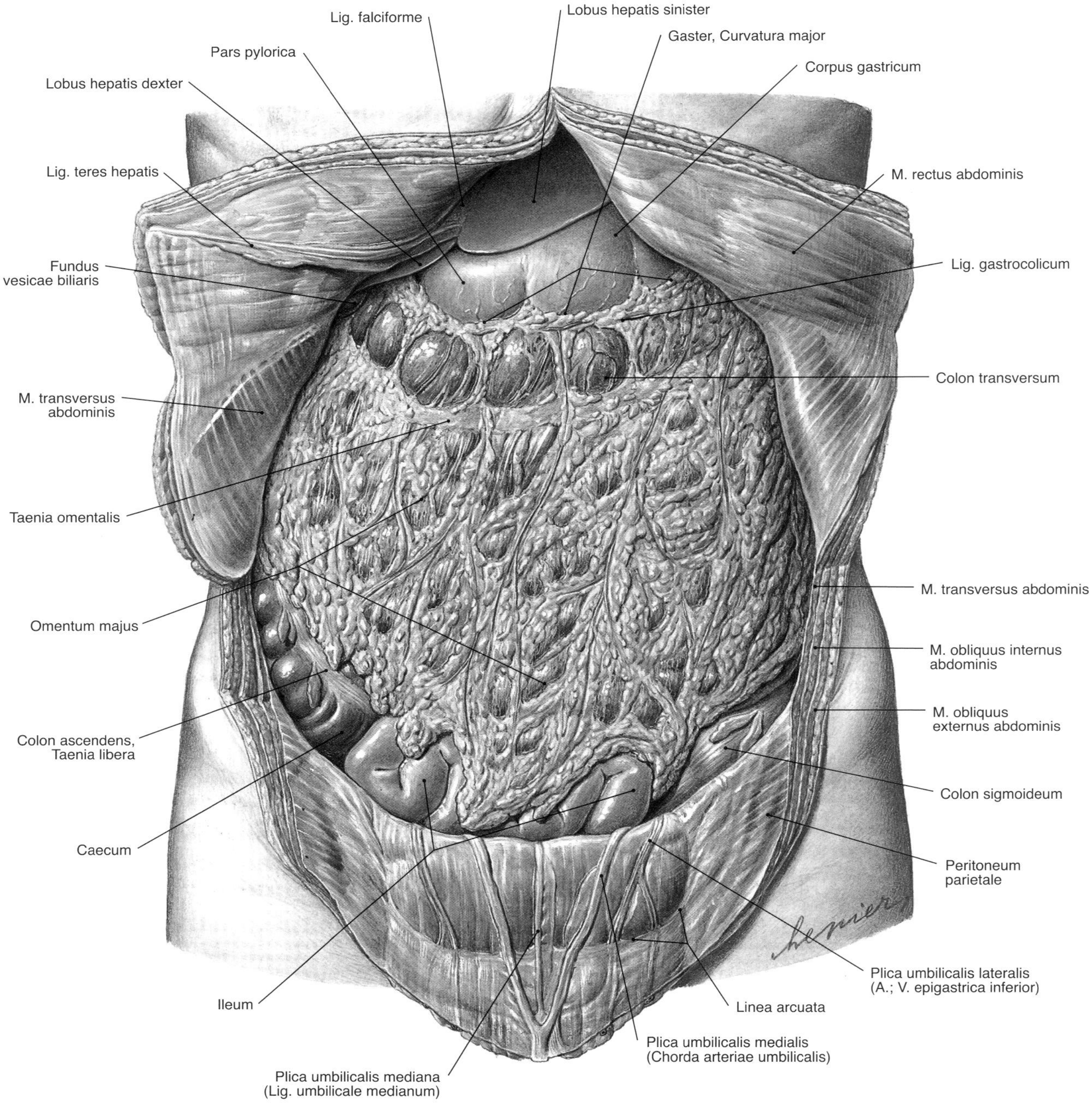

Lig. falciforme

Lobus hepatis sinister

Pars pylorica

Gaster, Curvatura major

Lobus hepatis dexter

Corpus gastricum

Lig. teres hepatis

M. rectus abdominis

Fundus
vesicae biliaris

Lig. gastrocolicum

M. transversus
abdominis

Colon transversum

Taenia omentalis

M. transversus abdominis

Omentum majus

M. obliquus internus
abdominis

M. obliquus
externus abdominis

Colon ascendens,
Taenia libera

Colon sigmoideum

Caecum

Peritoneum
parietale

Plica umbilicalis lateralis
(A.; V. epigastrica inferior)

Ileum

Linea arcuata

Plica umbilicalis medialis
(Chorda arteriae umbilicalis)

Plica umbilicalis mediana
(Lig. umbilicale medianum)

→ 846

Fig. 1048   Position of the abdominal viscera, Situs viscerum,
and greater omentum, Omentum majus.

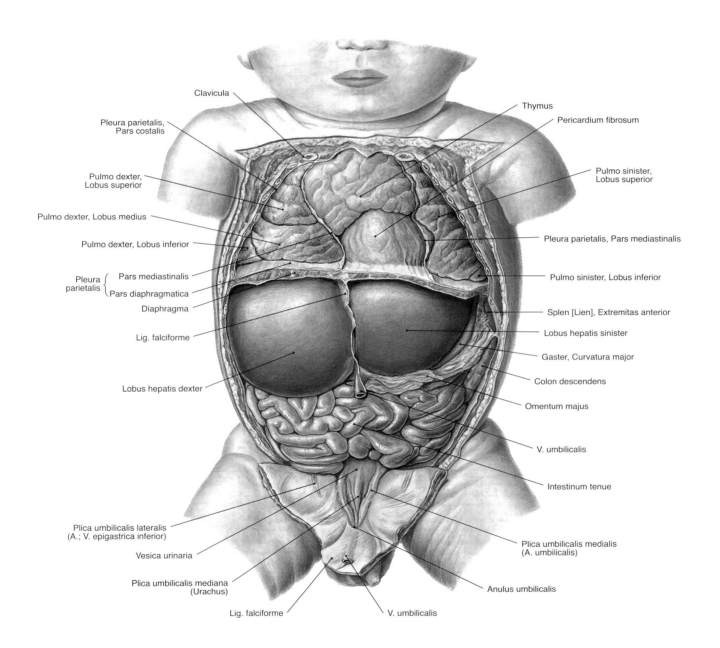

Clavicula

Thymus

Pleura parietalis, Pars costalis

Pericardium fibrosum

Pulmo dexter, Lobus superior

Pulmo sinister, Lobus superior

Pulmo dexter, Lobus medius

Pulmo dexter, Lobus inferior

Pleura parietalis, Pars mediastinalis

Pleura parietalis { Pars mediastinalis, Pars diaphragmatica

Pulmo sinister, Lobus inferior

Diaphragma

Splen [Lien], Extremitas anterior

Lig. falciforme

Lobus hepatis sinister

Gaster, Curvatura major

Colon descendens

Lobus hepatis dexter

Omentum majus

V. umbilicalis

Intestinum tenue

Plica umbilicalis lateralis (A.; V. epigastrica inferior)

Vesica urinaria

Plica umbilicalis medialis (A. umbilicalis)

Plica umbilicalis mediana (Urachus)

Anulus umbilicalis

Lig. falciforme

V. umbilicalis

Fig. 1049   Position of the abdominal viscera of the neonate.

Abdominal viscera in the upper abdomen

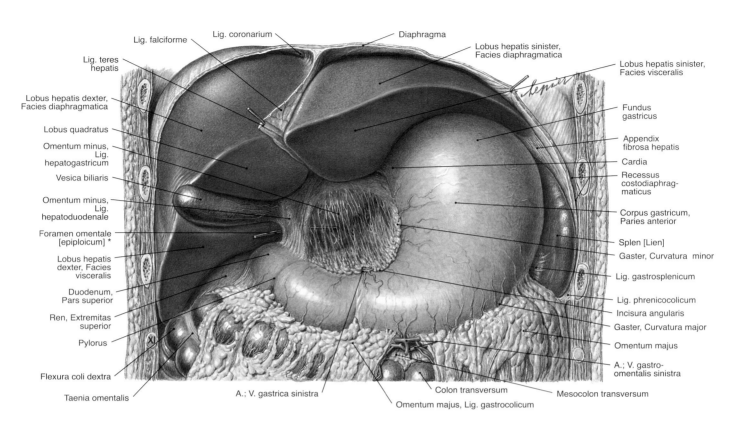

Fig. 1050 Position of the abdominal viscera in the upper abdomen; ventral view.

* Also: foramen of WINSLOW

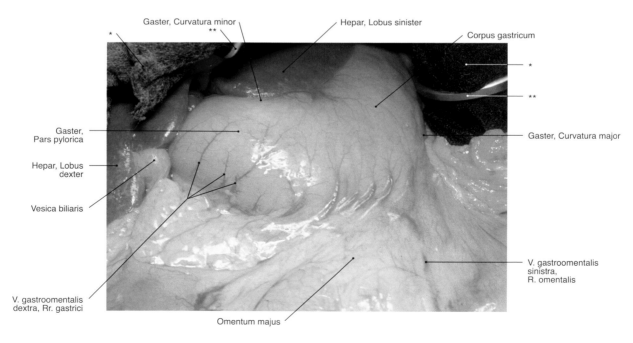

Fig. 1051 Stomach, Gaster, and greater omentum, Omentum majus; photograph taken during surgery; ventral view.

* Surgical drape
** Surgical retractor

Abdominal viscera in the upper abdomen

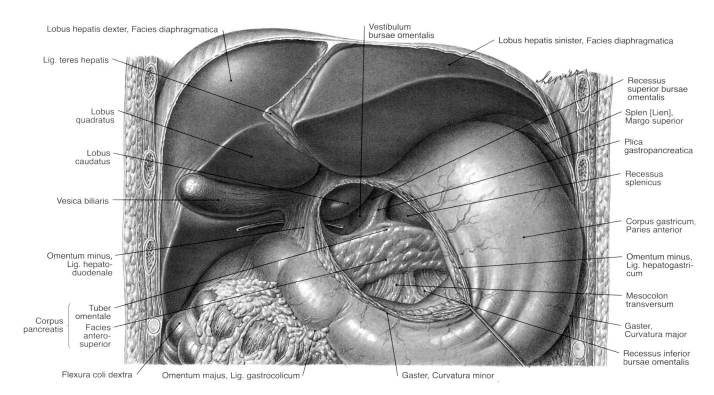

Lobus hepatis dexter, Facies diaphragmatica
Lig. teres hepatis
Lobus quadratus
Lobus caudatus
Vesica biliaris
Omentum minus, Lig. hepato-duodenale
Corpus pancreatis — Tuber omentale / Facies antero-superior
Flexura coli dextra
Omentum majus, Lig. gastrocolicum

Vestibulum bursae omentalis
Lobus hepatis sinister, Facies diaphragmatica
Recessus superior bursae omentalis
Splen [Lien], Margo superior
Plica gastropancreatica
Recessus splenicus
Corpus gastricum, Paries anterior
Omentum minus, Lig. hepatogastri-cum
Mesocolon transversum
Gaster, Curvatura major
Recessus inferior bursae omentalis
Gaster, Curvatura minor

Fig. 1052 Abdominal viscera in the upper abdomen;
parts of the lesser omentum have been removed to expose
the omental bursa and the pancreas;
oblique view from superior.

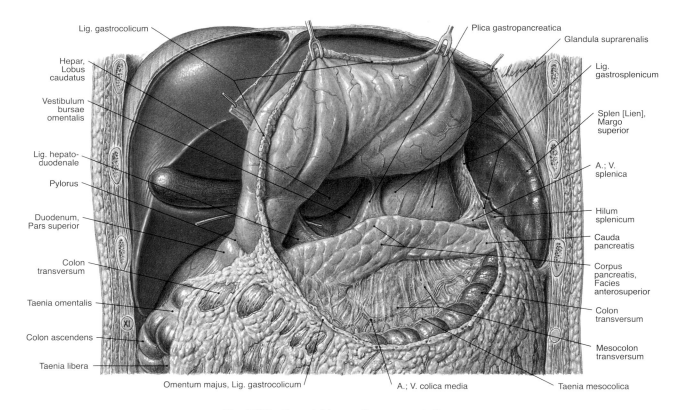

Lig. gastrocolicum
Hepar, Lobus caudatus
Vestibulum bursae omentalis
Lig. hepato-duodenale
Pylorus
Duodenum, Pars superior
Colon transversum
Taenia omentalis
Colon ascendens
Taenia libera
Omentum majus, Lig. gastrocolicum

Plica gastropancreatica
Glandula suprarenalis
Lig. gastrosplenicum
Splen [Lien], Margo superior
A.; V. splenica
Hilum splenicum
Cauda pancreatis
Corpus pancreatis, Facies anterosuperior
Colon transversum
Mesocolon transversum
Taenia mesocolica
A.; V. colica media

Fig. 1053 Omental bursa, Bursa omentalis;
after dissection of the gastrocolic ligament;
oblique view from inferior.

Abdominal viscera in the lower abdomen

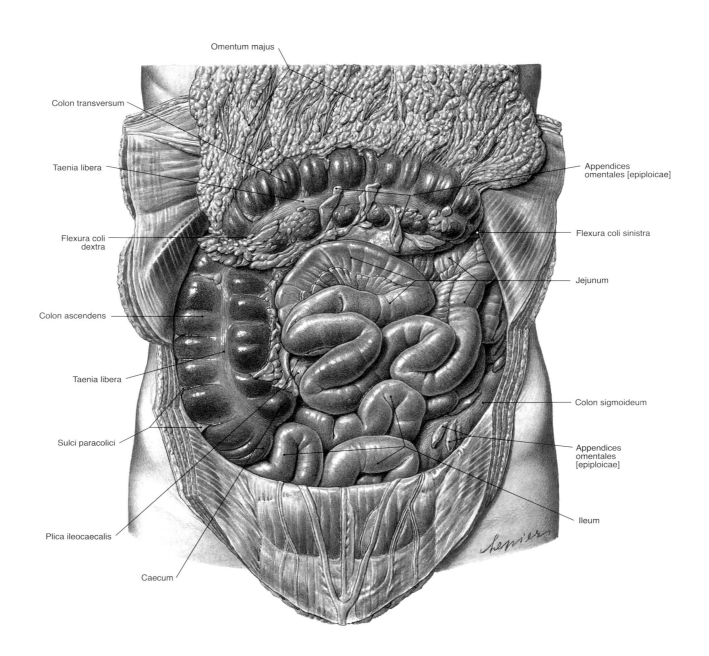

Omentum majus

Colon transversum

Taenia libera

Flexura coli dextra

Colon ascendens

Taenia libera

Sulci paracolici

Plica ileocaecalis

Caecum

Appendices omentales [epiploicae]

Flexura coli sinistra

Jejunum

Colon sigmoideum

Appendices omentales [epiploicae]

Ileum

Fig. 1054   Position of the abdominal viscera, Situs viscerum.

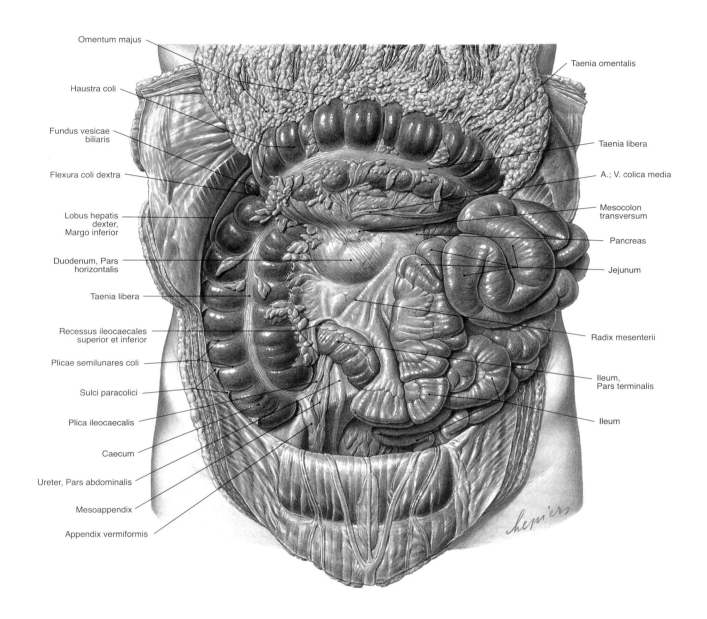

Omentum majus

Haustra coli

Fundus vesicae biliaris

Flexura coli dextra

Lobus hepatis dexter, Margo inferior

Duodenum, Pars horizontalis

Taenia libera

Recessus ileocaecales superior et inferior

Plicae semilunares coli

Sulci paracolici

Plica ileocaecalis

Caecum

Ureter, Pars abdominalis

Mesoappendix

Appendix vermiformis

Taenia omentalis

Taenia libera

A.; V. colica media

Mesocolon transversum

Pancreas

Jejunum

Radix mesenterii

Ileum, Pars terminalis

Ileum

Fig. 1055 Small intestine, Intestinum tenue, and large intestine, Intestinum crassum.

Abdominal viscera in the lower abdomen

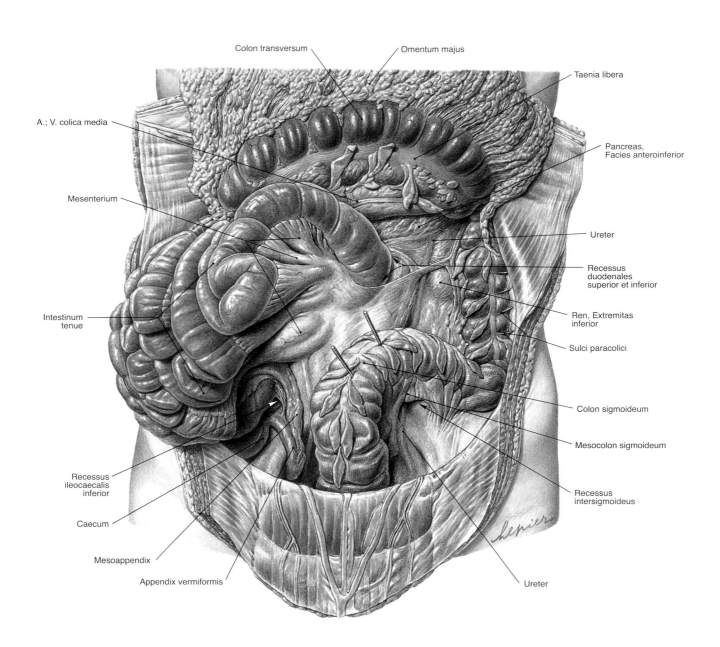

Colon transversum

Omentum majus

Taenia libera

A.; V. colica media

Pancreas, Facies anteroinferior

Mesenterium

Ureter

Recessus duodenales superior et inferior

Intestinum tenue

Ren, Extremitas inferior

Sulci paracolici

Colon sigmoideum

Mesocolon sigmoideum

Recessus ileocaecalis inferior

Recessus intersigmoideus

Caecum

Mesoappendix

Appendix vermiformis

Ureter

Fig. 1056 Small intestine, Intestinum tenue, and large intestine, Intestinum crassum.

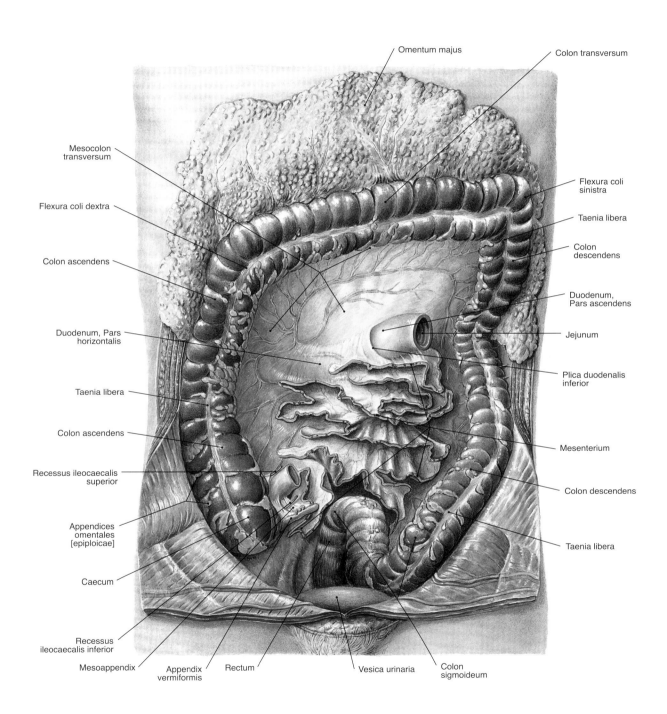

Omentum majus

Colon transversum

Mesocolon transversum

Flexura coli sinistra

Flexura coli dextra

Taenia libera

Colon ascendens

Colon descendens

Duodenum, Pars ascendens

Duodenum, Pars horizontalis

Jejunum

Taenia libera

Plica duodenalis inferior

Colon ascendens

Mesenterium

Recessus ileocaecalis superior

Colon descendens

Appendices omentales [epiploicae]

Taenia libera

Caecum

Recessus ileocaecalis inferior

Mesoappendix

Appendix vermiformis

Rectum

Vesica urinaria

Colon sigmoideum

Fig. 1057 Mesentery, Mesenterium, and large intestine, Intestinum crassum.

Mesenteric root and retroperitoneal space

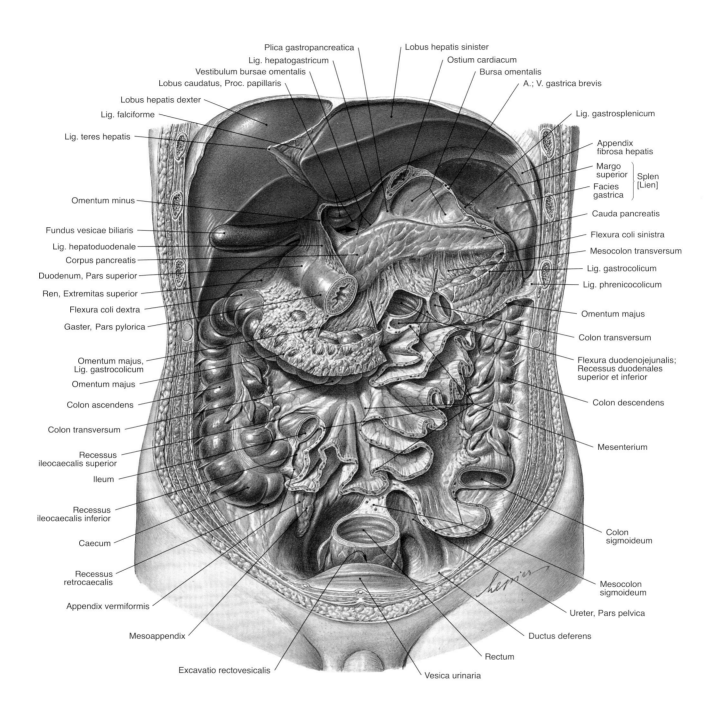

Fig. 1058 Position of the abdominal viscera, Situs viscerum, and the omental bursa, Bursa omentalis.
An arrow indicates the omental [epiploic] foramen.

Retroperitoneal space

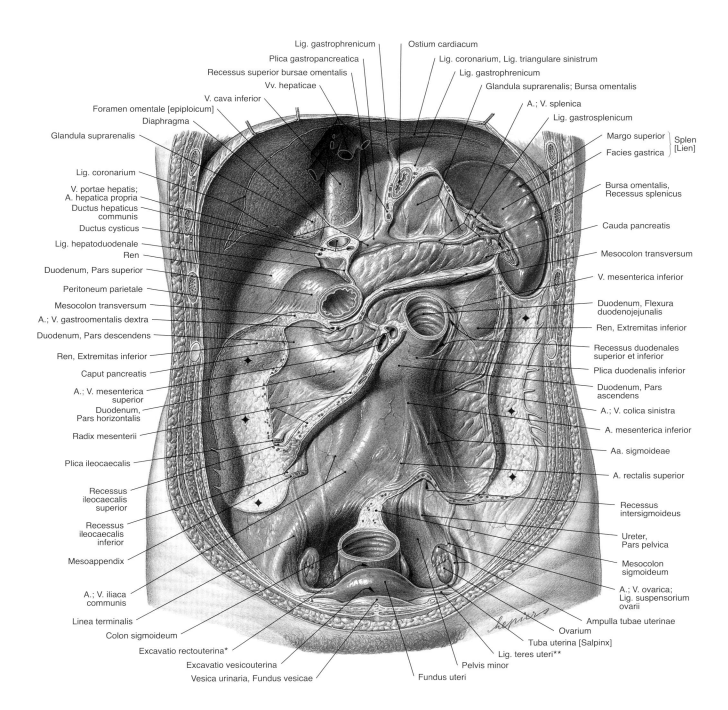

Lig. gastrophrenicum
Plica gastropancreatica
Recessus superior bursae omentalis
Vv. hepaticae
V. cava inferior
Foramen omentale [epiploicum]
Diaphragma
Glandula suprarenalis
Lig. coronarium
V. portae hepatis;
A. hepatica propria
Ductus hepaticus communis
Ductus cysticus
Lig. hepatoduodenale
Ren
Duodenum, Pars superior
Peritoneum parietale
Mesocolon transversum
A.; V. gastroomentalis dextra
Duodenum, Pars descendens
Ren, Extremitas inferior
Caput pancreatis
A.; V. mesenterica superior
Duodenum, Pars horizontalis
Radix mesenterii
Plica ileocaecalis
Recessus ileocaecalis superior
Recessus ileocaecalis inferior
Mesoappendix
A.; V. iliaca communis
Linea terminalis
Colon sigmoideum
Excavatio rectouterina*
Excavatio vesicouterina
Vesica urinaria, Fundus vesicae

Ostium cardiacum
Lig. coronarium, Lig. triangulare sinistrum
Lig. gastrophrenicum
Glandula suprarenalis; Bursa omentalis
A.; V. splenica
Lig. gastrosplenicum
Margo superior ⎫ Splen
Facies gastrica ⎭ [Lien]
Bursa omentalis, Recessus splenicus
Cauda pancreatis
Mesocolon transversum
V. mesenterica inferior
Duodenum, Flexura duodenojejunalis
Ren, Extremitas inferior
Recessus duodenales superior et inferior
Plica duodenalis inferior
Duodenum, Pars ascendens
A.; V. colica sinistra
A. mesenterica inferior
Aa. sigmoideae
A. rectalis superior
Recessus intersigmoideus
Ureter, Pars pelvica
Mesocolon sigmoideum
A.; V. ovarica; Lig. suspensorium ovarii
Ampulla tubae uterinae
Ovarium
Tuba uterina [Salpinx]
Lig. teres uteri**
Pelvis minor
Fundus uteri

Fig. 1059 Posterior wall of the peritoneal cavity, Cavitas peritonealis, and spleen, Splen [Lien], of the female. Sites of attachment of the ascending and descending colon are indicated (♦).

* Clinical term: pouch of DOUGLAS
** Clinical term: round ligament

Abdominal arteries, overview

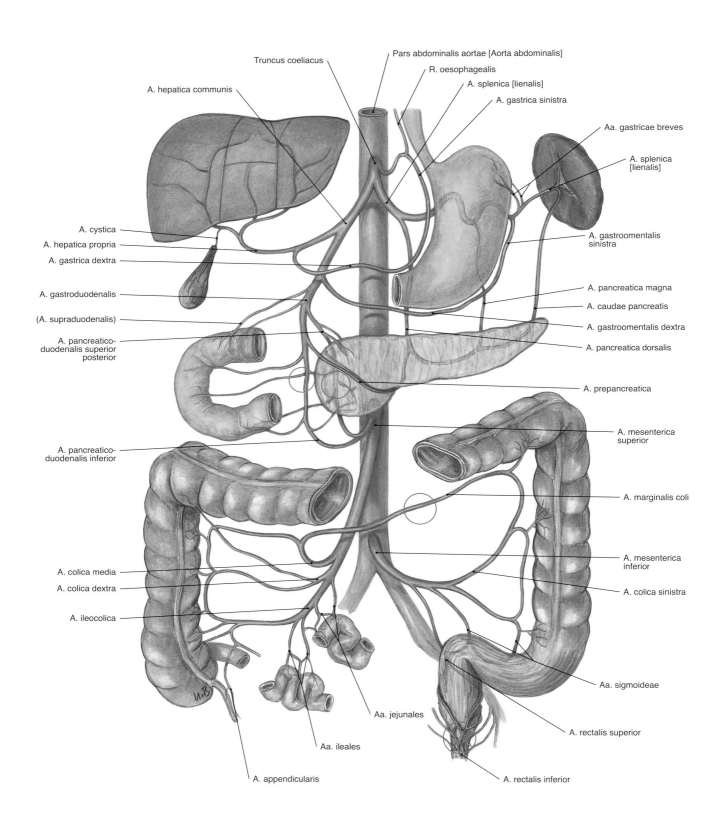

Truncus coeliacus

Pars abdominalis aortae [Aorta abdominalis]

R. oesophagealis

A. hepatica communis

A. splenica [lienalis]

A. gastrica sinistra

Aa. gastricae breves

A. splenica [lienalis]

A. cystica

A. hepatica propria

A. gastrica dextra

A. gastroomentalis sinistra

A. gastroduodenalis

(A. supraduodenalis)

A. pancreatico-duodenalis superior posterior

A. pancreatica magna

A. caudae pancreatis

A. gastroomentalis dextra

A. pancreatica dorsalis

A. prepancreatica

A. pancreatico-duodenalis inferior

A. mesenterica superior

A. marginalis coli

A. colica media

A. colica dextra

A. ileocolica

A. mesenterica inferior

A. colica sinistra

Aa. sigmoideae

A. rectalis superior

Aa. jejunales

Aa. ileales

A. appendicularis

A. rectalis inferior

Fig. 1060   Arteries of the abdominal viscera; semi-schematic; possible anastomoses are indicated (O).

Abdominal veins, overview

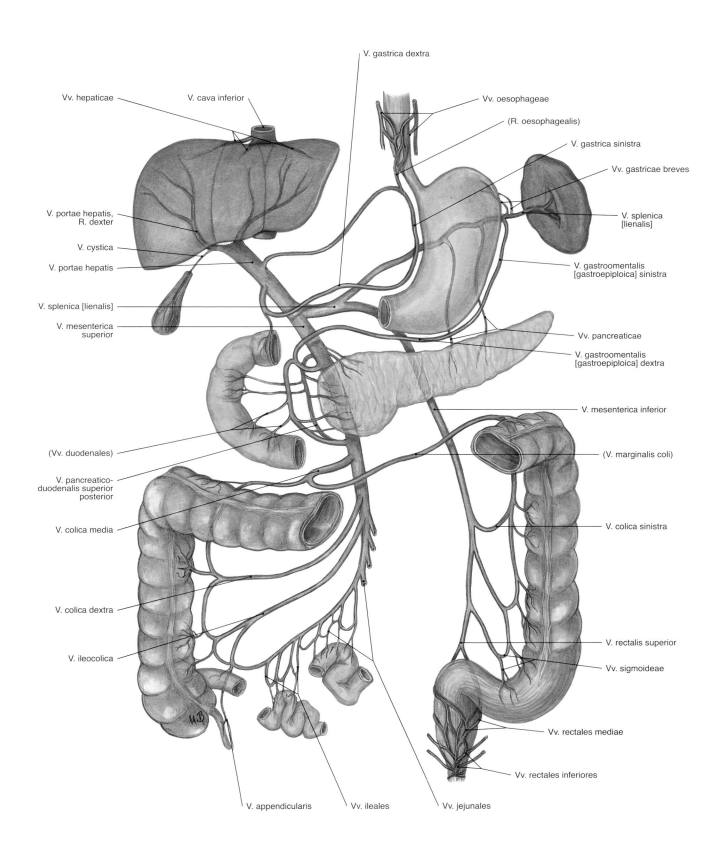

V. gastrica dextra

Vv. hepaticae

V. cava inferior

Vv. oesophageae

(R. oesophagealis)

V. gastrica sinistra

Vv. gastricae breves

V. portae hepatis, R. dexter

V. cystica

V. portae hepatis

V. splenica [lienalis]

V. gastroomentalis [gastroepiploica] sinistra

V. splenica [lienalis]

V. mesenterica superior

Vv. pancreaticae

V. gastroomentalis [gastroepiploica] dextra

V. mesenterica inferior

(Vv. duodenales)

(V. marginalis coli)

V. pancreatico-duodenalis superior posterior

V. colica media

V. colica sinistra

V. colica dextra

V. ileocolica

V. rectalis superior

Vv. sigmoideae

Vv. rectales mediae

Vv. rectales inferiores

V. appendicularis

Vv. ileales

Vv. jejunales

Fig. 1061 Hepatic portal vein, V. portae hepatis, with tributaries; semi-schematic.

Coeliac trunk

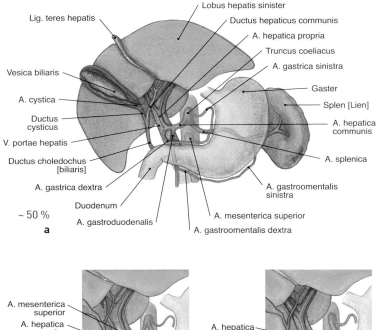

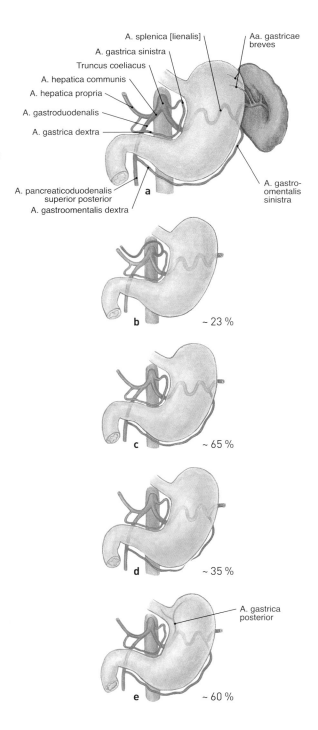

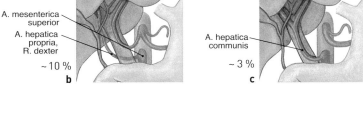

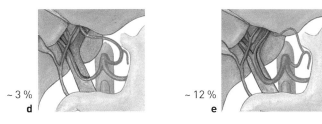

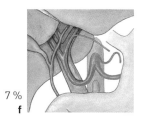

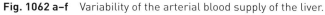

Fig. 1062 a–f   Variability of the arterial blood supply of the liver.
- **a** "Textbook case"
- **b** The superior mesenteric artery, A. mesenterica superior, participates in the supply of the right lobe of the liver.
- **c** The common hepatic artery, A. hepatica communis, arises from the superior mesenteric artery, A. mesenterica superior.
- **d** The left lobe of the liver is supplied by the left gastric artery, A. gastrica sinistra.
- **e** A branch of the left gastric artery, A. gastrica sinistra, supplies the left lobe of the liver along with the left branch of the hepatic artery proper, A. hepatica propria.
- **f** An accessory branch of the hepatic artery proper, A. hepatica propria, supplies the lesser curvature of the stomach.

Fig. 1063 a–e   Variability of the arterial blood supply of the stomach.
- **a** "Textbook case", closed arterial arcade supplying both the lesser and the greater curvature
- **b** The left gastric artery, A. gastrica sinistra, participates in the supply of the left lobe of the liver.
- **c** Anastomosis between the right and left gastro-omental arteries, Aa. gastroomentales dextra et sinistra, at the greater curvature
- **d** Absence of an anastomosis between the right and left gastro-omental arteries, Aa. gastroomentales dextra et sinistra, at the greater curvature
- **e** An accessory posterior gastric artery, A. gastrica posterior, arising from the splenic artery, A. splenica, supplies the posterior wall of the stomach.

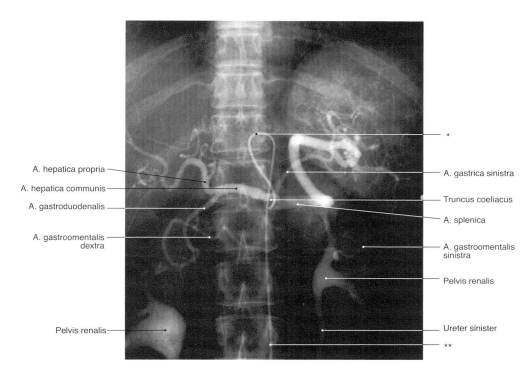

A. hepatica propria

A. hepatica communis

A. gastroduodenalis

A. gastroomentalis
dextra

Pelvis renalis

*

A. gastrica sinistra

Truncus coeliacus

A. splenica

A. gastroomentalis
sinistra

Pelvis renalis

Ureter sinister

**

Fig. 1064 Arteries of the stomach, Gaster; the spleen, Splen [Lien], and the liver, Hepar;
AP-radiograph after selective injection of a contrast medium into the coeliac trunk (coeliacography) with concomitant visualization of the renal pelvis due to the renal excretion of the medium; ventral view.

* Catheter loop in the aorta
** Catheter in the aorta

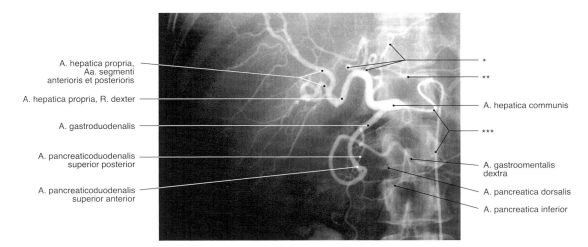

A. hepatica propria,
Aa. segmenti
anterioris et posterioris

A. hepatica propria, R. dexter

A. gastroduodenalis

A. pancreaticoduodenalis
superior posterior

A. pancreaticoduodenalis
superior anterior

*

**

A. hepatica communis

***

A. gastroomentalis
dextra

A. pancreatica dorsalis

A. pancreatica inferior

Fig. 1065 Common hepatic artery, A. hepatica communis;
AP-radiograph after selective injection of a contrast medium into the common hepatic artery;
ventral view.

* Branches to the left lobe of the liver replacing a single left branch of the hepatic artery proper
** An accessory branch of the hepatic artery to the lesser curvature of the stomach
*** Catheter in the aorta

Vessels of the upper abdomen

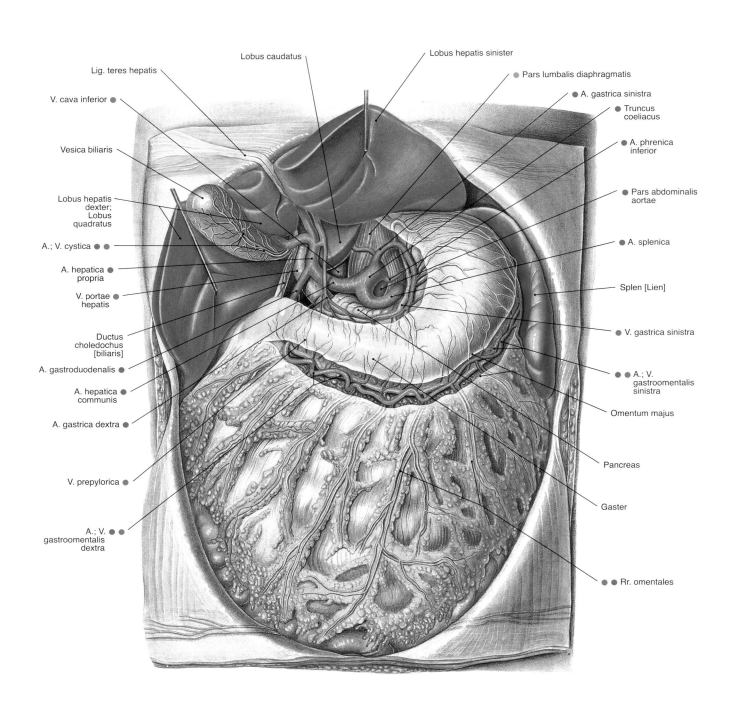

Lobus caudatus

Lobus hepatis sinister

Lig. teres hepatis

Pars lumbalis diaphragmatis

V. cava inferior

A. gastrica sinistra

Truncus coeliacus

Vesica biliaris

A. phrenica inferior

Lobus hepatis dexter; Lobus quadratus

Pars abdominalis aortae

A.; V. cystica

A. splenica

A. hepatica propria

Splen [Lien]

V. portae hepatis

V. gastrica sinistra

Ductus choledochus [biliaris]

A.; V. gastroomentalis sinistra

A. gastroduodenalis

Omentum majus

A. hepatica communis

A. gastrica dextra

Pancreas

V. prepylorica

Gaster

A.; V. gastroomentalis dextra

Rr. omentales

Fig. 1066 Vessels of the upper abdomen.

Vessels of the upper abdomen

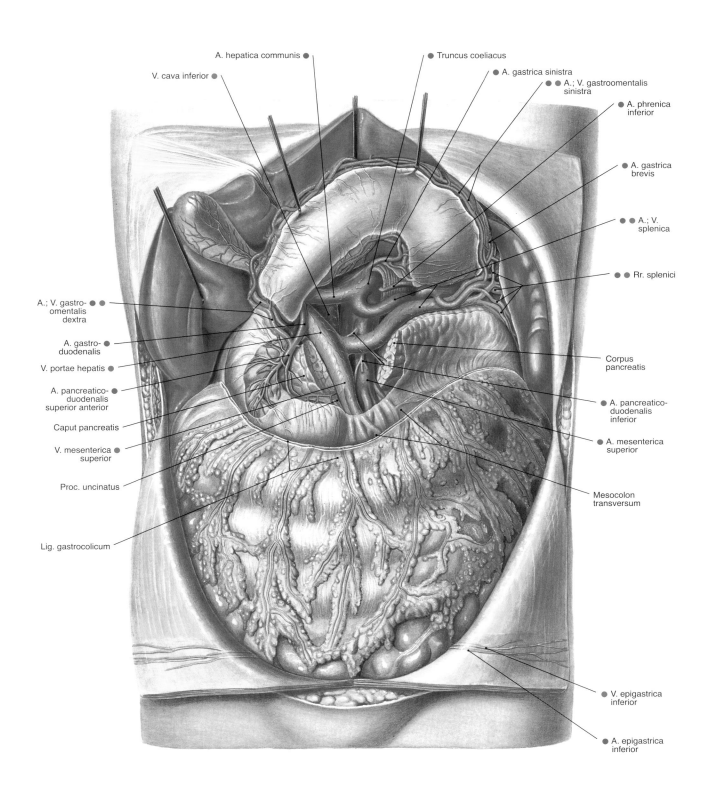

A. hepatica communis ●

V. cava inferior ●

● Truncus coeliacus

● A. gastrica sinistra

● ● A.; V. gastroomentalis sinistra

● A. phrenica inferior

● A. gastrica brevis

● ● A.; V. splenica

● ● Rr. splenici

A.; V. gastro- ● ●
omentalis
dextra

A. gastro- ●
duodenalis

V. portae hepatis ●

A. pancreatico- ●
duodenalis
superior anterior

Caput pancreatis

V. mesenterica ●
superior

Proc. uncinatus

Lig. gastrocolicum

Corpus pancreatis

● A. pancreatico-
duodenalis
inferior

● A. mesenterica
superior

Mesocolon
transversum

● V. epigastrica
inferior

● A. epigastrica
inferior

Fig. 1067   Vessels of the upper abdomen.

Superior mesenteric artery

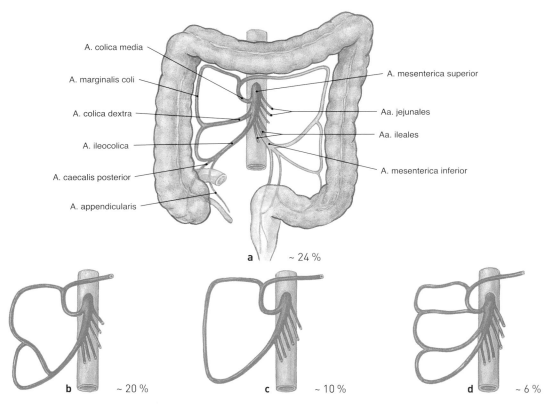

Fig. 1068 a–d Variability of the branches of the superior mesenteric artery, A. mesenterica superior, supplying the large intestine.

a "Textbook case", the ascending and the transverse colon, Colon ascendens et transversum, are supplied by three branches.

b The ileocolic artery, A. ileocolica, and the right colic artery, A. colica dextra, form a common trunk.

c Only two branches arise from the mesenteric artery while the right colic artery, A. colica dextra, is absent.

d Duplication of the right colic artery, A. colica dextra

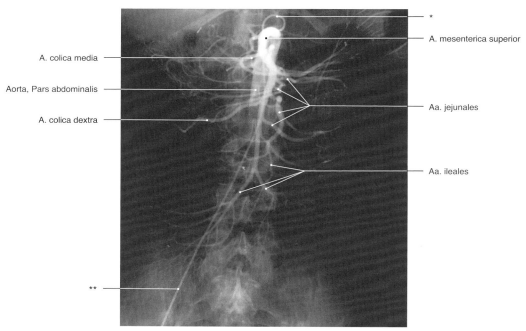

Fig. 1069 Superior mesenteric artery, A. mesenterica superior; AP-radiograph after injection of a contrast medium into the origin of the superior mesenteric artery; ventral view.

* Catheter in the aorta
** Catheter in the common iliac artery

Vessels of the lower abdomen

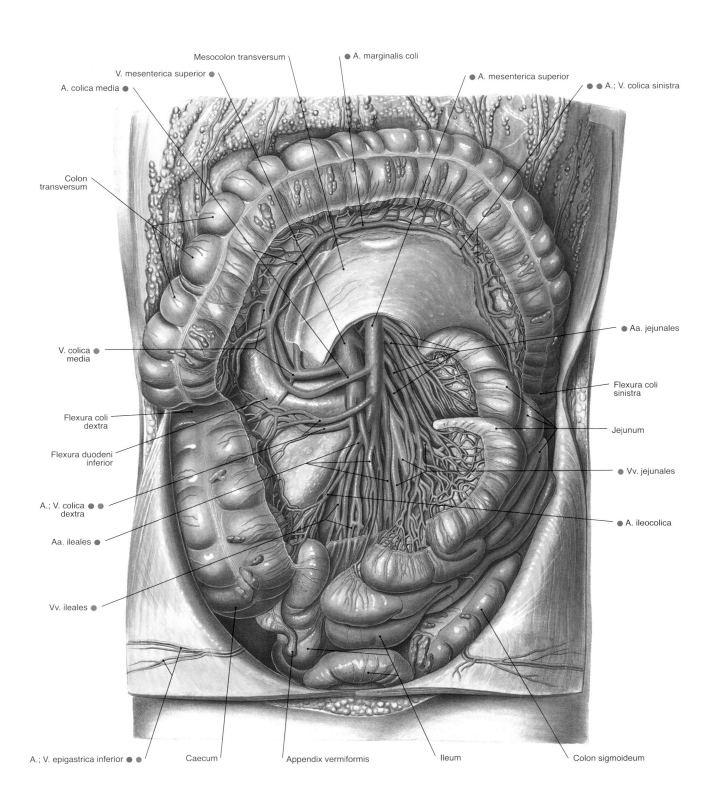

Mesocolon transversum

A. marginalis coli

V. mesenterica superior

A. mesenterica superior

A. colica media

A.; V. colica sinistra

Colon transversum

Aa. jejunales

V. colica media

Flexura coli sinistra

Flexura coli dextra

Jejunum

Flexura duodeni inferior

Vv. jejunales

A.; V. colica dextra

A. ileocolica

Aa. ileales

Vv. ileales

A.; V. epigastrica inferior

Caecum

Appendix vermiformis

Ileum

Colon sigmoideum

Fig. 1070 Superior mesenteric artery and vein, A. et V. mesenterica superior.
The arteries supplying the small intestine form a series of arcades.

Inferior mesenteric artery

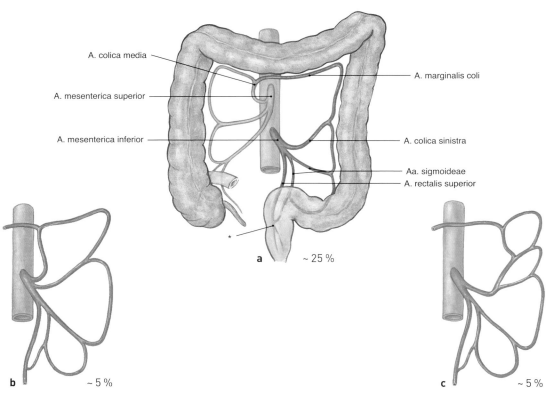

Fig. 1071 a–c Variations in the branches of the inferior mesenteric artery, A. mesenterica inferior.

a The inferior mesenteric artery, A. mesenterica inferior, divides into three parts supplying the descending and sigmoid colon, as well as the rectum.

b An accessory middle colic artery, A. colica media, arises from the inferior mesenteric artery, A. mesenterica inferior.

c An accessory middle colic artery, A. colica media, arises from the left colic artery, A. colica sinistra.

* Clinical term: SUDECK's point

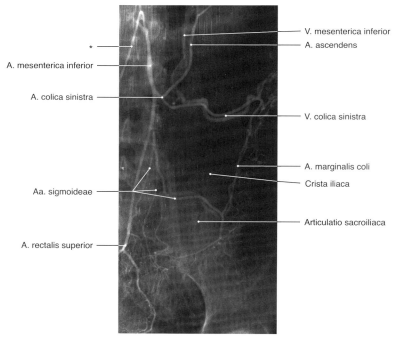

Fig. 1072 Inferior mesenteric artery, A. mesenterica inferior; AP-radiograph after selective injection of a contrast medium into the origin of the inferior mesenteric artery; ventral view.

* Catheter in the aorta

Vessels of the lower abdomen

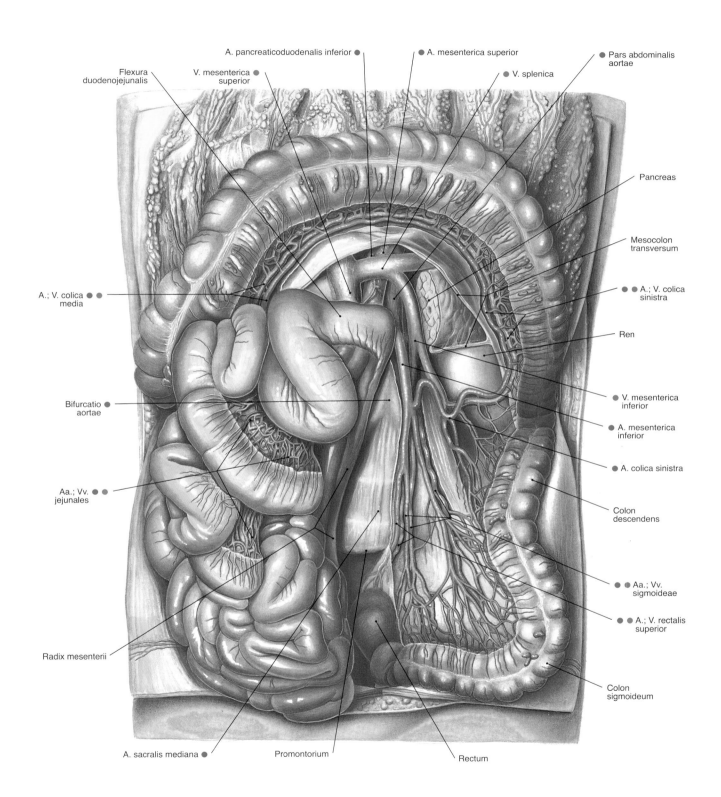

A. pancreaticoduodenalis inferior ●

● A. mesenterica superior

● Pars abdominalis aortae

Flexura duodenojejunalis

V. mesenterica ● superior

● V. splenica

Pancreas

Mesocolon transversum

A.; V. colica ● ● media

● ● A.; V. colica sinistra

Ren

Bifurcatio ● aortae

● V. mesenterica inferior

● A. mesenterica inferior

● A. colica sinistra

Colon descendens

Aa.; Vv. ● ● jejunales

● ● Aa.; Vv. sigmoideae

● ● A.; V. rectalis superior

Radix mesenterii

Colon sigmoideum

A. sacralis mediana ●

Promontorium

Rectum

Fig. 1073 Inferior mesenteric artery and vein,
A. et V. mesenterica inferior.

Coeliac trunk

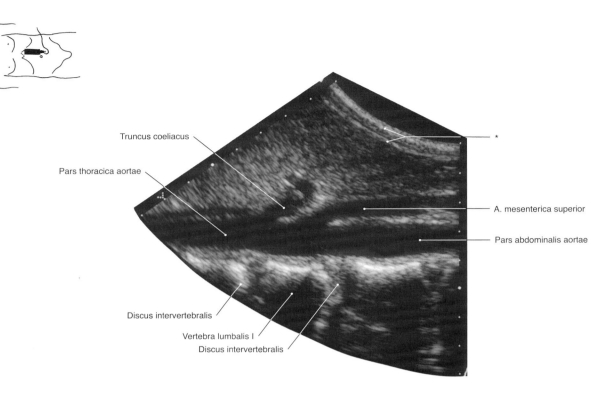

Fig. 1074 Abdominal aorta, Pars abdominalis aortae, with the coeliac trunk, Truncus coeliacus, and the superior mesenteric artery, A. mesenterica superior; ultrasound image; almost in the sagittal plane.
* Abdominal wall

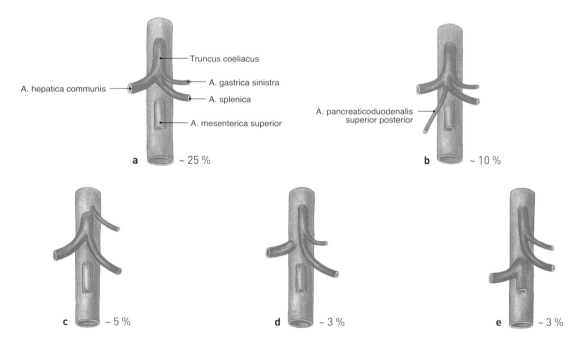

Fig. 1075 a–e Variability of the coeliac trunk, Truncus coeliacus.
a "Textbook case", division of the trunk into three branches
b Division of the trunk into four branches
c Development of a hepatosplenic trunk, Truncus hepatosplenicus

d Development of a gastrosplenic trunk, Truncus gastrosplenicus
e Development of a gastrosplenic trunk, Truncus gastrosplenicus, and a hepatomesenteric trunk, Truncus hepatomesentericus

Vessels of the retroperitoneal space

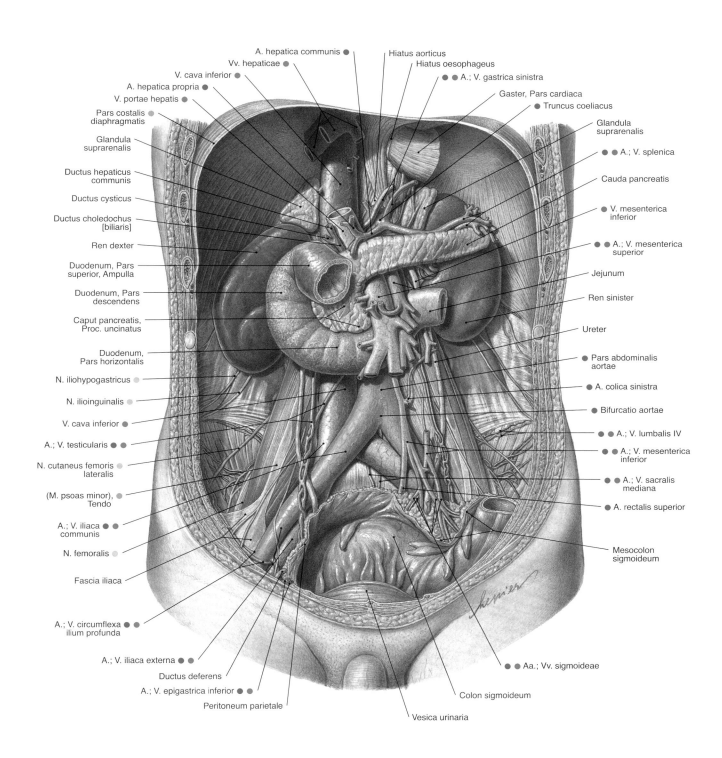

A. hepatica communis

Vv. hepaticae

V. cava inferior

A. hepatica propria

V. portae hepatis

Pars costalis
diaphragmatis

Glandula
suprarenalis

Ductus hepaticus
communis

Ductus cysticus

Ductus choledochus
[biliaris]

Ren dexter

Duodenum, Pars
superior, Ampulla

Duodenum, Pars
descendens

Caput pancreatis,
Proc. uncinatus

Duodenum,
Pars horizontalis

N. iliohypogastricus

N. ilioinguinalis

V. cava inferior

A.; V. testicularis

N. cutaneus femoris
lateralis

(M. psoas minor),
Tendo

A.; V. iliaca
communis

N. femoralis

Fascia iliaca

A.; V. circumflexa
ilium profunda

A.; V. iliaca externa

Ductus deferens

A.; V. epigastrica inferior

Peritoneum parietale

Hiatus aorticus

Hiatus oesophageus

A.; V. gastrica sinistra

Gaster, Pars cardiaca

Truncus coeliacus

Glandula
suprarenalis

A.; V. splenica

Cauda pancreatis

V. mesenterica
inferior

A.; V. mesenterica
superior

Jejunum

Ren sinister

Ureter

Pars abdominalis
aortae

A. colica sinistra

Bifurcatio aortae

A.; V. lumbalis IV

A.; V. mesenterica
inferior

A.; V. sacralis
mediana

A. rectalis superior

Mesocolon
sigmoideum

Aa.; Vv. sigmoideae

Colon sigmoideum

Vesica urinaria

Fig. 1076 Vessels of the retroperitoneal space,
Situs retroperitonealis, of the male.

Hepatic portal vein, overview

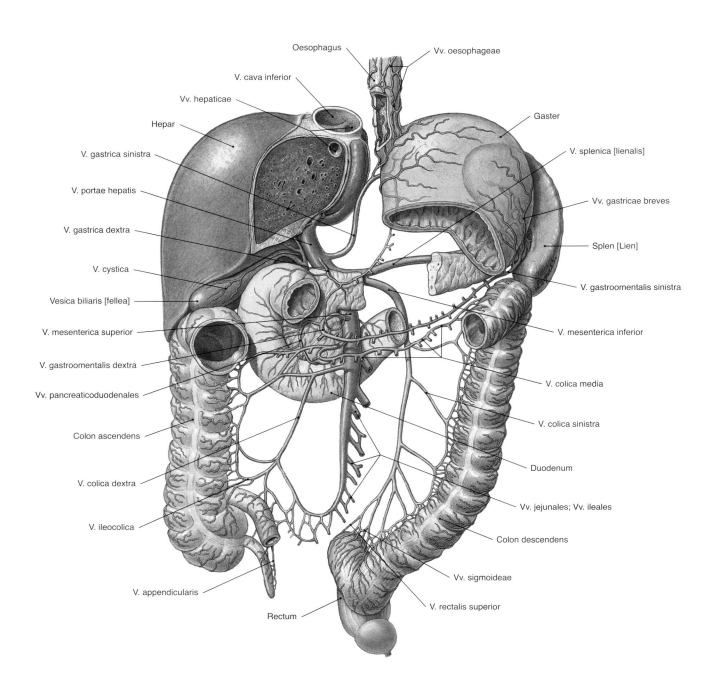

Oesophagus

Vv. oesophageae

V. cava inferior

Vv. hepaticae

Hepar

Gaster

V. gastrica sinistra

V. splenica [lienalis]

V. portae hepatis

Vv. gastricae breves

V. gastrica dextra

Splen [Lien]

V. cystica

Vesica biliaris [fellea]

V. gastroomentalis sinistra

V. mesenterica superior

V. mesenterica inferior

V. gastroomentalis dextra

Vv. pancreaticoduodenales

V. colica media

Colon ascendens

V. colica sinistra

V. colica dextra

Duodenum

V. ileocolica

Vv. jejunales; Vv. ileales

Colon descendens

V. appendicularis

Vv. sigmoideae

Rectum

V. rectalis superior

Fig. 1077   Hepatic portal vein, V. portae hepatis;
ventral view.

Portocaval anastomoses

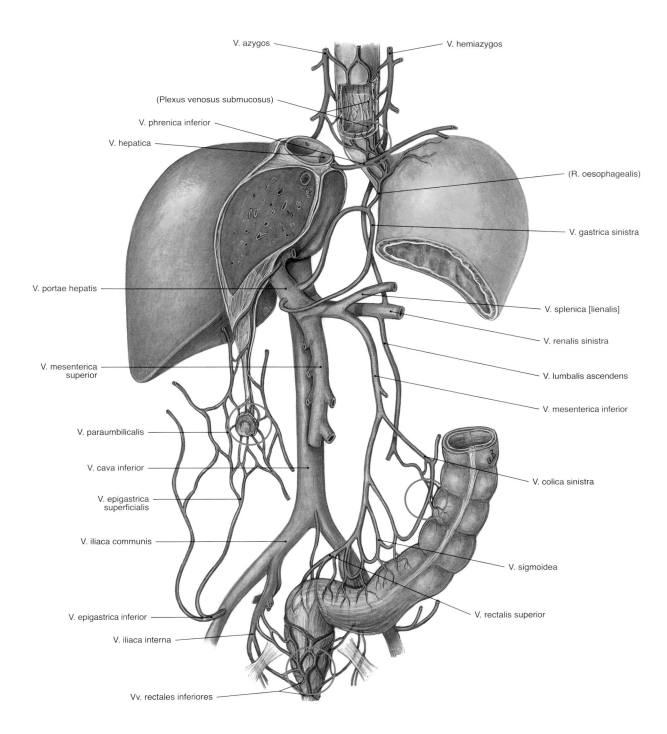

V. azygos

V. hemiazygos

(Plexus venosus submucosus)

V. phrenica inferior

V. hepatica

(R. oesophagealis)

V. gastrica sinistra

V. portae hepatis

V. splenica [lienalis]

V. renalis sinistra

V. mesenterica superior

V. lumbalis ascendens

V. mesenterica inferior

V. paraumbilicalis

V. cava inferior

V. colica sinistra

V. epigastrica superficialis

V. iliaca communis

V. sigmoidea

V. epigastrica inferior

V. iliaca interna

V. rectalis superior

Vv. rectales inferiores

Fig. 1078 Hepatic portal vein, V. portae hepatis,
and inferior vena cava, V. cava inferior;
semi-schematic;
tributaries of the inferior vena cava in blue;
tributaries of the hepatic portal vein in purple;
potential portocaval anastomoses are indicated
by circles.

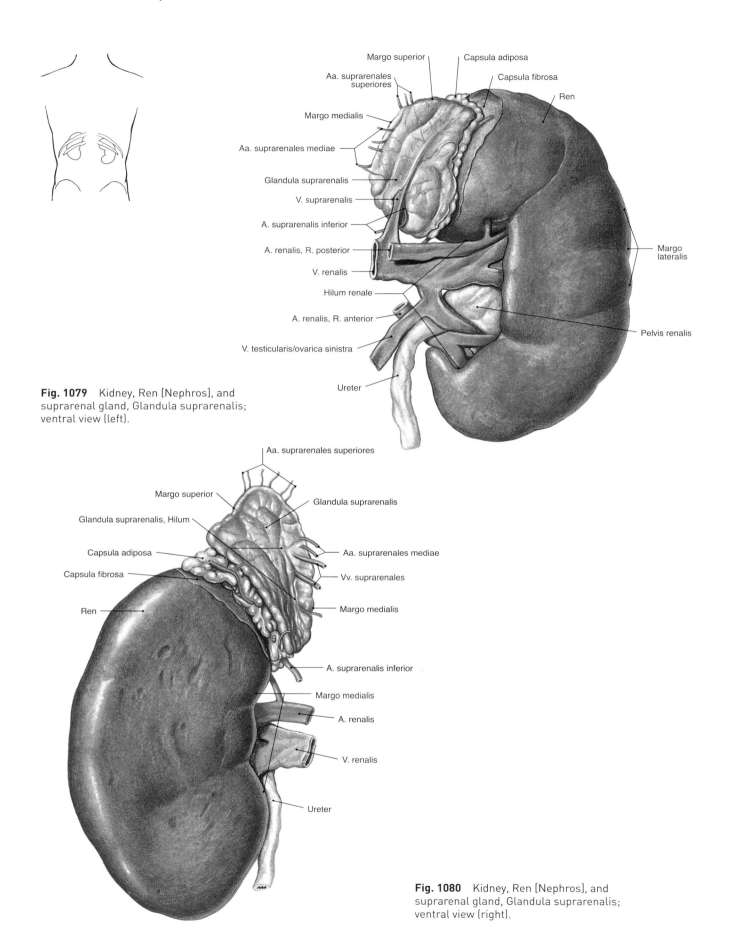

Margo superior

Aa. suprarenales
superiores

Margo medialis

Aa. suprarenales mediae

Glandula suprarenalis

V. suprarenalis

A. suprarenalis inferior

A. renalis, R. posterior

V. renalis

Hilum renale

A. renalis, R. anterior

V. testicularis/ovarica sinistra

Ureter

Capsula adiposa

Capsula fibrosa

Ren

Margo
lateralis

Pelvis renalis

Fig. 1079 Kidney, Ren [Nephros], and
suprarenal gland, Glandula suprarenalis;
ventral view (left).

Aa. suprarenales superiores

Margo superior

Glandula suprarenalis, Hilum

Capsula adiposa

Capsula fibrosa

Ren

Glandula suprarenalis

Aa. suprarenales mediae

Vv. suprarenales

Margo medialis

A. suprarenalis inferior

Margo medialis

A. renalis

V. renalis

Ureter

Fig. 1080 Kidney, Ren [Nephros], and
suprarenal gland, Glandula suprarenalis;
ventral view (right).

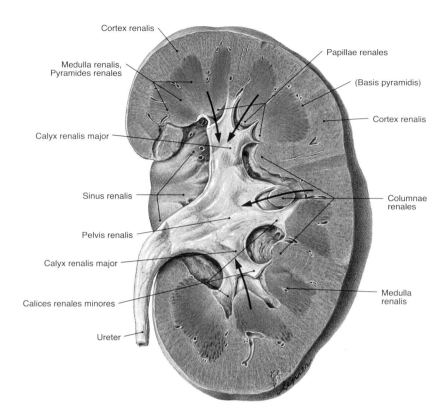

Cortex renalis

Medulla renalis,
Pyramides renales

Calyx renalis major

Sinus renalis

Pelvis renalis

Calyx renalis major

Calices renales minores

Ureter

Papillae renales

(Basis pyramidis)

Cortex renalis

Columnae
renales

Medulla
renalis

Fig. 1081 Kidney, Ren [Nephros];
oblique and vertical hemisection
displaying the renal cortex, the medulla
and the pelvis;
ventral view (left).
Arrows point from the pyramids to the
calyces.

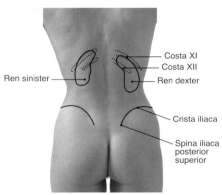

Ren sinister

Costa XI
Costa XII
Ren dexter

Crista iliaca

Spina iliaca
posterior
superior

Fig. 1082 Projection of the kidneys
onto the back.

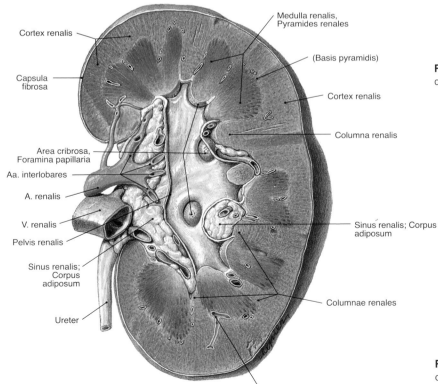

Cortex renalis

Capsula
fibrosa

Area cribrosa,
Foramina papillaria

Aa. interlobares

A. renalis

V. renalis

Pelvis renalis

Sinus renalis;
Corpus
adiposum

Ureter

Medulla renalis,
Pyramides renales

(Basis pyramidis)

Cortex renalis

Columna renalis

Sinus renalis; Corpus
adiposum

Columnae renales

A. arcuata

Fig. 1083 Kidney, Ren [Nephros];
oblique and vertical hemisection;
ventral view (left).

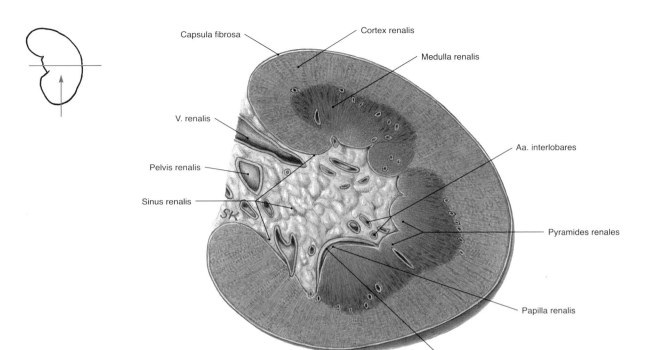

Fig. 1084 Kidney, Ren [Nephros];
transverse section through the renal sinus;
inferior view (left).

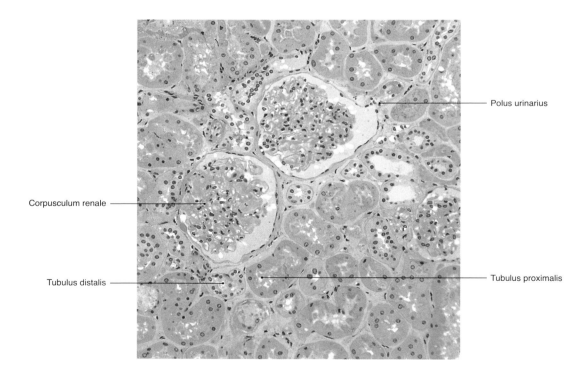

Fig. 1085 Kidney, Ren [Nephros];
microscopic section of the cortex (100×).

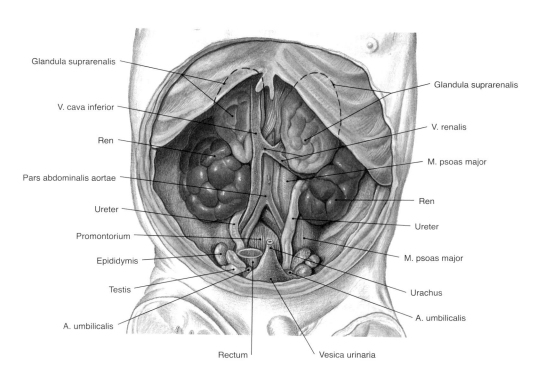

Glandula suprarenalis
V. cava inferior
Ren
Pars abdominalis aortae
Ureter
Promontorium
Epididymis
Testis
A. umbilicalis

Glandula suprarenalis
V. renalis
M. psoas major
Ren
Ureter
M. psoas major
Urachus
A. umbilicalis

Rectum
Vesica urinaria

Fig. 1086 Kidney, Ren [Nephros], and the suprarenal gland, Glandula suprarenalis, of a ~ 5-month-old foetus.

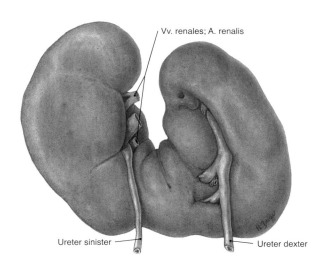

Vv. renales; A. renalis

Ureter sinister
Ureter dexter

Fig. 1087 Kidney, Ren [Nephros]; dorsal view.
The lower poles of both kidneys are fused (= horseshoe kidney).

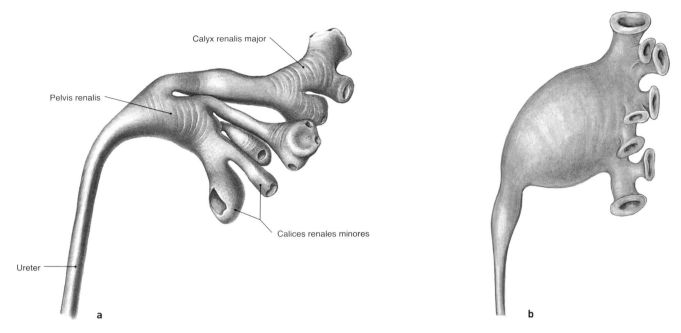

Calyx renalis major

Pelvis renalis

Calices renales minores

Ureter

a

b

Fig. 1088 a, b   Renal pelvis, Pelvis renalis;
corrosion casts;
ventral view (left).
a Dendritic type
b Ampullar type

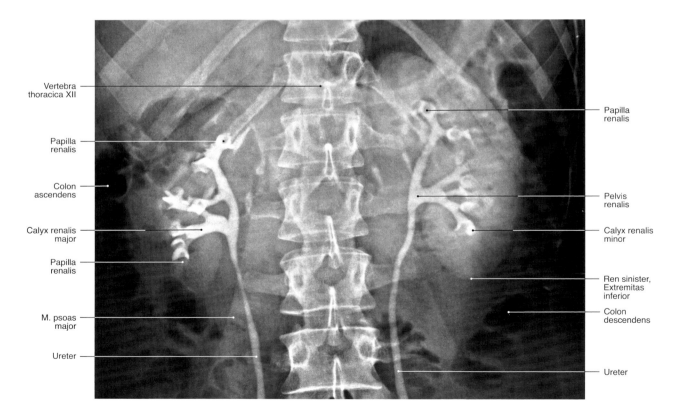

Vertebra
thoracica XII

Papilla
renalis

Colon
ascendens

Calyx renalis
major

Papilla
renalis

M. psoas
major

Ureter

Papilla
renalis

Pelvis
renalis

Calyx renalis
minor

Ren sinister,
Extremitas
inferior

Colon
descendens

Ureter

Fig. 1089   Kidney, Ren [Nephros];
renal pelvis, Pelvis renalis, and ureter, Ureter;
AP-radiograph after retrograde injection of a
contrast medium via both ureters.

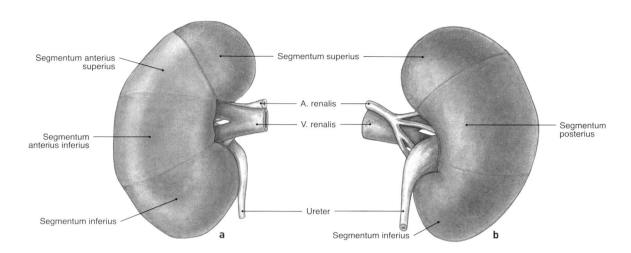

Segmentum anterius superius

Segmentum superius

A. renalis

V. renalis

Segmentum posterius

Segmentum anterius inferius

Segmentum inferius

Ureter

Segmentum inferius

a

b

Fig. 1090 a, b Renal segments, Segmenta renalia.

a Ventral view (right)
b Dorsal view (right)

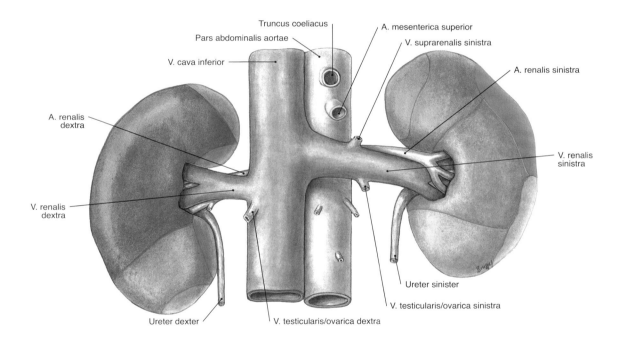

Truncus coeliacus

Pars abdominalis aortae

A. mesenterica superior

V. suprarenalis sinistra

V. cava inferior

A. renalis sinistra

A. renalis dextra

V. renalis sinistra

V. renalis dextra

Ureter sinister

V. testicularis/ovarica sinistra

Ureter dexter

V. testicularis/ovarica dextra

Fig. 1091 Kidney, Ren; areas of contact with adjacent organs; ventral view.

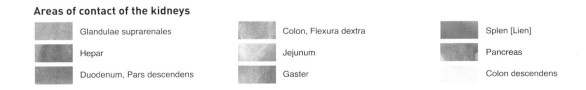

Areas of contact of the kidneys

Glandulae suprarenales

Colon, Flexura dextra

Splen [Lien]

Hepar

Jejunum

Pancreas

Duodenum, Pars descendens

Gaster

Colon descendens

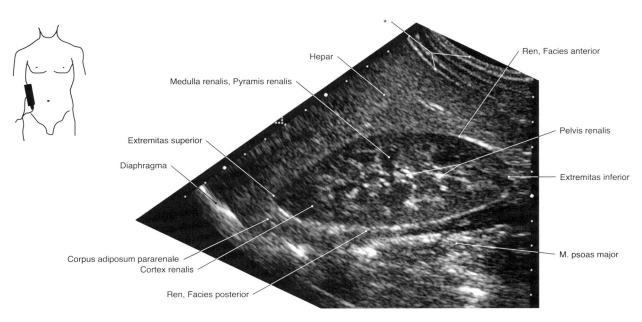

Hepar

Medulla renalis, Pyramis renalis

Extremitas superior

Diaphragma

Corpus adiposum pararenale

Cortex renalis

Ren, Facies posterior

Ren, Facies anterior

Pelvis renalis

Extremitas inferior

M. psoas major

Fig. 1092 Kidney, Ren [Nephros];
ultrasound image;
the transducer is directed from ventroinferior to dorsosuperior;
lateral view (right).
* Abdominal wall

Colon

Hepar, Lobus dexter

Cutis

Ren

Mm. abdominales

*

Ren, Capsula adiposa

Fascia renalis

Costa XII

V. cava inferior

Pars abdominalis
aortae

V. renalis dextra

Corpus vertebrae

Proc. spinosus

Sinus renalis | M. erector spinae

→ 1196

Fig. 1093 Kidney, Ren [Nephros];
puncture of the right kidney;
computed tomographic cross-section (CT);
inferior view.
* Guidance of a needle for kidney biopsy

Suprarenal gland

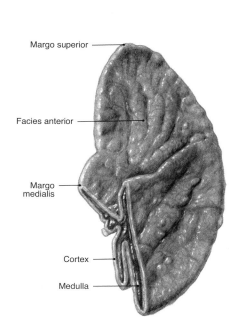

Margo superior

Facies anterior

Margo medialis

Cortex

Medulla

Fig. 1094 Suprarenal gland, Glandula suprarenalis; ventral view (right).

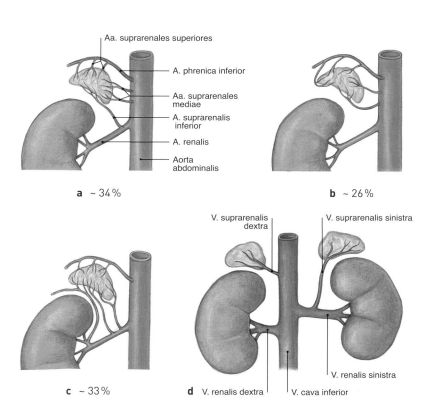

Aa. suprarenales superiores

A. phrenica inferior

Aa. suprarenales mediae

A. suprarenalis inferior

A. renalis

Aorta abdominalis

a ~ 34 %

b ~ 26 %

V. suprarenalis dextra

V. suprarenalis sinistra

c ~ 33 %

d V. renalis dextra

V. renalis sinistra

V. cava inferior

Fig. 1095 a–d Variability of the suprarenal arteries, Aa. suprarenales, and course of the suprarenal veins, Vv. suprarenales.
a Arterial supply by three arteries ("textbook case")
b Arterial supply without a branch from the renal artery, A. renalis
c Arterial supply without a direct branch from the aorta, Aorta
d Course of the suprarenal veins, Vv. suprarenales

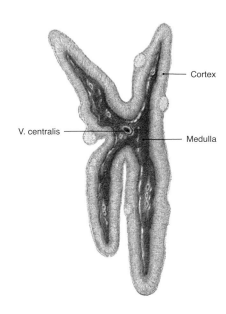

Cortex

V. centralis

Medulla

Fig. 1096 Suprarenal gland, Glandula suprarenalis; sagittal section; lateral view (right).

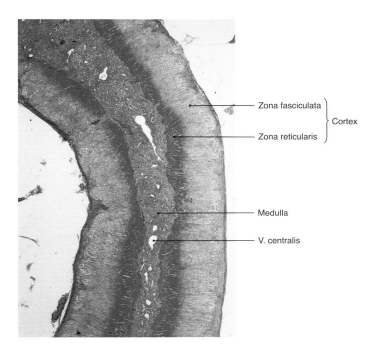

Zona fasciculata

Cortex

Zona reticularis

Medulla

V. centralis

Fig. 1097 Suprarenal gland, Glandula suprarenalis; microscopic enlargement at low magnification.

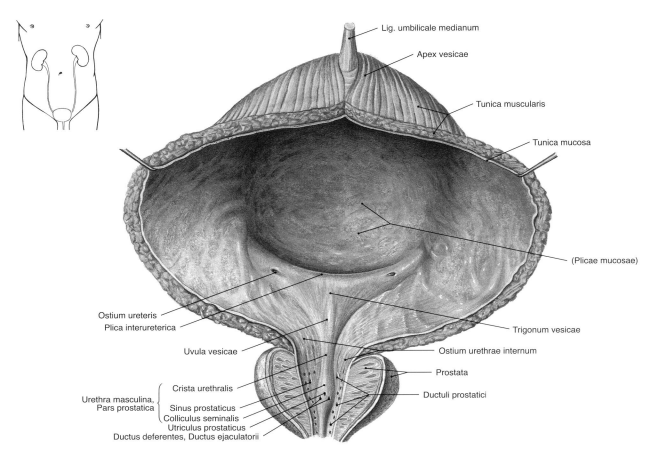

Lig. umbilicale medianum

Apex vesicae

Tunica muscularis

Tunica mucosa

(Plicae mucosae)

Ostium ureteris

Plica interureterica

Uvula vesicae

Trigonum vesicae

Ostium urethrae internum

Prostata

Crista urethralis

Urethra masculina, Pars prostatica

Sinus prostaticus

Colliculus seminalis

Utriculus prostaticus

Ductus deferentes, Ductus ejaculatorii

Ductuli prostatici

Fig. 1098   Urinary bladder, Vesica urinaria; prostate, Prostata, and urethra, Urethra; ventral view.

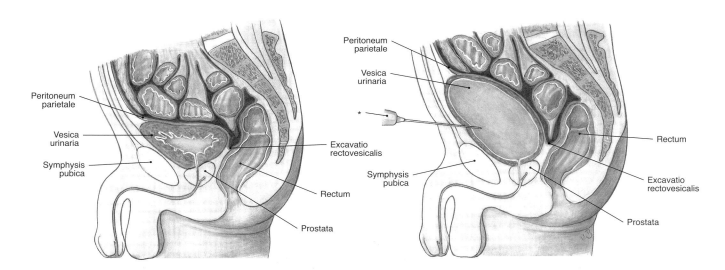

Peritoneum parietale

Vesica urinaria

Symphysis pubica

Excavatio rectovesicalis

Rectum

Prostata

Peritoneum parietale

Vesica urinaria

*

Symphysis pubica

Rectum

Excavatio rectovesicalis

Prostata

Fig. 1099   Urinary bladder, Vesica urinaria, almost completely voided.

Fig. 1100   Urinary bladder, Vesica urinaria, filled. In this situation, the bladder can be punctured from just above the pubic bone without passing through the peritoneal cavity.

* Puncture needle

Urinary bladder, ductus deferens and seminal vesicle

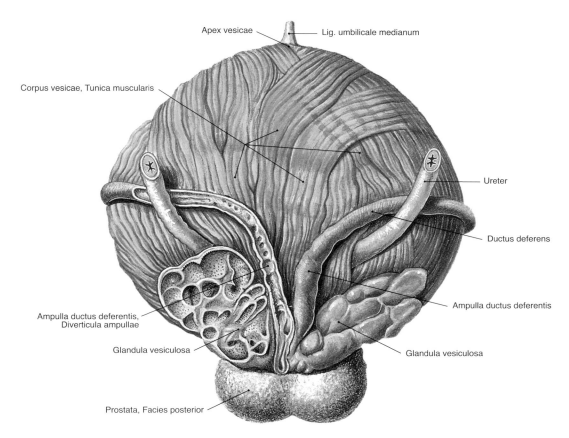

Apex vesicae — Lig. umbilicale medianum

Corpus vesicae, Tunica muscularis

Ureter

Ductus deferens

Ampulla ductus deferentis

Ampulla ductus deferentis,
Diverticula ampullae

Glandula vesiculosa

Glandula vesiculosa

Prostata, Facies posterior

Fig. 1101 Urinary bladder, Vesica urinaria; ductus deferentes,
Ductus deferentes; seminal vesicles, Glandulae vesiculosae,
and prostate, Prostata;
dorsal view.

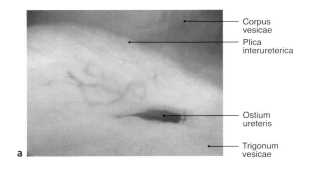

Corpus
vesicae

Plica
interureterica

Ostium
ureteris

Trigonum
vesicae

a

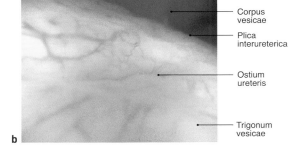

Corpus
vesicae

Plica
interureterica

Ostium
ureteris

Trigonum
vesicae

b

Fig. 1102 a, b Urinary bladder, Vesica urinaria;
endoscopic view of the opening of the ureter
(cystoscopy).
a Open ostium of the ureter with a peristaltic
wave transporting urine into the bladder
b Closed ostium of the ureter

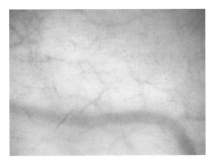

Fig. 1103 Urinary bladder, Vesica urinaria;
endoscopic view of the mucosa in the body of
the bladder (cystoscopy);
inferior view.

192

► **Pelvic viscera
and retroperitoneal space**

Male urinary and genital organs, overview

►► | Kidney | Suprarenal gland | Urinary bladd

►►► **Male genita**

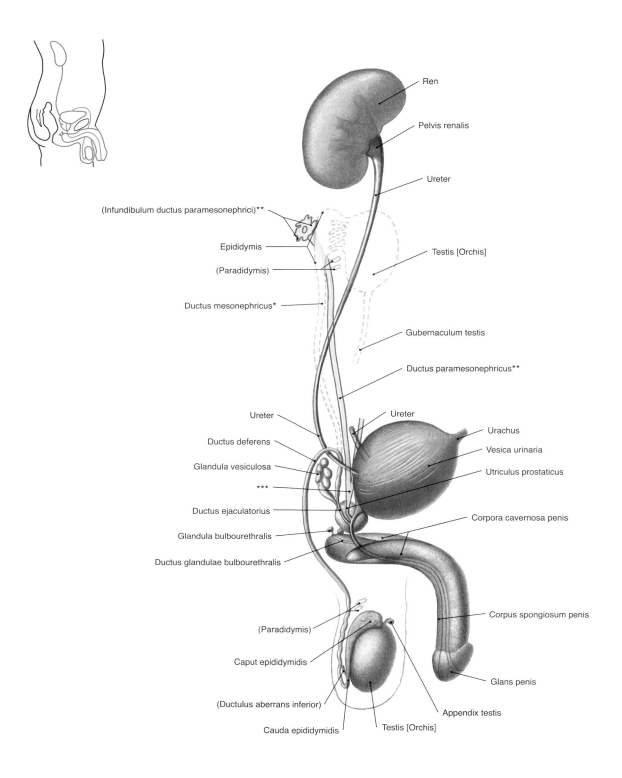

Ren

Pelvis renalis

Ureter

(Infundibulum ductus paramesonephrici)**

Epididymis

(Paradidymis)

Testis [Orchis]

Ductus mesonephricus*

Gubernaculum testis

Ductus paramesonephricus**

Ureter

Ureter

Ductus deferens

Urachus

Glandula vesiculosa

Vesica urinaria

***

Utriculus prostaticus

Ductus ejaculatorius

Glandula bulbourethralis

Corpora cavernosa penis

Ductus glandulae bulbourethralis

(Paradidymis)

Corpus spongiosum penis

Caput epididymidis

Glans penis

(Ductulus aberrans inferior)

Cauda epididymidis

Testis [Orchis]

Appendix testis

→ 1119

Fig. 1104   Male urinary and genital organs;
Organa urogenitalia masculina;
diagram of the development: the parts that degenerate are
displayed in pale pink, and the reposition of the testis prior to its
descent is indicated by the dashed line;
viewed from the right.

Epididymis = genital part of the mesonephros;
Paradidymis = remnants of tubules of the mesonephros
*   WOLFFian duct
**   MÜLLERian duct
*** Junction of the MÜLLERian ducts,
      Ductus paramesonephrici

Testis and epididymis

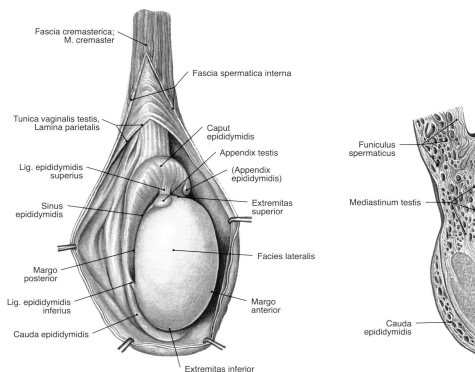

Fascia cremasterica; M. cremaster

Fascia spermatica interna

Tunica vaginalis testis, Lamina parietalis

Caput epididymidis

Appendix testis

Lig. epididymidis superius

(Appendix epididymidis)

Sinus epididymidis

Extremitas superior

Facies lateralis

Margo posterior

Lig. epididymidis inferius

Margo anterior

Cauda epididymidis

Extremitas inferior

Fig. 1105 Testis, Testis [Orchis], and epididymis, Epididymis; viewed from the right.

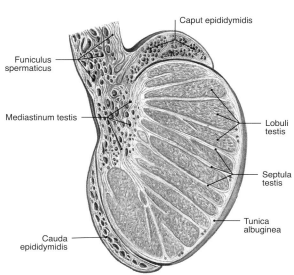

Caput epididymidis

Funiculus spermaticus

Mediastinum testis

Lobuli testis

Septula testis

Tunica albuginea

Cauda epididymidis

Fig. 1106 Testis, Testis [Orchis], and epididymis, Epididymis; viewed from the right.

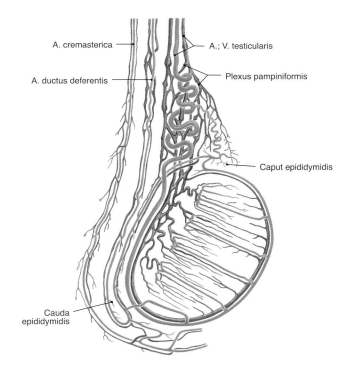

A. cremasterica

A.; V. testicularis

A. ductus deferentis

Plexus pampiniformis

Caput epididymidis

Cauda epididymidis

Fig. 1107 Blood vessels of the testis, Testis, the epididymis, Epididymis, and the spermatic cord, Funiculus spermaticus; viewed from the right.

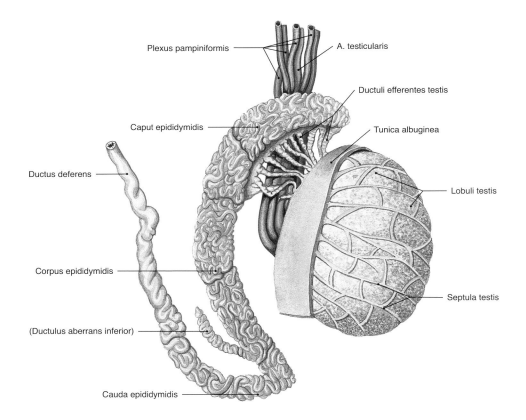

Plexus pampiniformis

A. testicularis

Ductuli efferentes testis

Caput epididymidis

Tunica albuginea

Ductus deferens

Lobuli testis

Corpus epididymidis

Septula testis

(Ductulus aberrans inferior)

Cauda epididymidis

Fig. 1108 Testis, Testis; epididymis, Epididymis, and ductus deferens (vas deferens), Ductus deferens; lateral view.

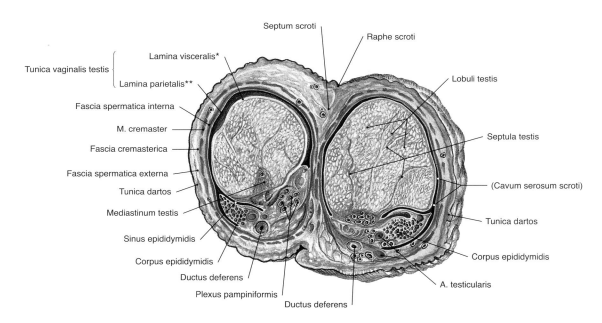

Septum scroti

Raphe scroti

Lamina visceralis*

Tunica vaginalis testis { Lamina parietalis**

Lobuli testis

Fascia spermatica interna

M. cremaster

Septula testis

Fascia cremasterica

Fascia spermatica externa

Tunica dartos

(Cavum serosum scroti)

Mediastinum testis

Tunica dartos

Sinus epididymidis

Corpus epididymidis

Corpus epididymidis

A. testicularis

Ductus deferens

Plexus pampiniformis

Ductus deferens

Fig. 1109 Testis, Testis; epididymis, Epididymis, and scrotum, Scrotum; superior view.
* Also: Epiorchium
** Also: Periorchium

Ductus deferens and seminal vesicle

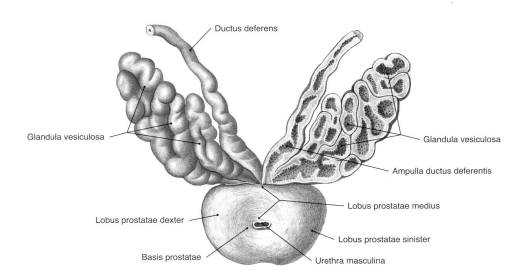

Fig. 1110 Ductus deferentes, Ductus deferentes, seminal vesicles, Glandulae vesiculosae, and prostate, Prostata; superior view.

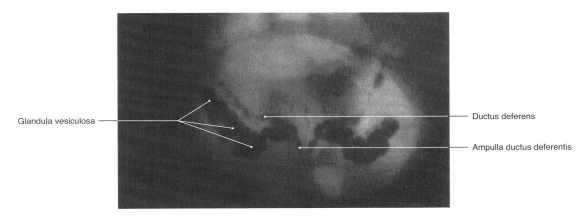

Fig. 1111 Ductus deferentes, Ductus deferentes, and seminal vesicles, Glandulae vesiculosae; AP-radiograph after injection of a contrast medium via the ejaculatory ducts; ventral view.

Though this technique demonstrates size and position of the seminal vesicles, it is no more applied under clinical circumstances.

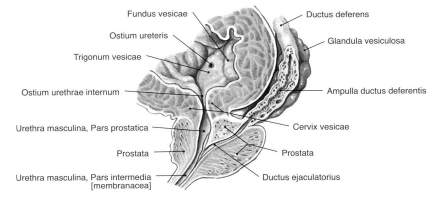

Fig. 1112 Urinary bladder, Vesica urinaria; prostate, Prostata; ductus deferens (vas deferens), Ductus deferens, and seminal vesicle, Glandula vesiculosa; viewed from the right.

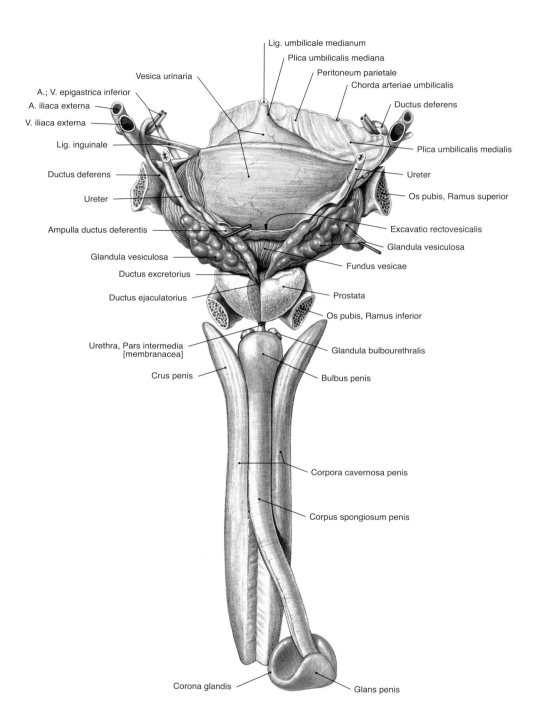

Fig. 1113   Urinary bladder, Vesica urinaria; ductus deferentes, Ductus deferentes; seminal vesicles, Glandulae vesiculosae; prostate, Prostata, and male urethra, Urethra masculina; dorsal view.

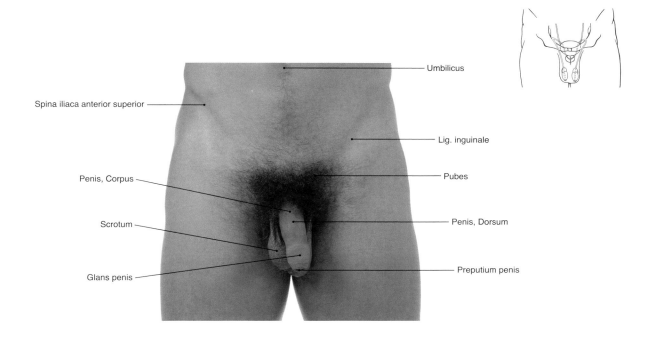

Umbilicus

Spina iliaca anterior superior

Lig. inguinale

Pubes

Penis, Corpus

Scrotum

Penis, Dorsum

Glans penis

Preputium penis

Fig. 1114 Male external genitalia, Organa genitalia masculina externa.

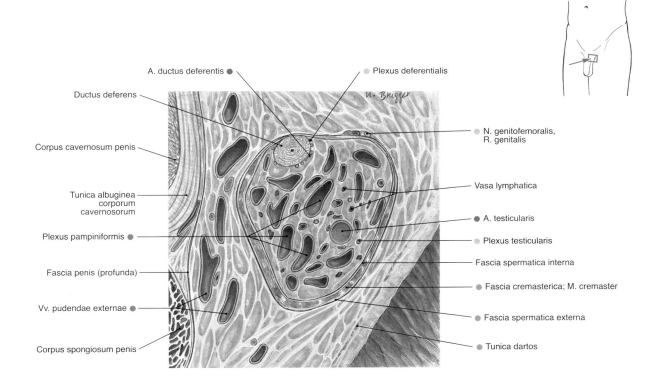

A. ductus deferentis ●

● Plexus deferentialis

Ductus deferens

N. genitofemoralis, R. genitalis

Corpus cavernosum penis

Tunica albuginea corporum cavernosorum

Vasa lymphatica

Plexus pampiniformis ●

● A. testicularis

● Plexus testicularis

Fascia penis (profunda)

Fascia spermatica interna

● Fascia cremasterica; M. cremaster

Vv. pudendae externae ●

● Fascia spermatica externa

Corpus spongiosum penis

● Tunica dartos

Fig. 1115 Spermatic cord, Funiculus spermaticus; frontal section; ventral view (left, 250%).

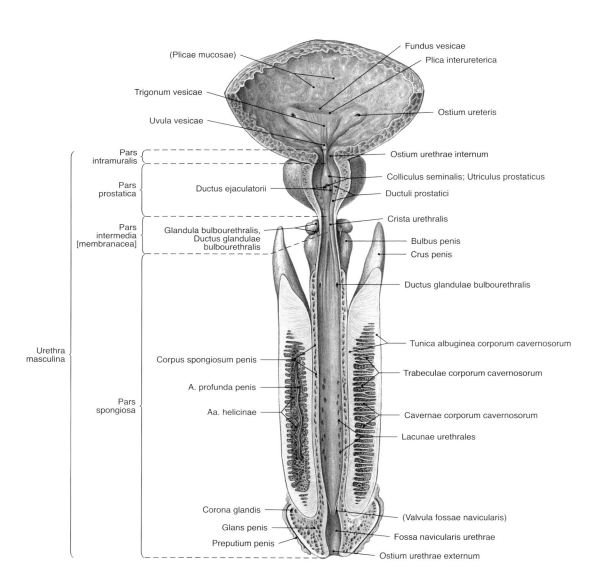

(Plicae mucosae)

Fundus vesicae

Plica interureterica

Trigonum vesicae

Uvula vesicae

Ostium ureteris

Pars intramuralis

Ostium urethrae internum

Pars prostatica

Colliculus seminalis; Utriculus prostaticus

Ductus ejaculatorii

Ductuli prostatici

Pars intermedia [membranacea]

Crista urethralis

Glandula bulbourethralis, Ductus glandulae bulbourethralis

Bulbus penis

Crus penis

Ductus glandulae bulbourethralis

Urethra masculina

Tunica albuginea corporum cavernosorum

Corpus spongiosum penis

Trabeculae corporum cavernosorum

A. profunda penis

Pars spongiosa

Aa. helicinae

Cavernae corporum cavernosorum

Lacunae urethrales

Corona glandis

(Valvula fossae navicularis)

Glans penis

Fossa navicularis urethrae

Preputium penis

Ostium urethrae externum

→ 1199

Fig. 1116   Urinary bladder, Vesica urinaria; prostate, Prostata, and male urethra, Urethra masculina; ventral view.

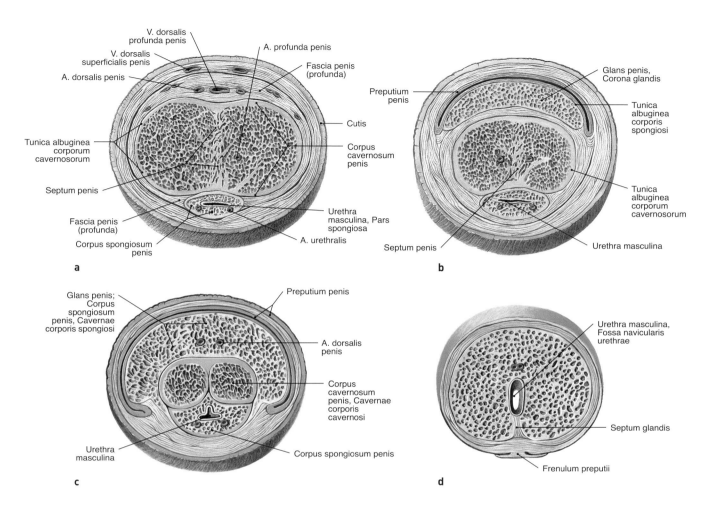

Fig. 1117 a–d Penis, Penis;
cross-sections; planes indicated in Fig. 1118;
ventral view.

a Cross-section through the middle of the shaft
b Cross-section at the level of the proximal part of the glans penis
c Cross-section through the middle of the glans penis
d Cross-section at the level of the distal part of the glans penis

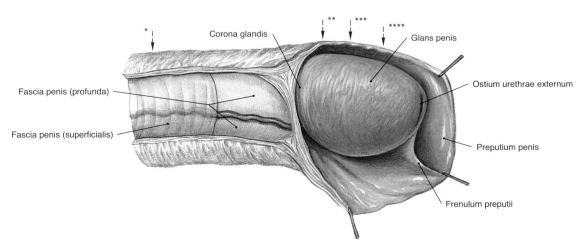

Fig. 1118 Penis, Penis, with glans penis, Glans penis,
and prepuce, Preputium penis.

*   Level of section of Fig. 1117a
**   Level of section of Fig. 1117b
***   Level of section of Fig. 1117c
**** Level of section of Fig. 1117d

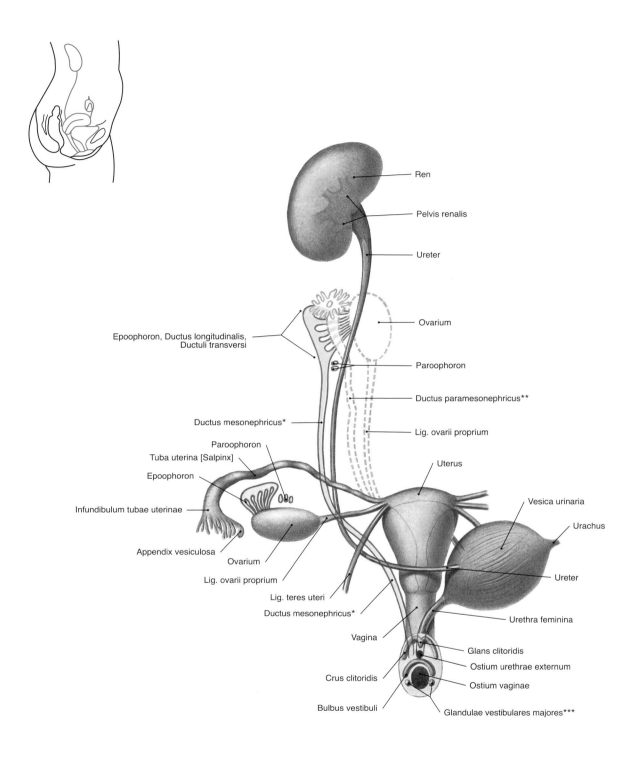

Ren

Pelvis renalis

Ureter

Ovarium

Epoophoron, Ductus longitudinalis, Ductuli transversi

Paroophoron

Ductus paramesonephricus**

Ductus mesonephricus*

Lig. ovarii proprium

Paroophoron

Uterus

Tuba uterina [Salpinx]

Epoophoron

Vesica urinaria

Urachus

Infundibulum tubae uterinae

Ureter

Appendix vesiculosa

Ovarium

Lig. ovarii proprium

Lig. teres uteri

Ductus mesonephricus*

Urethra feminina

Vagina

Glans clitoridis

Ostium urethrae externum

Crus clitoridis

Ostium vaginae

Bulbus vestibuli

Glandulae vestibulares majores***

→ 1104

Fig. 1119 Female urinary and genital organs, Organa urogenitalia feminina; diagram of the development: the parts that degenerate are displayed in pale pink, and rhe position of the ovary prior to its descent is indicated by the dashed line; ventral view.

Epoophoron = genital part of the mesonephros;
Paroophoron = remnants of the tubules of the mesonephros

*   WOLFFian duct
** MÜLLERian duct
***BARTHOLIN's glands

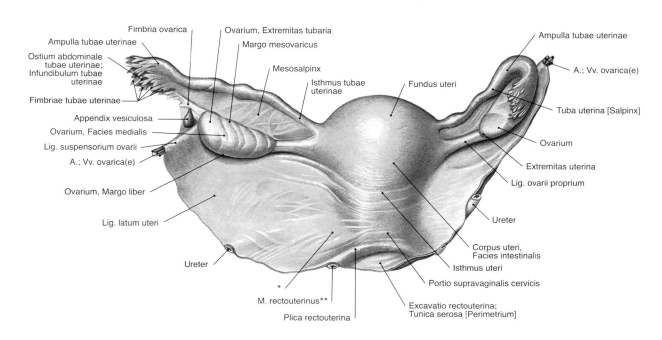

Fimbria ovarica
Ovarium, Extremitas tubaria
Margo mesovaricus
Ampulla tubae uterinae
Ostium abdominale tubae uterinae; Infundibulum tubae uterinae
Mesosalpinx
Isthmus tubae uterinae
Fundus uteri
Ampulla tubae uterinae
A.; Vv. ovarica(e)
Fimbriae tubae uterinae
Tuba uterina [Salpinx]
Appendix vesiculosa
Ovarium, Facies medialis
Ovarium
Lig. suspensorium ovarii
A.; Vv. ovarica(e)
Extremitas uterina
Lig. ovarii proprium
Ovarium, Margo liber
Ureter
Lig. latum uteri
Corpus uteri, Facies intestinalis
Isthmus uteri
Ureter
Portio supravaginalis cervicis
*
M. rectouterinus**
Excavatio rectouterina; Tunica serosa [Perimetrium]
Plica rectouterina

Fig. 1120 Uterus, Uterus; ovary, Ovar, and uterine tube, Tuba uterina; dorsal view.

* Clinical term: cardinal ligament
** Clinical term: sacrouterine ligament

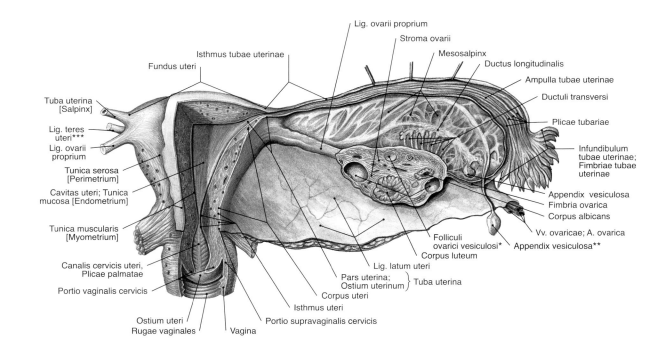

Lig. ovarii proprium
Stroma ovarii
Isthmus tubae uterinae
Mesosalpinx
Fundus uteri
Ductus longitudinalis
Ampulla tubae uterinae
Tuba uterina [Salpinx]
Ductuli transversi
Lig. teres uteri***
Plicae tubariae
Lig. ovarii proprium
Tunica serosa [Perimetrium]
Infundibulum tubae uterinae; Fimbriae tubae uterinae
Cavitas uteri; Tunica mucosa [Endometrium]
Appendix vesiculosa
Fimbria ovarica
Corpus albicans
Tunica muscularis [Myometrium]
Vv. ovaricae; A. ovarica
Folliculi ovarici vesiculosi*
Appendix vesiculosa**
Canalis cervicis uteri, Plicae palmatae
Corpus luteum
Portio vaginalis cervicis
Pars uterina; Ostium uterinum } Tuba uterina
Lig. latum uteri
Ostium uteri
Rugae vaginales
Vagina
Corpus uteri
Isthmus uteri
Portio supravaginalis cervicis

Fig. 1121 Uterus, Uterus; ovary, Ovar, and uterine tube, Tuba uterina; dorsal view.

*   Clinical term: GRAAFian follicle
** Stalked hydatid
*** Clinical term: round ligament

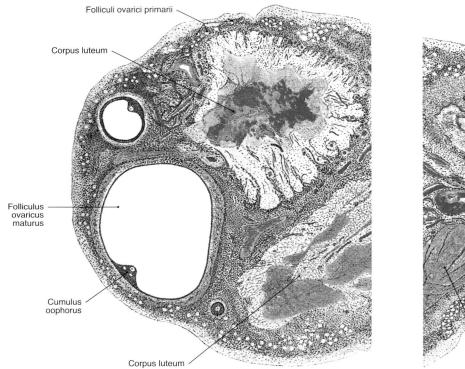

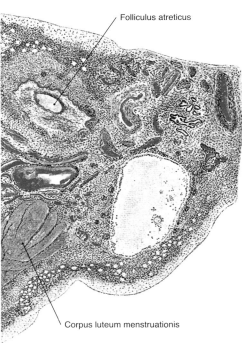

Folliculi ovarici primarii

Corpus luteum

Folliculus ovaricus maturus

Cumulus oophorus

Corpus luteum

Folliculus atreticus

Corpus luteum menstruationis

Fig. 1122 Ovary, Ovar;
microscopic enlargement at low magnification.

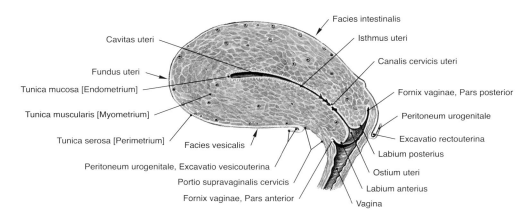

Cavitas uteri

Fundus uteri

Tunica mucosa [Endometrium]

Tunica muscularis [Myometrium]

Tunica serosa [Perimetrium]

Facies vesicalis

Peritoneum urogenitale, Excavatio vesicouterina

Portio supravaginalis cervicis

Fornix vaginae, Pars anterior

Facies intestinalis

Isthmus uteri

Canalis cervicis uteri

Fornix vaginae, Pars posterior

Peritoneum urogenitale

Excavatio rectouterina

Labium posterius

Ostium uteri

Labium anterius

Vagina

Fig. 1123 Uterus, Uterus, and vagina, Vagina;
viewed from the right.

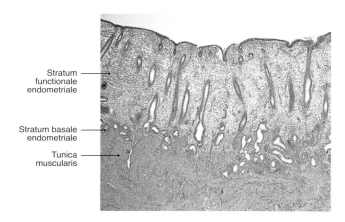

Stratum functionale endometriale

Stratum basale endometriale

Tunica muscularis

Fig. 1124 Mucosa of the uterus, Uterus;
early phase of proliferation.

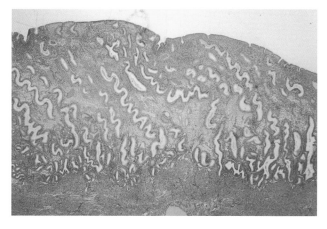

Fig. 1125 Mucosa of the uterus, Uterus;
late phase of proliferation with excretory glands.

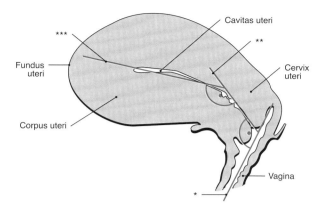

Fundus uteri

Corpus uteri

Cavitas uteri

Cervix uteri

Vagina

***

**

*

Fig. 1126 Uterus, Uterus, and vagina, Vagina; normal angles between the vagina, the cervix, and the body of uterus; viewed from the right.
* * Longitudinal axis of the vagina
* ** Longitudinal axis of the cervix of uterus
* *** Longitudinal axis of the body of uterus
Angle between vagina and cervix of uterus = version
Angle between cervix and body of uterus = flexion
Normal topographical situation of the uterus: anteversion, anteflexion
Relation to the median plane = position

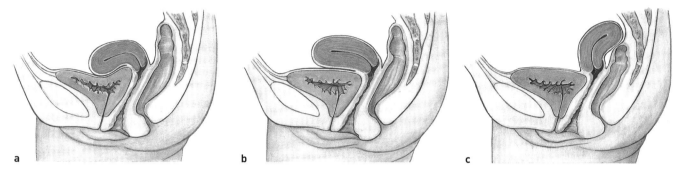

a   b   c

Fig. 1127 a–c Uterus, Uterus, and vagina, Vagina.
a Anteversion, anteflexion = normal position
b Anteversion, but no anteflexion
c Retroversion, retroflexion

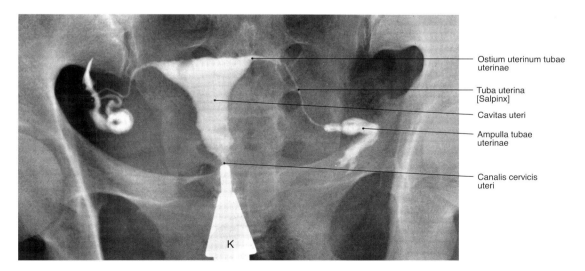

Ostium uterinum tubae uterinae

Tuba uterina [Salpinx]

Cavitas uteri

Ampulla tubae uterinae

Canalis cervicis uteri

K

Fig. 1128 Uterus, Uterus, and uterine tube, Tuba uterina; AP-radiograph after injection of to contrast medium into the cervix of uterus (hysterosalpingography); uterus in dextroposition; ventral view.

This formerly clinically applied technique allows to determine the position of the organs and the patency of the tubes.
K = tube adaptor for injection of the contrast medium

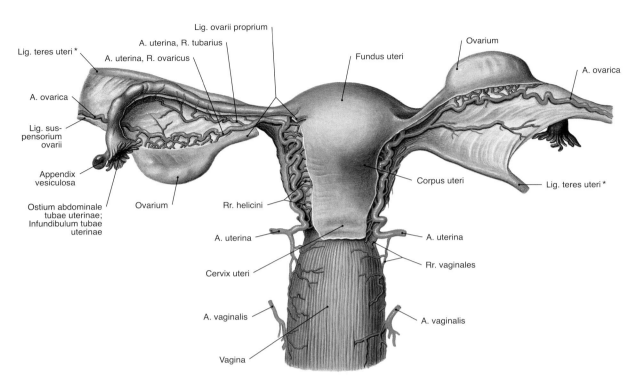

Fig. 1129 Arteries of the female internal genitalia, Organa genitalia feminina interna; dorsal view.

* Clinical term: round ligament

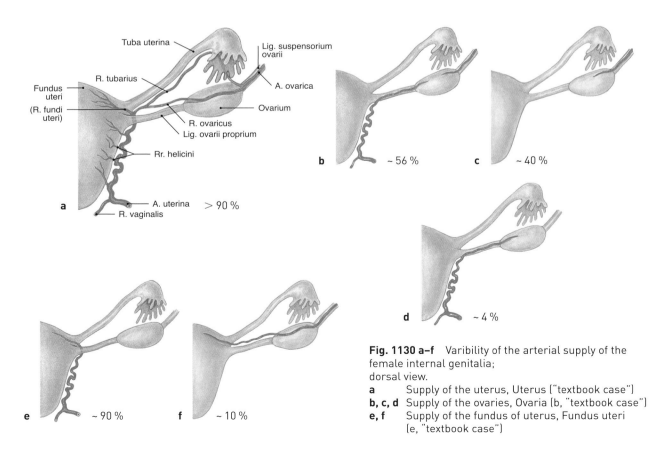

Fig. 1130 a–f Varibility of the arterial supply of the female internal genitalia; dorsal view.

a Supply of the uterus, Uterus ("textbook case")

b, c, d Supply of the ovaries, Ovaria (b, "textbook case")

e, f Supply of the fundus of uterus, Fundus uteri (e, "textbook case")

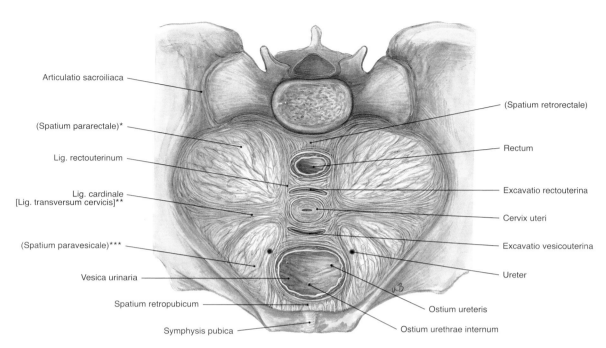

Articulatio sacroiliaca

(Spatium pararectale)*

Lig. rectouterinum

Lig. cardinale
[Lig. transversum cervicis]**

(Spatium paravesicale)***

Vesica urinaria

Spatium retropubicum

Symphysis pubica

(Spatium retrorectale)

Rectum

Excavatio rectouterina

Cervix uteri

Excavatio vesicouterina

Ureter

Ostium ureteris

Ostium urethrae internum

Fig. 1131 Uterus, Uterus;
uterine ligaments and connective tissue spaces;
semi-schematic transverse section at the
level of the cervix of uterus;
superior view.

*   Clinical term: Paraproctium
**   Clinical term: Parametrium
      (existence of this structure is controversial)
*** Clinical term: Paracystium

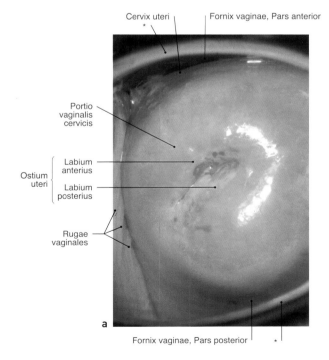

Cervix uteri

Fornix vaginae, Pars anterior

Portio
vaginalis
cervicis

Ostium
uteri

Labium
anterius

Labium
posterius

Rugae
vaginales

a

Fornix vaginae, Pars posterior

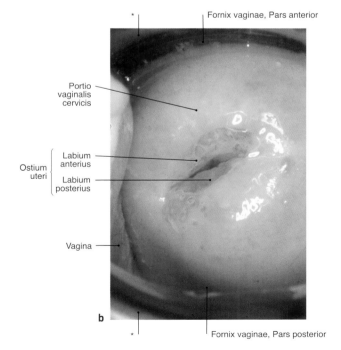

*

Fornix vaginae, Pars anterior

Portio
vaginalis
cervicis

Ostium
uteri

Labium
anterius

Labium
posterius

Vagina

b

*

Fornix vaginae, Pars posterior

Fig. 1132 a, b Vaginal portion of the cervix of uterus, Portio
vaginalis cervicis.
a Photograph of the cervix of a young nulliparous woman
b Photograph of the cervix of a young woman who has given
birth to two children

For the inspection of the vaginal portion of the cervix the
normally slit-like vagina is spreaded by means of a bivalve
speculum (*);
inferior view.

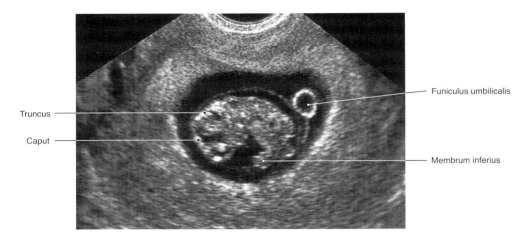

Truncus

Caput

Funiculus umbilicalis

Membrum inferius

Fig. 1133 Uterus, Uterus, with an embryo; ultrasound image taken in the eighth week of pregnancy; lateral view (right).

The embryo is immersed in the amniotic fluid of the chorionic cavity.

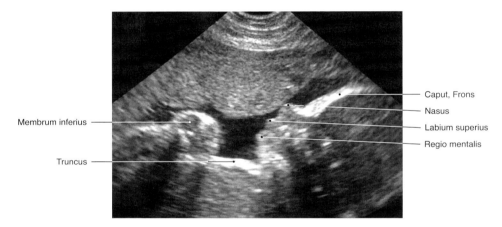

Membrum inferius

Truncus

Caput, Frons

Nasus

Labium superius

Regio mentalis

Fig. 1134 Uterus, Uterus, with a foetus; ultrasound image taken in the 28th week of pregnancy; lateral view (left).

Ultrasound examination allows the visualization of movements of the extremities and the opening of the mouth.

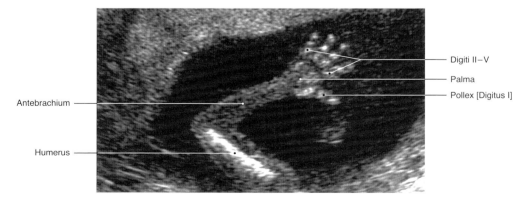

Antebrachium

Humerus

Digiti II–V

Palma

Pollex [Digitus I]

Fig. 1135 Hand, Manus, of a foetus; ultrasound image taken in the 18th week of pregnancy; lateral view.

Details such as fingers can be observed.

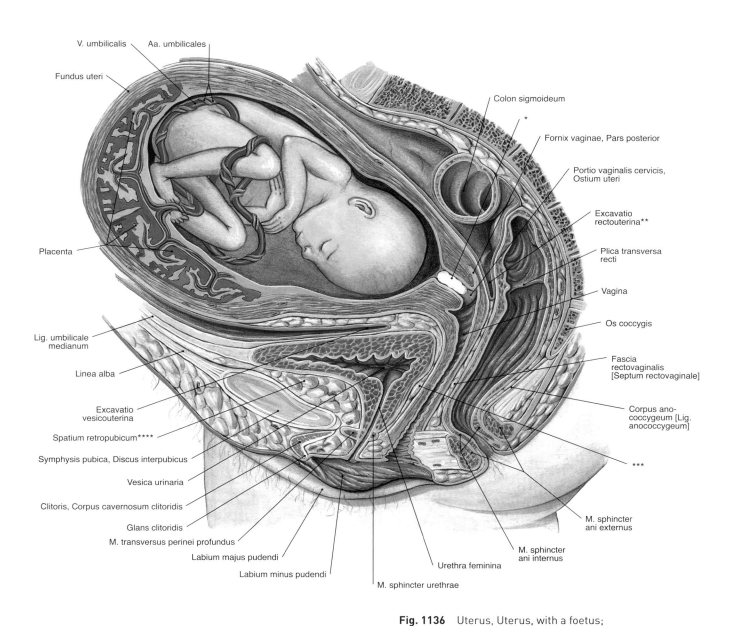

V. umbilicalis   Aa. umbilicales

Fundus uteri

Colon sigmoideum

*

Fornix vaginae, Pars posterior

Portio vaginalis cervicis, Ostium uteri

Excavatio rectouterina**

Plica transversa recti

Placenta

Vagina

Os coccygis

Lig. umbilicale medianum

Fascia rectovaginalis [Septum rectovaginale]

Linea alba

Corpus ano-coccygeum [Lig. anococcygeum]

Excavatio vesicouterina

***

Spatium retropubicum****

Symphysis pubica, Discus interpubicus

Vesica urinaria

M. sphincter ani externus

Clitoris, Corpus cavernosum clitoridis

Glans clitoridis

M. sphincter ani internus

M. transversus perinei profundus

Labium majus pudendi

M. sphincter urethrae

Urethra feminina

Labium minus pudendi

M. sphincter urethrae

Fig. 1136   Uterus, Uterus, with a foetus;
the pelvis has been sectioned in the median plane.

*   Mucous plug (of KRISTELLER) in the cervical canal of the uterus
**   Clinical term: pouch of DOUGLAS
*** Clinical term: vesicovaginal septum
**** Clinical term: cave of RETZIUS

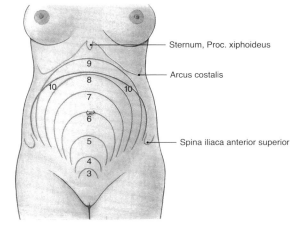

Sternum, Proc. xiphoideus

Arcus costalis

Spina iliaca anterior superior

Fig. 1137   Uterus, Uterus;
position of the fundus of uterus during pregnancy.
Numbers refer to the end of the respective
month of pregnancy (= 28 days).

208

► **Pelvic viscera
and retroperitoneal space**

Placenta

►► Kidney | Suprarenal gland | Urinary bladd

►►► Male genit

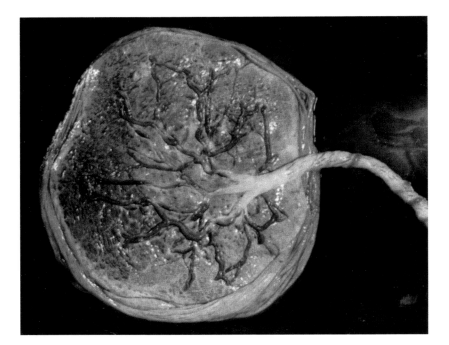

a

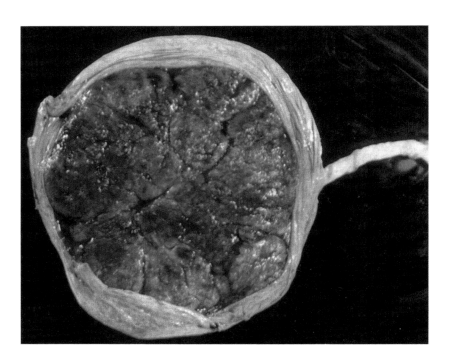

b

Fig. 1138 a, b   Placenta, Placenta, and
umbilical cord, Funiculus umbilicalis.
a View of the foetal surface
b View of the maternal surface of a
   parturient placenta

Ovaries and uterine tubes

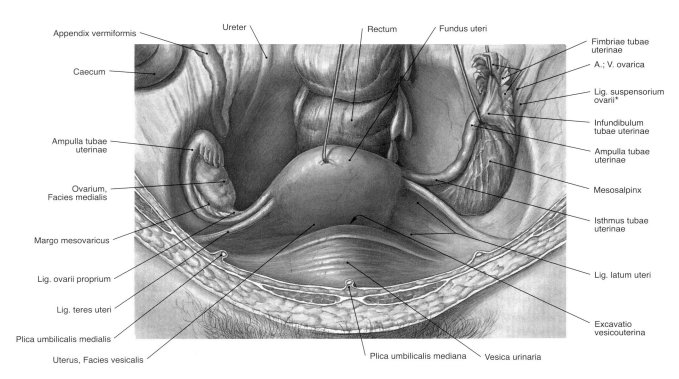

Appendix vermiformis

Caecum

Ampulla tubae uterinae

Ovarium, Facies medialis

Margo mesovaricus

Lig. ovarii proprium

Lig. teres uteri

Plica umbilicalis medialis

Uterus, Facies vesicalis

Ureter

Rectum

Fundus uteri

Fimbriae tubae uterinae

A.; V. ovarica

Lig. suspensorium ovarii*

Infundibulum tubae uterinae

Ampulla tubae uterinae

Mesosalpinx

Isthmus tubae uterinae

Lig. latum uteri

Excavatio vesicouterina

Plica umbilicalis mediana

Vesica urinaria

Fig. 1139 Female internal genitalia, Organa genitalia feminina interna; ventral view.

* Clinical term: infundibulopelvic ligament

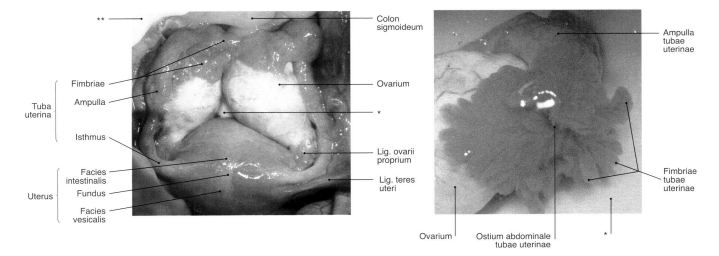

**

Tuba uterina
{ Fimbriae
Ampulla
Isthmus }

Uterus
{ Facies intestinalis
Fundus
Facies vesicalis }

Colon sigmoideum

Ovarium

*

Lig. ovarii proprium

Lig. teres uteri

Ampulla tubae uterinae

Fimbriae tubae uterinae

Ovarium

Ostium abdominale tubae uterinae

*

Fig. 1140 Female internal genitalia, Organa genitalia feminina interna; surgical exposure in a young woman; ovaries displaced both medially and superiorly by compresses (*) in the pouch of DOUGLAS; ventrosuperior view.

** Swab

Fig. 1141 Abdominal ostium of the uterine tube, Ostium abdominale tubae uterinae; surgical exposure in a young woman; the pelvic cavity is filled with saline to demonstrate the fimbria; dorsosuperior view.

* Plastic tray to support the uterine tube

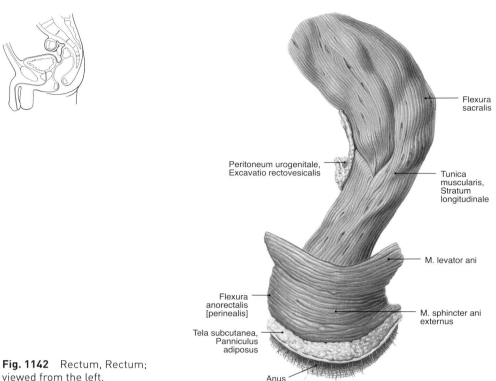

Flexura sacralis

Peritoneum urogenitale, Excavatio rectovesicalis

Tunica muscularis, Stratum longitudinale

M. levator ani

Flexura anorectalis [perinealis]

M. sphincter ani externus

Tela subcutanea, Panniculus adiposus

Anus

Fig. 1142 Rectum, Rectum; viewed from the left.

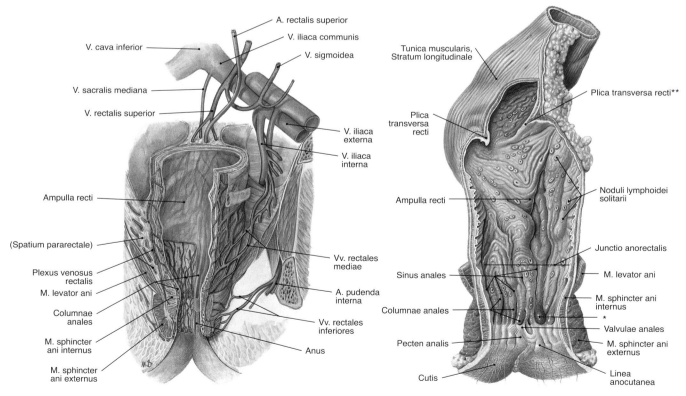

A. rectalis superior

V. iliaca communis

V. cava inferior

V. sigmoidea

V. sacralis mediana

V. rectalis superior

V. iliaca externa

V. iliaca interna

Ampulla recti

(Spatium pararectale)

Plexus venosus rectalis

M. levator ani

Columnae anales

M. sphincter ani internus

M. sphincter ani externus

Vv. rectales mediae

A. pudenda interna

Vv. rectales inferiores

Anus

Tunica muscularis, Stratum longitudinale

Plica transversa recti**

Plica transversa recti

Noduli lymphoidei solitarii

Ampulla recti

Junctio anorectalis

Sinus anales

M. levator ani

Columnae anales

M. sphincter ani internus

Pecten analis

*

Valvulae anales

M. sphincter ani externus

Cutis

Linea anocutanea

Fig. 1143 Rectum, Rectum; blood supply; the mucosa and the pararectal adipose tissues have been partly removed; openings into the hepatic portal vein in purple.

Fig. 1144 Rectum, Rectum, and anus, Anus; ventral view.

* Haemorrhoidal node
** KOHLRAUSCH's fold

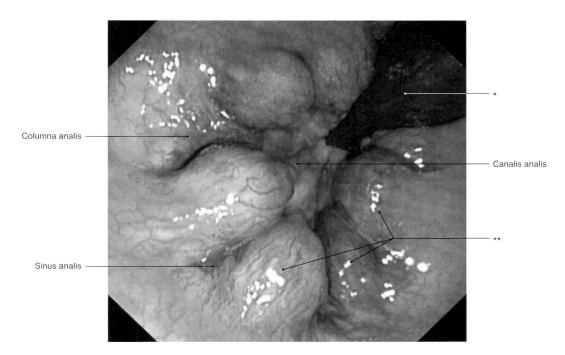

Columna analis

Canalis analis

Sinus analis

*

**

Fig. 1145 Rectum, Rectum;
endoscopic image of the anal canal with six enlarged
nodes of the cavernous rectal body, haemorrhoids;
superior view.
* Colonoscope
** Three haemorrhoidal nodes

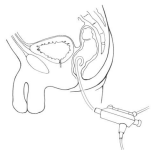

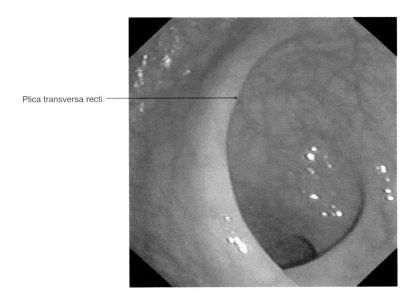

Plica transversa recti

Fig. 1146 Rectum, Rectum;
endoscopic image of the rectal ampulla (rectoscopy);
inferior view.

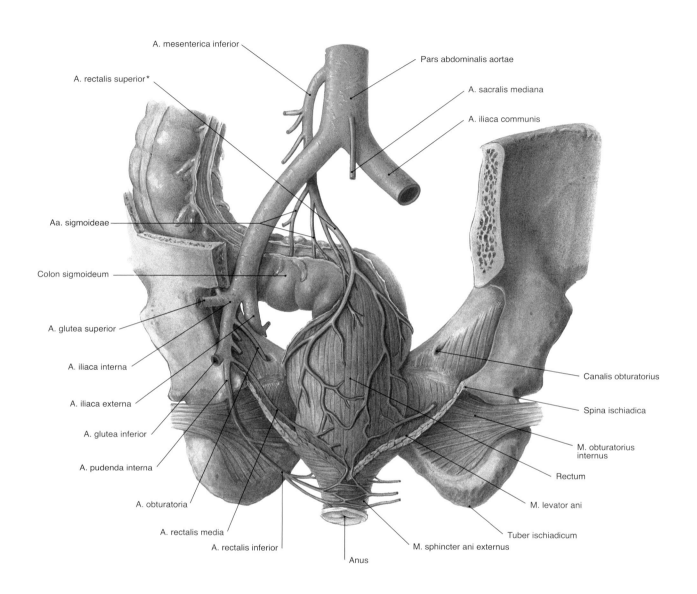

A. mesenterica inferior

A. rectalis superior*

Pars abdominalis aortae

A. sacralis mediana

A. iliaca communis

Aa. sigmoideae

Colon sigmoideum

A. glutea superior

A. iliaca interna

A. iliaca externa

A. glutea inferior

A. pudenda interna

A. obturatoria

A. rectalis media

A. rectalis inferior

Anus

Canalis obturatorius

Spina ischiadica

M. obturatorius internus

Rectum

M. levator ani

Tuber ischiadicum

M. sphincter ani externus

Fig. 1147   Rectal arteries, Aa. rectales;
dorsal view.

* Clinical term: SUDECK's point (from this point on there are
  no further anastomoses with the sigmoid arteries)

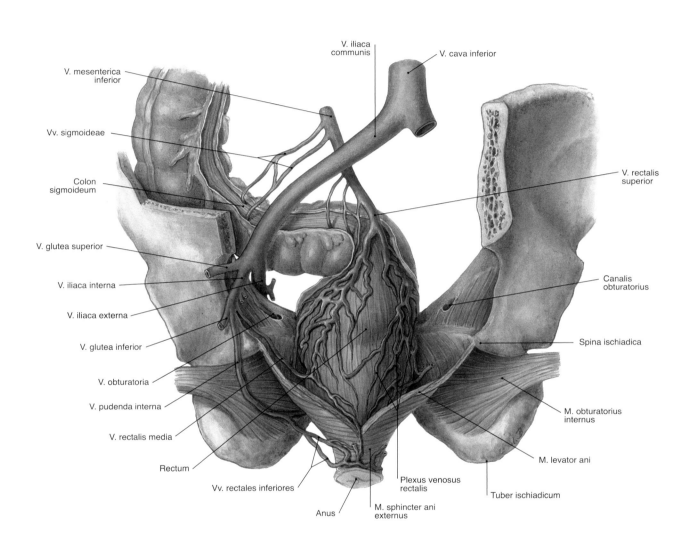

V. iliaca communis

V. cava inferior

V. mesenterica inferior

Vv. sigmoideae

Colon sigmoideum

V. glutea superior

V. iliaca interna

V. iliaca externa

V. glutea inferior

V. obturatoria

V. pudenda interna

V. rectalis media

Rectum

Vv. rectales inferiores

Anus

M. sphincter ani externus

Plexus venosus rectalis

V. rectalis superior

Canalis obturatorius

Spina ischiadica

M. obturatorius internus

M. levator ani

Tuber ischiadicum

Fig. 1148 Rectal veins, Vv. rectales; diagram with parts of the pelvis and the pelvic diaphragm; dorsal view.
There are numerous connections between the veins draining into the hepatic portal vein (superior rectal vein) and those draining into the inferior vena cava (middle and inferior rectal veins). They form the portocaval anastomoses, which are of particular clinical importance.

→ 1077, 1078

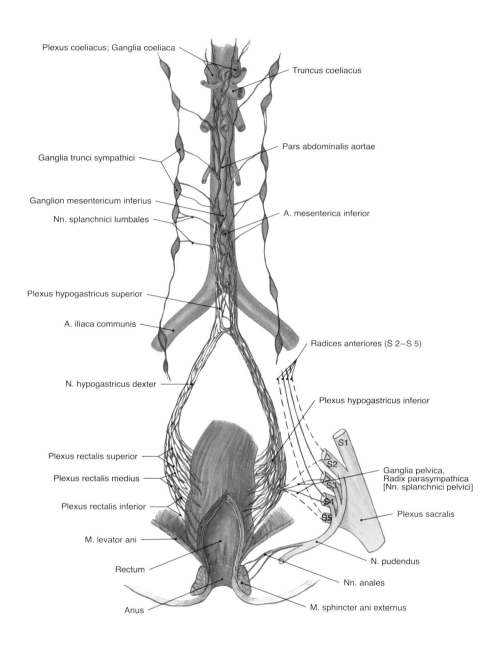

Plexus coeliacus; Ganglia coeliaca

Truncus coeliacus

Ganglia trunci sympathici

Pars abdominalis aortae

Ganglion mesentericum inferius

Nn. splanchnici lumbales

A. mesenterica inferior

Plexus hypogastricus superior

A. iliaca communis

Radices anteriores (S 2–S 5)

N. hypogastricus dexter

Plexus hypogastricus inferior

S1
S2
S3
S4
S5

Plexus rectalis superior

Plexus rectalis medius

Ganglia pelvica,
Radix parasympathica
[Nn. splanchnici pelvici]

Plexus rectalis inferior

Plexus sacralis

M. levator ani

Rectum

N. pudendus

Nn. anales

Anus

M. sphincter ani externus

Fig. 1149 Rectum, Rectum;
schematic overview of the innervation;
ventral view.
Green = sympathetic nervous system
Purple = parasympathetic nervous system

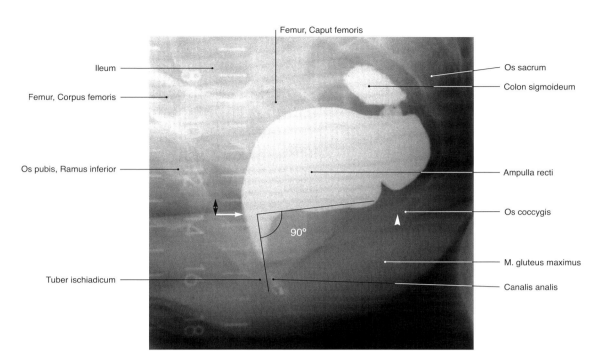

Fig. 1150 Rectum, Rectum;
lateral radiograph in voluntary closure of the anus after filling with a contrast medium (defaecography).

The transitional zone between the anus and the rectum (arrow) is located at the level of the tip of the coccyx (triangle). The angle between the axes of the anus and the rectum (∢) is approximately 90° and depends upon the curvature of the levator ani muscle (puborectal muscle). Scale in cm.

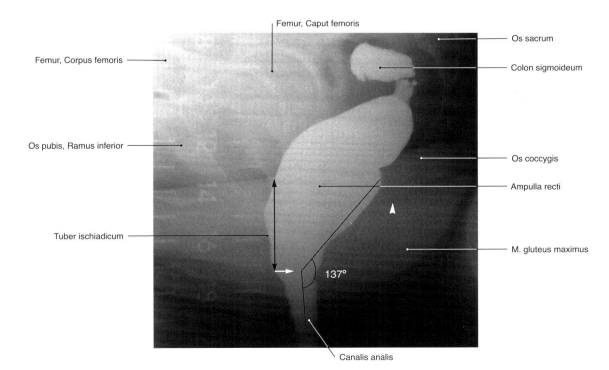

Fig. 1151 Rectum, Rectum;
lateral radiograph of the defaecation after filling with a contrast medium (defaecography).

In comparison to Fig. 1150, the anorectal transitional zone has descended and the angle (∢) increased to 137° due to the relaxation of the curvature of the levator ani muscle. As the bending acts like a valve, the elongation results in an unimpeded pressure of the faeces on the anal canal leading to defaecation.

Arterial supply of the kidney

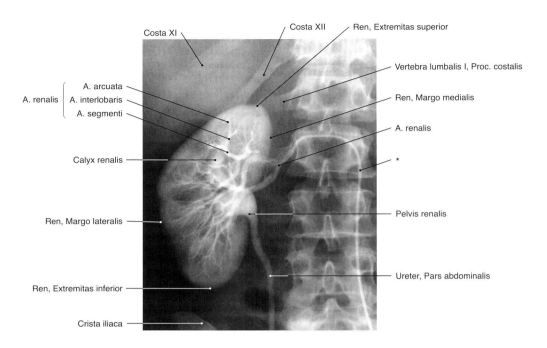

Fig. 1152 Kidney, Ren;
AP-radiograph after intravenous injection of a contrast medium which is excreted via the kidneys to demonstrate the renal pelvis and the ureters (intravenous pyelography); concomitant visualization of the arteries by injection of a contrast medium into the renal artery through a catheter* introduced into the aorta (arteriography).

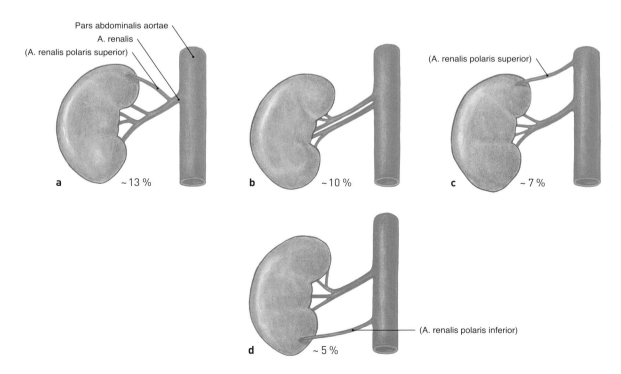

Fig. 1153 a–d Variations in the arterial supply of the kidney.
a One renal artery, A. renalis, with a branch to the superior pole
b Two renal arteries to the renal hilum
c Two renal arteries, one of which supplies the superior pole
d Two renal arteries, one of which supplies the inferior pole

Retroperitoneal space, overview

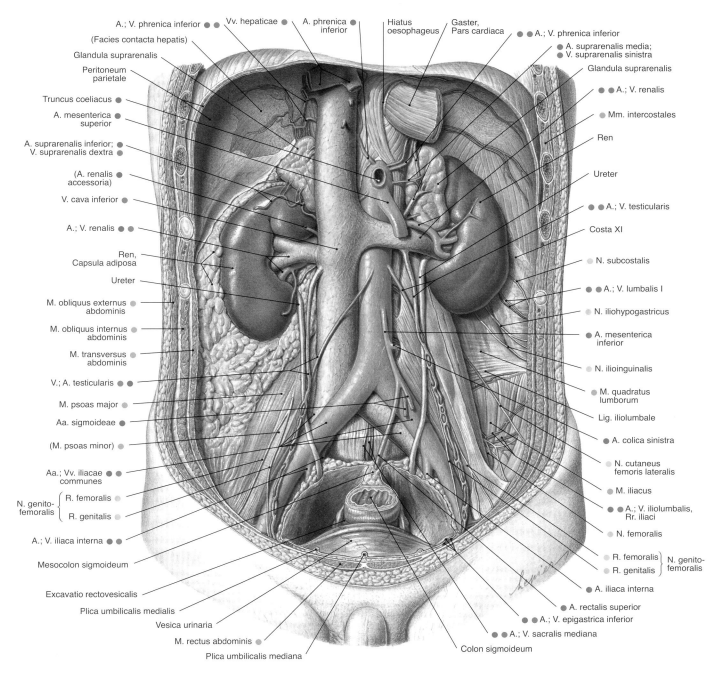

A.; V. phrenica inferior — Vv. hepaticae — A. phrenica inferior — Hiatus oesophageus — Gaster, Pars cardiaca — A.; V. phrenica inferior

(Facies contacta hepatis)

Glandula suprarenalis

A. suprarenalis media; V. suprarenalis sinistra

Peritoneum parietale

Glandula suprarenalis

Truncus coeliacus

A.; V. renalis

A. mesenterica superior

Mm. intercostales

A. suprarenalis inferior; V. suprarenalis dextra

Ren

(A. renalis accessoria)

Ureter

V. cava inferior

A.; V. testicularis

A.; V. renalis

Costa XI

Ren, Capsula adiposa

N. subcostalis

Ureter

A.; V. lumbalis I

M. obliquus externus abdominis

N. iliohypogastricus

M. obliquus internus abdominis

A. mesenterica inferior

M. transversus abdominis

N. ilioinguinalis

V.; A. testicularis

M. quadratus lumborum

M. psoas major

Lig. iliolumbale

Aa. sigmoideae

A. colica sinistra

(M. psoas minor)

N. cutaneus femoris lateralis

Aa.; Vv. iliacae communes

M. iliacus

N. genito-femoralis { R. femoralis / R. genitalis }

A.; V. iliolumbalis, Rr. iliaci

N. femoralis

A.; V. iliaca interna

R. femoralis } N. genito-femoralis
R. genitalis }

Mesocolon sigmoideum

A. iliaca interna

Excavatio rectovesicalis

A. rectalis superior

Plica umbilicalis medialis

A.; V. epigastrica inferior

Vesica urinaria

A.; V. sacralis mediana

M. rectus abdominis

Colon sigmoideum

Plica umbilicalis mediana

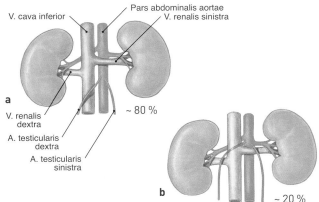

V. cava inferior — Pars abdominalis aortae — V. renalis sinistra

a

V. renalis dextra

A. testicularis dextra

A. testicularis sinistra

~ 80 %

b

~ 20 %

Fig. 1154 Position of the retroperitoneal structures, Situs retroperitonealis, of the male.
Whereas the left testicular vein opens into the left renal vein, the right testicular vein drains directly into the inferior vena cava. The same applies to the ovarian veins.

Fig. 1155 a, b Variability of the course of the testicular arteries, Aa. testiculares.
a "Textbook case"
b Both testicular arteries, Aa. testiculares, branch off cranially to the renal veins, Vv. renales; the right artery passes posterior to the inferior vena cava, V. cava inferior, and the left artery passes anterior to the left renal vein, V. renalis sinistra.

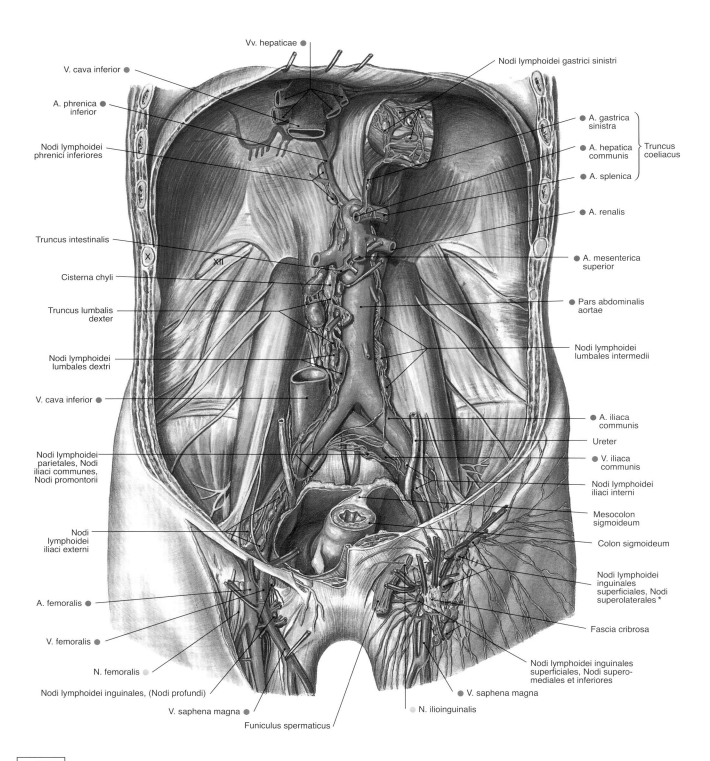

Vv. hepaticae ●

V. cava inferior ●

A. phrenica ● inferior

Nodi lymphoidei phrenici inferiores

Truncus intestinalis

Cisterna chyli

Truncus lumbalis dexter

Nodi lymphoidei lumbales dextri

V. cava inferior ●

Nodi lymphoidei parietales, Nodi iliaci communes, Nodi promontorii

Nodi lymphoidei iliaci externi

A. femoralis ●

V. femoralis ●

N. femoralis ●

Nodi lymphoidei inguinales, (Nodi profundi)

V. saphena magna ●

Funiculus spermaticus

Nodi lymphoidei gastrici sinistri

A. gastrica sinistra ●
A. hepatica ● communis ┃ Truncus coeliacus
A. splenica ●

A. renalis ●

A. mesenterica ● superior

Pars abdominalis ● aortae

Nodi lymphoidei lumbales intermedii

A. iliaca ● communis
Ureter
V. iliaca ● communis
Nodi lymphoidei iliaci interni
Mesocolon sigmoideum
Colon sigmoideum
Nodi lymphoidei inguinales superficiales, Nodi superolaterales *
Fascia cribrosa
Nodi lymphoidei inguinales superficiales, Nodi supero- mediales et inferiores
V. saphena magna ●
N. ilioinguinalis

→ 1389

Fig. 1156 Lymph nodes, Nodi lymphoidei, and lymphatics, Vasa lymphatica, of the posterior abdominal wall and the inguinal region; ventral view.

The numbers X and XII indicate the respective ribs.
* Clinical term: "horizontal chain", draining the lower abdominal wall, the gluteal region, the perineum and the external genital

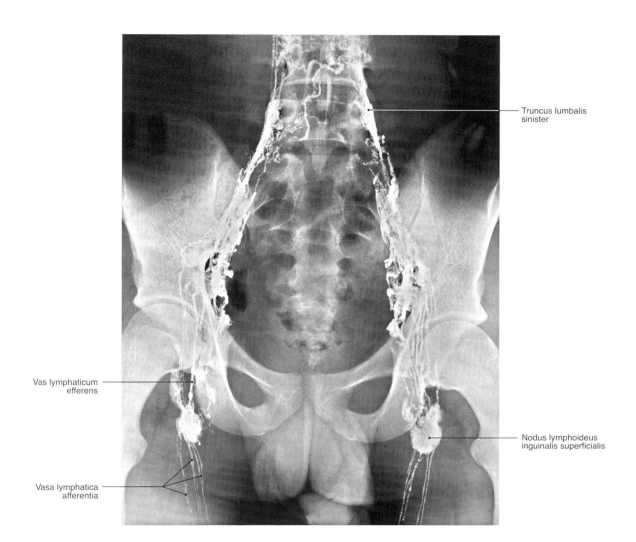

Truncus lumbalis
sinister

Vas lymphaticum
efferens

Nodus lymphoideus
inguinalis superficialis

Vasa lymphatica
afferentia

Fig. 1157   Lymphatics, Vasa lymphatica, and lymph nodes,
Nodi lymphoidei, of the inguinal, the pelvic and the
lumbar region;
AP-radiograph after bilateral injection of a contrast
medium into lymphatics of the foot (lymphography).
This formerly applied technique visualizes the position and
size of lymphatics and lymph nodes.

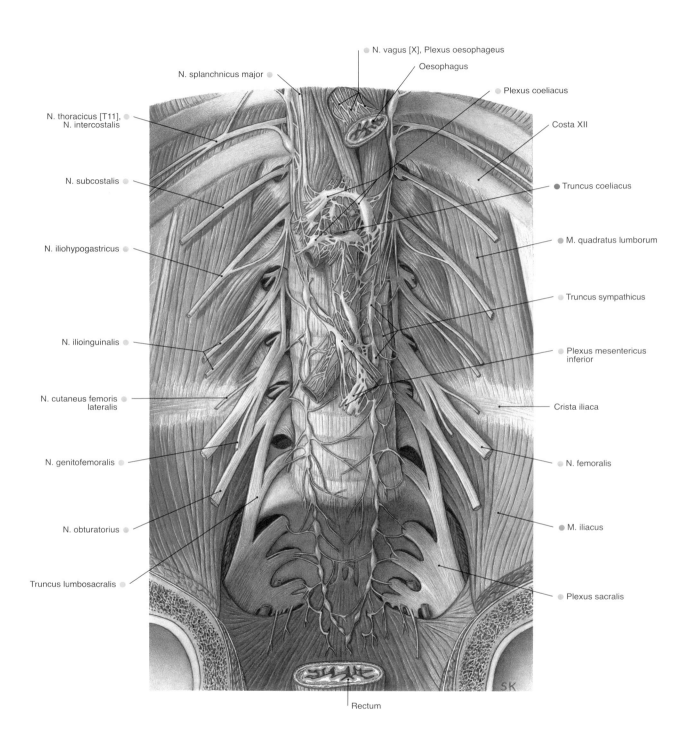

N. vagus [X], Plexus oesophageus

N. splanchnicus major

Oesophagus

Plexus coeliacus

N. thoracicus [T11], N. intercostalis

Costa XII

N. subcostalis

Truncus coeliacus

N. iliohypogastricus

M. quadratus lumborum

Truncus sympathicus

N. ilioinguinalis

Plexus mesentericus inferior

N. cutaneus femoris lateralis

Crista iliaca

N. genitofemoralis

N. femoralis

N. obturatorius

M. iliacus

Truncus lumbosacralis

Plexus sacralis

Rectum

→ 47, 49, 50

Fig. 1158 Nerves of the posterior abdominal wall, the lumbosacral plexus, Plexus lumbosacralis, and the abdominal part of the autonomous nervous system, Pars abdominalis autonomica; ventral view.

Vessels and nerves of the retroperitoneal space

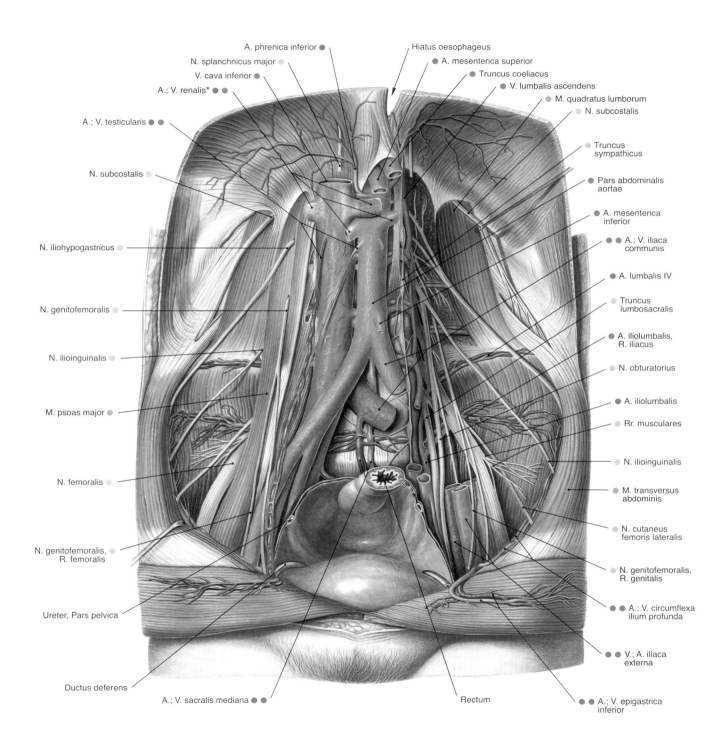

A. phrenica inferior ●
N. splanchnicus major ●
V. cava inferior ●
A.; V. renalis* ● ●
A.; V. testicularis ● ●
N. subcostalis ●
N. iliohypogastricus ●
N. genitofemoralis ●
N. ilioinguinalis ●
M. psoas major ●
N. femoralis ●
N. genitofemoralis, ●
R. femoralis
Ureter, Pars pelvica
Ductus deferens
A.; V. sacralis mediana ● ●

Hiatus oesophageus
A. mesenterica superior ●
Truncus coeliacus ●
V. lumbalis ascendens ●
M. quadratus lumborum ●
N. subcostalis ●
Truncus sympathicus ●
Pars abdominalis aortae ●
A. mesenterica inferior ●
A.; V. iliaca communis ● ●
A. lumbalis IV ●
Truncus lumbosacralis ●
A. iliolumbalis, R. iliacus ●
N. obturatorius ●
A. iliolumbalis ●
Rr. musculares ●
N. ilioinguinalis ●
M. transversus abdominis ●
N. cutaneus femoris lateralis ●
N. genitofemoralis, R. genitalis ●
A.; V. circumflexa ilium profunda ● ●
V.; A. iliaca externa ● ●
A.; V. epigastrica inferior ● ●
Rectum

Fig. 1159 Vessels and nerves of the posterior abdominal wall of the male.
* In ~10% the left renal vein passes posterior to the aorta.

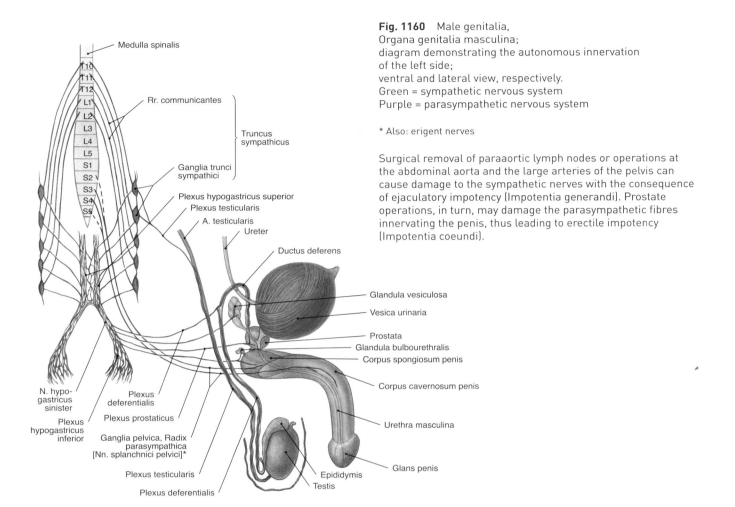

Fig. 1160 Male genitalia,
Organa genitalia masculina;
diagram demonstrating the autonomous innervation
of the left side;
ventral and lateral view, respectively.
Green = sympathetic nervous system
Purple = parasympathetic nervous system

* Also: erigent nerves

Surgical removal of paraaortic lymph nodes or operations at
the abdominal aorta and the large arteries of the pelvis can
cause damage to the sympathetic nerves with the consequence
of ejaculatory impotency (Impotentia generandi). Prostate
operations, in turn, may damage the parasympathetic fibres
innervating the penis, thus leading to erectile impotency
(Impotentia coeundi).

Innervation of the male genitalia

	Origin	Course	Organ	Function
Parasympathetic	Sacral part of the spinal cord (S2 – S4)	Ganglia pelvica, Radix parasympathica [Nn. splanchnici pelvici]	Penis Corpus cavernosum	Vasodilatation Erection
Sympathetic	Thoracic part of the spinal cord (T10 – T12)	Plexus mesenterici superior et inferior ↓ Truncus sympathicus ↓ Plexus testicularis ↓	Testis	Regulation of blood flow
	Lumbar part of the spinal cord (L1 – L2)	Plexus hypogastricus superior ↓ N. hypogastricus ↓		
		Plexus hypogastricus inferior	Glandula bulbo-urethralis	Expulsion of its fluid
			Ductus (vas) deferens	Contraction, transport of the sperms into the urethra
			Glandula vesiculosa Prostata	Expulsion of its content into the urethra
Somatomotor, somatosensory	Sacral part of the spinal cord (S2 – S4)	N. pudendus	(M. sphincter vesicae)	Closure of the urinary bladder to prevent retrograde ejaculation
			M. ischiocavernosus M. bulbospongiosus	Expulsion of the ejaculate out of the urethra
		Nn. scrotales posteriores N. dorsalis penis	Scrotal skin Penile skin	

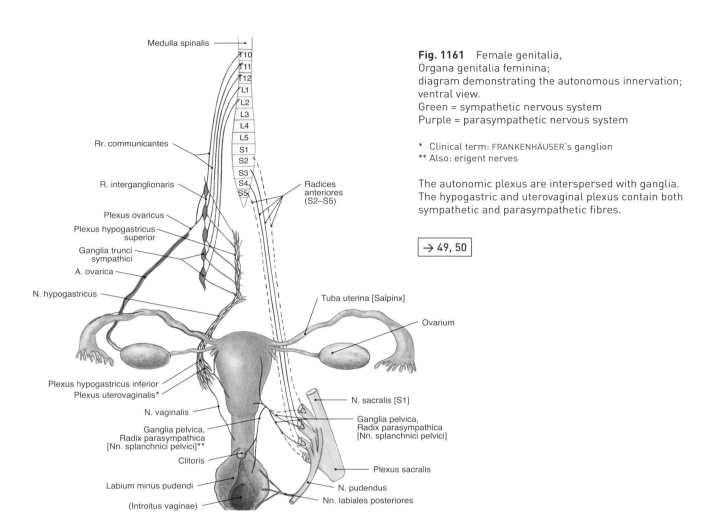

Fig. 1161 Female genitalia,
Organa genitalia feminina;
diagram demonstrating the autonomous innervation;
ventral view.
Green = sympathetic nervous system
Purple = parasympathetic nervous system

* Clinical term: FRANKENHÄUSER's ganglion
** Also: erigent nerves

The autonomic plexus are interspersed with ganglia.
The hypogastric and uterovaginal plexus contain both
sympathetic and parasympathetic fibres.

→ 49, 50

Innervation of the female genitalia

	Origin	Course	Organ	Function
Parasympathetic	Sacral part of the spinal cord (S2 – S4)	Ganglia pelvica, Radix parasympathica [Nn. splanchnici pelvici] ↓ Nn. cavernosi clitoridis	Tuba uterina Uterus Vagina Clitoris	Vasodilatation Vasodilatation Transsudation Erection
Sympathetic	Thoracic part of the spinal cord (T10 – T12)	Plexus mesentericus superior ↘ Plexus ovaricus ↗ Plexus renalis Truncus sympathicus ↓	Ovar	Vasoconstriction
	Lumbar part of the spinal cord (L1 – L2)	Plexus hypogastricus superior ↓ N. hypogastricus Plexus hypogastricus inferior ↓ Plexus uterovaginalis (FRANKENHÄUSER's ganglion)	- Tuba uterina Uterus Vagina	Contraction
Somatomotor, somatosensory	Sacral part of the spinal cord (S2 – S4)	N. dorsalis ↗ clitoridis N. pudendus ↘ Nn. labiales posteriores	Clitoris Labia majora M. ischiocavernosus M. bulbospongiosus	Contraction

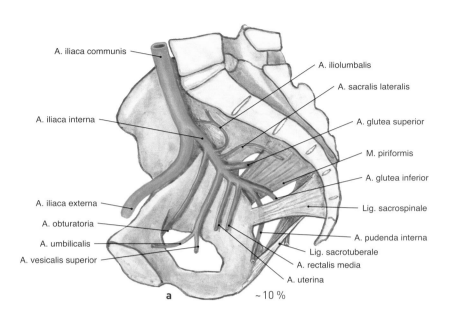

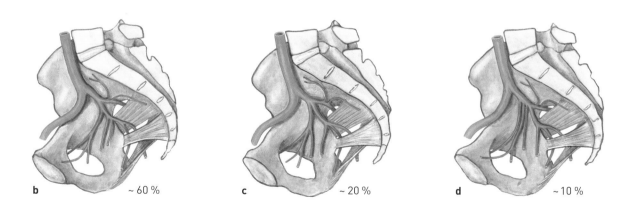

Fig. 1162 a–d Variability of the branching pattern of the internal iliac artery, A. iliaca interna; viewed from the left.

a All branches arise from the same stem.
b The internal iliac artery, A. iliaca interna, divides into two major branches ("textbook case").
c The internal iliac artery, A. iliaca interna, divides into three major branches.
d The internal iliac artery, A. iliaca interna, divides into more than three major branches.

Vessels and nerves of the pelvic wall

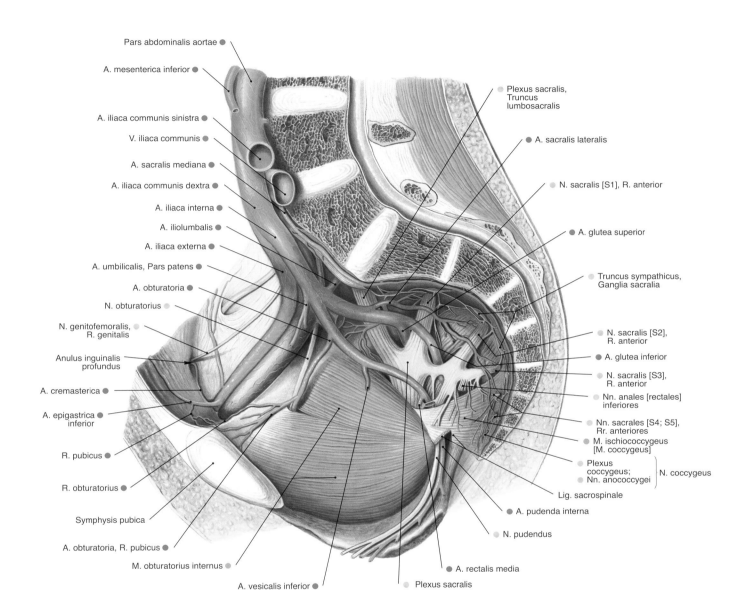

Pars abdominalis aortae ●

A. mesenterica inferior ●

A. iliaca communis sinistra ●

V. iliaca communis ●

A. sacralis mediana ●

A. iliaca communis dextra ●

A. iliaca interna ●

A. iliolumbalis ●

A. iliaca externa ●

A. umbilicalis, Pars patens ●

A. obturatoria ●

N. obturatorius ●

N. genitofemoralis, ●
R. genitalis

Anulus inguinalis
profundus

A. cremasterica ●

A. epigastrica ●
inferior

R. pubicus ●

R. obturatorius ●

Symphysis pubica

A. obturatoria, R. pubicus ●

M. obturatorius internus ●

A. vesicalis inferior ●

● Plexus sacralis,
Truncus
lumbosacralis

● A. sacralis lateralis

● N. sacralis [S1], R. anterior

● A. glutea superior

● Truncus sympathicus,
Ganglia sacralia

● N. sacralis [S2],
R. anterior

● A. glutea inferior

● N. sacralis [S3],
R. anterior

● Nn. anales [rectales]
inferiores

● Nn. sacrales [S4; S5],
Rr. anteriores

● M. ischiococcygeus
[M. coccygeus]

● Plexus
coccygeus;   } N. coccygeus
● Nn. anococcygei

Lig. sacrospinale

● A. pudenda interna

● N. pudendus

● A. rectalis media

● Plexus sacralis

Fig. 1163 Internal iliac artery, A. iliaca interna,
and sacral plexus, Plexus sacralis;
viewed from the left.

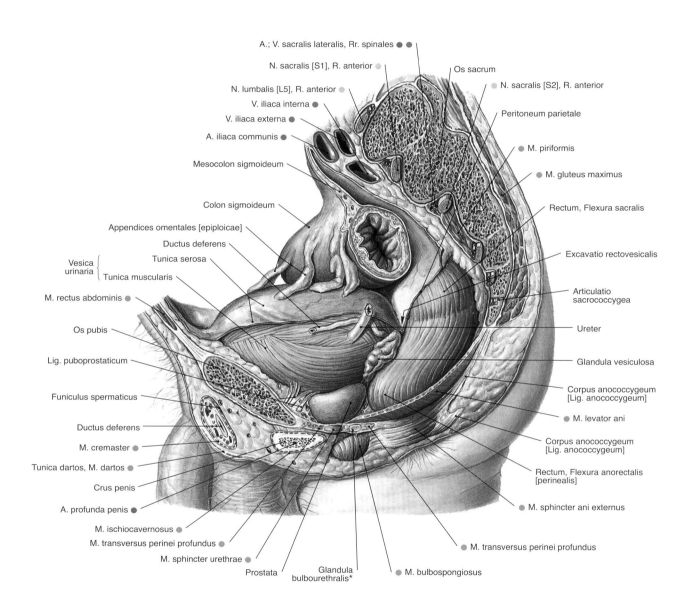

A.; V. sacralis lateralis, Rr. spinales ● ●

N. sacralis [S1], R. anterior ●

N. lumbalis [L5], R. anterior ●

V. iliaca interna ●

V. iliaca externa ●

A. iliaca communis ●

Mesocolon sigmoideum

Colon sigmoideum

Appendices omentales [epiploicae]

Ductus deferens

Vesica urinaria ⎰ Tunica serosa

⎱ Tunica muscularis

M. rectus abdominis ●

Os pubis

Lig. puboprostaticum

Funiculus spermaticus

Ductus deferens

M. cremaster ●

Tunica dartos, M. dartos ●

Crus penis

A. profunda penis ●

M. ischiocavernosus ●

M. transversus perinei profundus ●

M. sphincter urethrae ●

Prostata

Glandula bulbourethralis*

Os sacrum

N. sacralis [S2], R. anterior ●

Peritoneum parietale

● M. piriformis

● M. gluteus maximus

Rectum, Flexura sacralis

Excavatio rectovesicalis

Articulatio sacrococcygea

Ureter

Glandula vesiculosa

Corpus anococcygeum [Lig. anococcygeum]

● M. levator ani

Corpus anococcygeum [Lig. anococcygeum]

Rectum, Flexura anorectalis [perinealis]

● M. sphincter ani externus

● M. transversus perinei profundus

● M. bulbospongiosus

Fig. 1164 Organs of the male pelvis.
* Clinical term: COWPER's gland

Vessels of the male pelvis

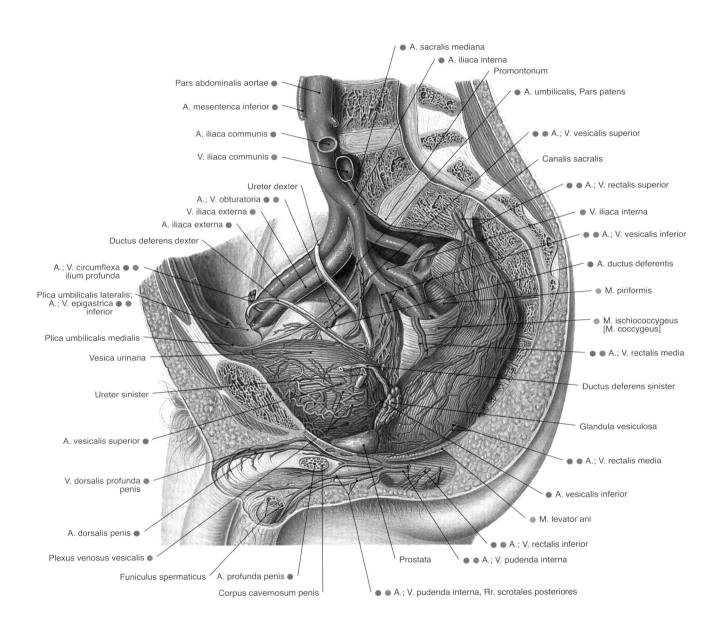

A. sacralis mediana
A. iliaca interna
Promontorium
Pars abdominalis aortae
A. umbilicalis, Pars patens
A. mesenterica inferior
A.; V. vesicalis superior
A. iliaca communis
Canalis sacralis
V. iliaca communis
A.; V. rectalis superior
Ureter dexter
V. iliaca interna
A.; V. obturatoria
V. iliaca externa
A.; V. vesicalis inferior
A. iliaca externa
A. ductus deferentis
Ductus deferens dexter
M. piriformis
A.; V. circumflexa
ilium profunda
M. ischiococcygeus
[M. coccygeus]
Plica umbilicalis lateralis;
A.; V. epigastrica
inferior
A.; V. rectalis media
Plica umbilicalis medialis
Ductus deferens sinister
Vesica urinaria
Glandula vesiculosa
Ureter sinister
A.; V. rectalis media
A. vesicalis superior
A. vesicalis inferior
V. dorsalis profunda
penis
M. levator ani
A. dorsalis penis
A.; V. rectalis inferior
Plexus venosus vesicalis
A.; V. pudenda interna
Funiculus spermaticus
A. profunda penis
Prostata
Corpus cavernosum penis
A.; V. pudenda interna, Rr. scrotales posteriores

Fig. 1165 Blood supply of the male pelvis.

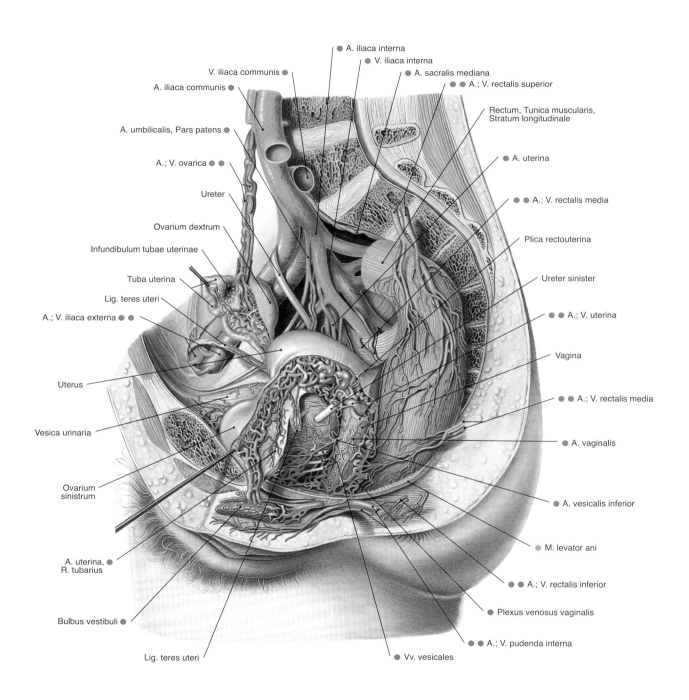

A. iliaca interna

V. iliaca interna

V. iliaca communis

A. sacralis mediana

A. iliaca communis

A.; V. rectalis superior

A. umbilicalis, Pars patens

Rectum, Tunica muscularis, Stratum longitudinale

A.; V. ovarica

A. uterina

Ureter

A.; V. rectalis media

Ovarium dextrum

Plica rectouterina

Infundibulum tubae uterinae

Tuba uterina

Ureter sinister

Lig. teres uteri

A.; V. iliaca externa

A.; V. uterina

Vagina

Uterus

A.; V. rectalis media

Vesica urinaria

A. vaginalis

Ovarium sinistrum

A. vesicalis inferior

M. levator ani

A. uterina, R. tubarius

A.; V. rectalis inferior

Plexus venosus vaginalis

Bulbus vestibuli

A.; V. pudenda interna

Lig. teres uteri

Vv. vesicales

Fig. 1166 Blood supply of the female pelvis.

Vessels of the female pelvis

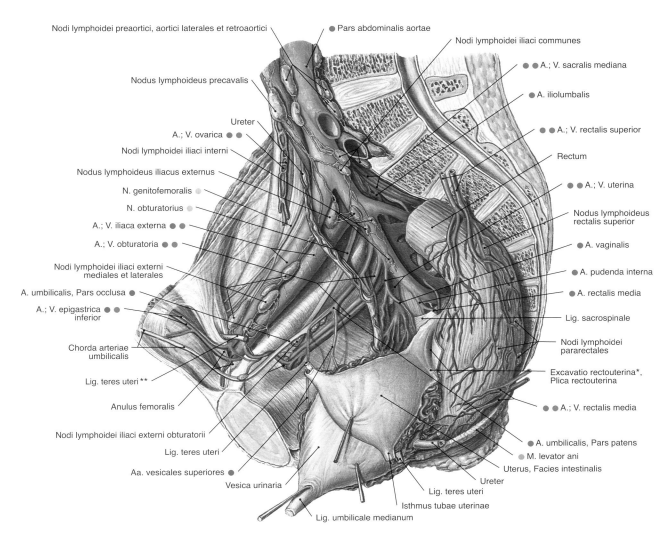

Nodi lymphoidei preaortici, aortici laterales et retroaortici
Nodus lymphoideus precavalis
Ureter
A.; V. ovarica ● ●
Nodi lymphoidei iliaci interni
Nodus lymphoideus iliacus externus
N. genitofemoralis ●
N. obturatorius ●
A.; V. iliaca externa ● ●
A.; V. obturatoria ● ●
Nodi lymphoidei iliaci externi mediales et laterales
A. umbilicalis, Pars occlusa ●
A.; V. epigastrica ● ● inferior
Chorda arteriae umbilicalis
Lig. teres uteri **
Anulus femoralis
Nodi lymphoidei iliaci externi obturatorii
Lig. teres uteri
Aa. vesicales superiores ●
Vesica urinaria

Pars abdominalis aortae
Nodi lymphoidei iliaci communes
● ● A.; V. sacralis mediana
● A. iliolumbalis
● ● A.; V. rectalis superior
Rectum
● ● A.; V. uterina
Nodus lymphoideus rectalis superior
● A. vaginalis
● A. pudenda interna
● A. rectalis media
Lig. sacrospinale
Nodi lymphoidei pararectales
Excavatio rectouterina*, Plica rectouterina
● ● A.; V. rectalis media
● A. umbilicalis, Pars patens
● M. levator ani
Uterus, Facies intestinalis
Ureter
Lig. teres uteri
Isthmus tubae uterinae
Lig. umbilicale medianum

Fig. 1167 Lymphatics, Vasa lymphatica, and lymph nodes, Nodi lymphoidei, of the pelvic wall of the female.

The lymph nodes are frequently much smaller than illustrated but they are always present. Tumour cells from the uterus can reach the superficial inguinal lymph nodes via lymphatics of the round ligament of uterus.

* Clinical term: pouch of DOUGLAS
** Clinical term: round ligament

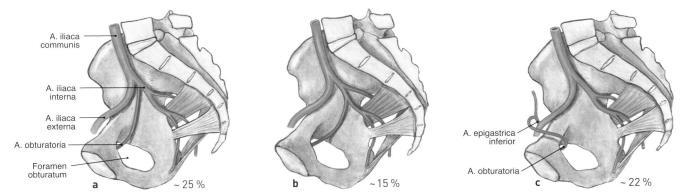

A. iliaca communis
A. iliaca interna
A. iliaca externa
A. obturatoria
Foramen obturatum

a ~ 25 %
b ~ 15 %

A. epigastrica inferior
A. obturatoria

c ~ 22 %

Fig. 1168 a–c Variability of the origin of the obturator artery, A. obturatoria; medial view.
a Origin from the anterior branch of the internal iliac artery, A. iliaca interna ("textbook case")

b Origin as an independent branch from the internal iliac artery, A. iliaca interna
c Origin from the external iliac artery, A. iliaca externa
Only in 75% of the cases, the obturator artery originates from the trunk of the internal iliac artery.

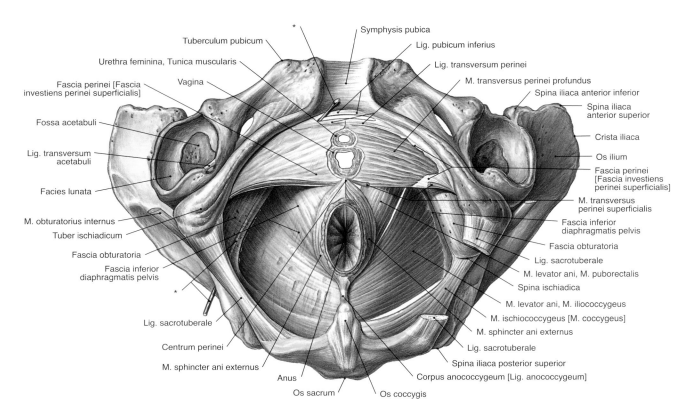

Fig. 1169 Perineal muscles, Mm. perinei, and the pelvic diaphragm, Diaphragma pelvis, of the female; inferior view.

* Probe in the pudendal canal (ALCOCK's canal)

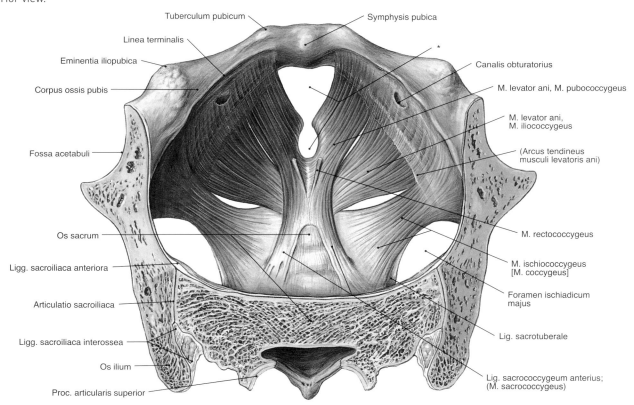

Fig. 1170 Pelvic diaphragm, Diaphragma pelvis, of the female; superior view.

* Clinical term: levator hiatus (Hiatus urogenitalis et ani)

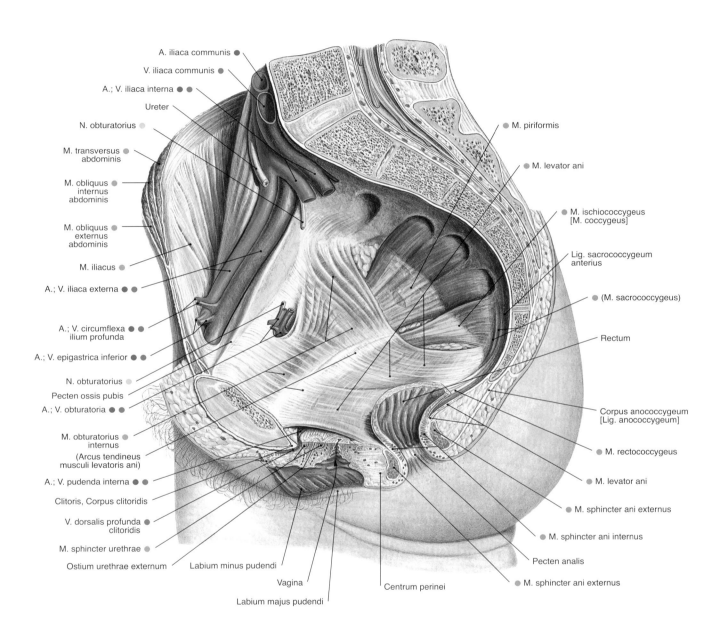

A. iliaca communis ●

V. iliaca communis ●

A.; V. iliaca interna ● ●

Ureter

N. obturatorius ○

M. transversus abdominis ●

M. obliquus internus abdominis ●

M. obliquus externus abdominis ●

M. iliacus ●

A.; V. iliaca externa ● ●

A.; V. circumflexa ilium profunda ● ●

A.; V. epigastrica inferior ● ●

N. obturatorius ○

Pecten ossis pubis

A.; V. obturatoria ● ●

M. obturatorius internus ●

(Arcus tendineus musculi levatoris ani)

A.; V. pudenda interna ● ●

Clitoris, Corpus clitoridis

V. dorsalis profunda clitoridis ●

M. sphincter urethrae ○

Ostium urethrae externum

Labium minus pudendi

Vagina

Labium majus pudendi

Centrum perinei

M. piriformis ●

M. levator ani ●

M. ischiococcygeus [M. coccygeus] ●

Lig. sacrococcygeum anterius

(M. sacrococcygeus) ●

Rectum

Corpus anococcygeum [Lig. anococcygeum]

M. rectococcygeus ●

M. levator ani ●

M. sphincter ani externus ●

M. sphincter ani internus ●

Pecten analis

M. sphincter ani externus ●

Fig. 1171   Muscles of the pelvic diaphragm, Diaphragma pelvis, of the female.

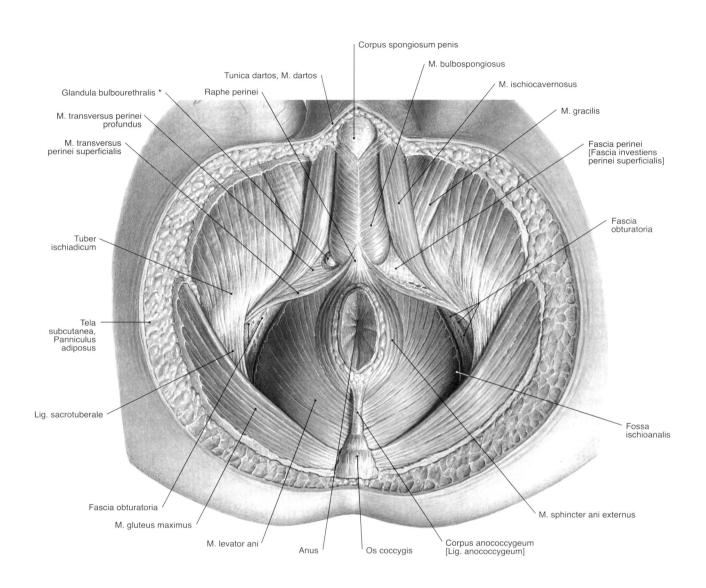

Corpus spongiosum penis

M. bulbospongiosus

M. ischiocavernosus

M. gracilis

Tunica dartos, M. dartos

Raphe perinei

Glandula bulbourethralis *

M. transversus perinei profundus

M. transversus perinei superficialis

Fascia perinei [Fascia investiens perinei superficialis]

Fascia obturatoria

Tuber ischiadicum

Tela subcutanea, Panniculus adiposus

Lig. sacrotuberale

Fossa ischioanalis

Fascia obturatoria

M. gluteus maximus

M. levator ani

Anus

Os coccygis

Corpus anococcygeum [Lig. anococcygeum]

M. sphincter ani externus

→ T 22

Fig. 1172   Perineum, Perineum, and pelvic diaphragm, Diaphragma pelvis, of the male; inferior view.

* Clinical term: COWPER's gland

Female pelvic diaphragm

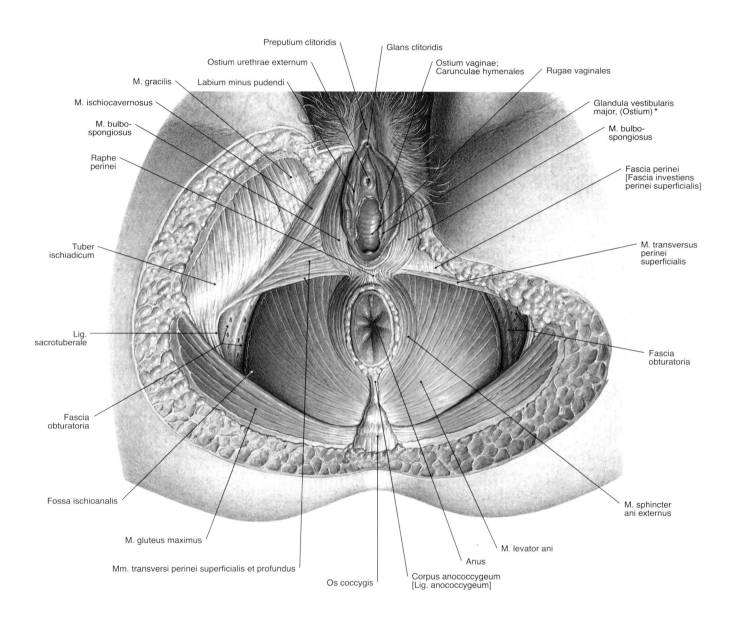

Preputium clitoridis

Ostium urethrae externum

Glans clitoridis

Ostium vaginae;
Carunculae hymenales

Rugae vaginales

M. gracilis

Labium minus pudendi

M. ischiocavernosus

Glandula vestibularis
major, (Ostium) *

M. bulbo-
spongiosus

M. bulbo-
spongiosus

Raphe
perinei

Fascia perinei
[Fascia investiens
perinei superficialis]

Tuber
ischiadicum

M. transversus
perinei
superficialis

Lig.
sacrotuberale

Fascia
obturatoria

Fascia
obturatoria

Fossa ischioanalis

M. sphincter
ani externus

M. gluteus maximus

M. levator ani

Mm. transversi perinei superficialis et profundus

Anus

Os coccygis

Corpus anococcygeum
[Lig. anococcygeum]

Fig. 1173 Perineum, Perineum; pelvic diaphragm,
Diaphragma pelvis, and female external genitalia,
Organa genitalia feminina externa;
inferior view.
* Clinical term: BARTHOLIN's gland

→ T 22

The vaginal and the anal orifices are located in close proximity.
During delivery the skin and muscles of the perineum can
rupture up to the sphincter muscles of the anus (I. – III. degree
perineal lacerations). These can be prevented by surgical
incisions directed either laterally or in the median plane
(perineal incision = lateral or medial episiotomy).

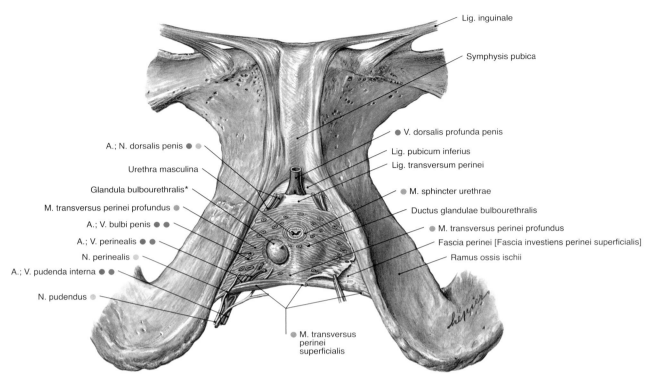

Lig. inguinale

Symphysis pubica

● V. dorsalis profunda penis

A.; N. dorsalis penis ● ●

Lig. pubicum inferius

Lig. transversum perinei

Urethra masculina

● M. sphincter urethrae

Glandula bulbourethralis*

Ductus glandulae bulbourethralis

M. transversus perinei profundus ●

● M. transversus perinei profundus

A.; V. bulbi penis ● ●

Fascia perinei [Fascia investiens perinei superficialis]

A.; V. perinealis ● ●

Ramus ossis ischii

N. perinealis ●

A.; V. pudenda interna ● ●

N. pudendus ●

● M. transversus perinei superficialis

Fig. 1174 Urogenital diaphragm, Diaphragma urogenitale, of the male; inferior view.
* Clinical term: COWPER's gland

→ T 22

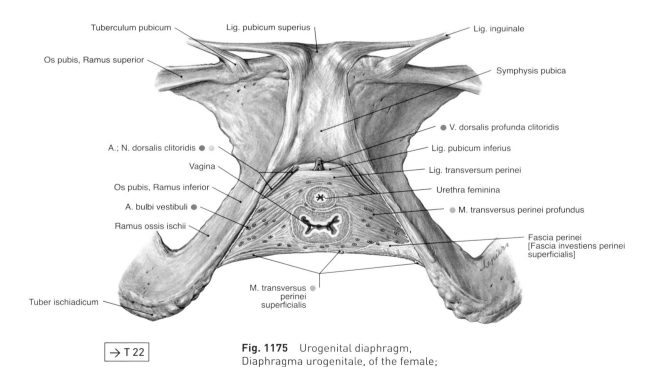

Tuberculum pubicum

Lig. pubicum superius

Lig. inguinale

Os pubis, Ramus superior

Symphysis pubica

● V. dorsalis profunda clitoridis

A.; N. dorsalis clitoridis ● ●

Lig. pubicum inferius

Vagina

Lig. transversum perinei

Os pubis, Ramus inferior

Urethra feminina

A. bulbi vestibuli ●

● M. transversus perinei profundus

Ramus ossis ischii

Fascia perinei [Fascia investiens perinei superficialis]

Tuber ischiadicum

M. transversus ● perinei superficialis

Fig. 1175 Urogenital diaphragm, Diaphragma urogenitale, of the female; inferior view.

→ T 22

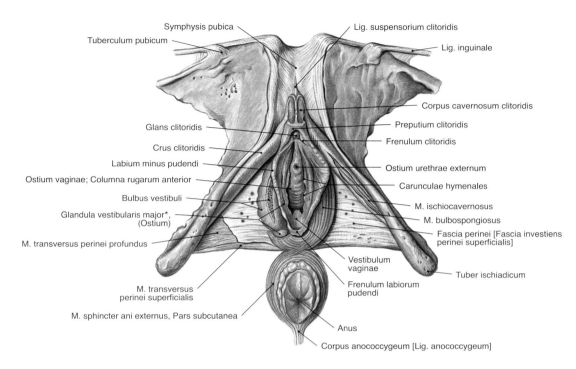

Symphysis pubica
Tuberculum pubicum
Lig. suspensorium clitoridis
Lig. inguinale
Corpus cavernosum clitoridis
Glans clitoridis
Preputium clitoridis
Frenulum clitoridis
Crus clitoridis
Labium minus pudendi
Ostium urethrae externum
Ostium vaginae; Columna rugarum anterior
Carunculae hymenales
Bulbus vestibuli
M. ischiocavernosus
Glandula vestibularis major*, (Ostium)
M. bulbospongiosus
M. transversus perinei profundus
Fascia perinei [Fascia investiens perinei superficialis]
Vestibulum vaginae
Tuber ischiadicum
M. transversus perinei superficialis
Frenulum labiorum pudendi
M. sphincter ani externus, Pars subcutanea
Anus
Corpus anococcygeum [Lig. anococcygeum]

Fig. 1176 Female external genitalia,
Organa genitalia feminina externa;
ventroinferior view.
* Clinical term: BARTHOLIN's gland

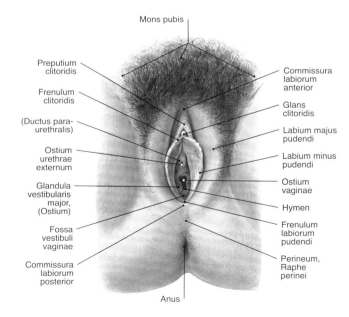

Mons pubis
Preputium clitoridis
Frenulum clitoridis
(Ductus para-urethralis)
Ostium urethrae externum
Glandula vestibularis major, (Ostium)
Fossa vestibuli vaginae
Commissura labiorum posterior
Anus
Commissura labiorum anterior
Glans clitoridis
Labium majus pudendi
Labium minus pudendi
Ostium vaginae
Hymen
Frenulum labiorum pudendi
Perineum, Raphe perinei

Fig. 1177 Female external genitalia,
Organa genitalia feminina externa;
inferior view.

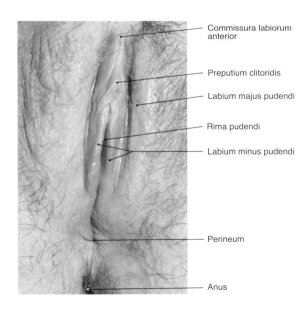

Commissura labiorum anterior
Preputium clitoridis
Labium majus pudendi
Rima pudendi
Labium minus pudendi
Perineum
Anus

Fig. 1178 Female external genitalia,
Organa genitalia feminina externa;
inferior view.

Male pelvic organs and retroperitoneal space

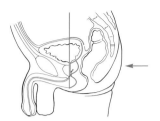

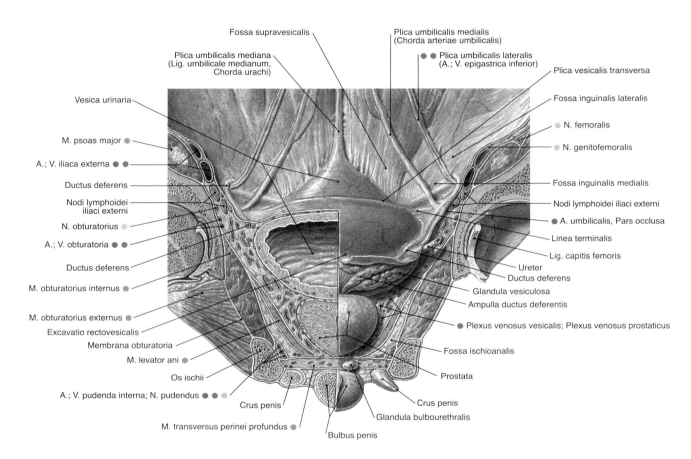

Fossa supravesicalis

Plica umbilicalis mediana
(Lig. umbilicale medianum,
Chorda urachi)

Plica umbilicalis medialis
(Chorda arteriae umbilicalis)

Plica umbilicalis lateralis
(A.; V. epigastrica inferior)

Plica vesicalis transversa

Vesica urinaria

Fossa inguinalis lateralis

M. psoas major

N. femoralis

A.; V. iliaca externa

N. genitofemoralis

Ductus deferens

Fossa inguinalis medialis

Nodi lymphoidei
iliaci externi

Nodi lymphoidei iliaci externi

N. obturatorius

A. umbilicalis, Pars occlusa

A.; V. obturatoria

Linea terminalis

Ductus deferens

Lig. capitis femoris

M. obturatorius internus

Ureter

Ductus deferens

Glandula vesiculosa

M. obturatorius externus

Ampulla ductus deferentis

Excavatio rectovesicalis

Plexus venosus vesicalis; Plexus venosus prostaticus

Membrana obturatoria

M. levator ani

Fossa ischioanalis

Os ischii

Prostata

A.; V. pudenda interna; N. pudendus

Crus penis

Crus penis

M. transversus perinei profundus

Glandula bulbourethralis

Bulbus penis

Fig. 1179   Pelvic diaphragm, Diaphragma pelvis;
pelvic organs and anterior abdominal wall,
Organa abdominis et pelvis, of the male;
frontal section through the head of the femur
and the urinary bladder on the left;
dorsal view.

Female pelvic organs and retroperitoneal space

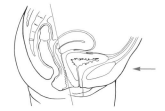

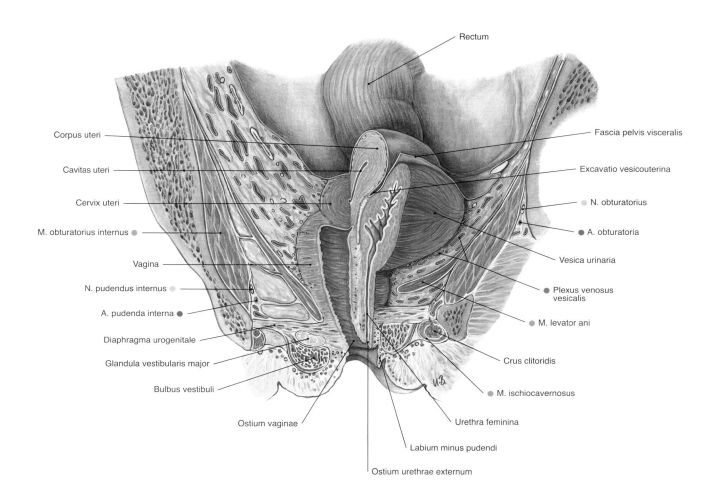

Rectum

Corpus uteri

Cavitas uteri

Cervix uteri

M. obturatorius internus

Vagina

N. pudendus internus

A. pudenda interna

Diaphragma urogenitale

Glandula vestibularis major

Bulbus vestibuli

Ostium vaginae

Fascia pelvis visceralis

Excavatio vesicouterina

N. obturatorius

A. obturatoria

Vesica urinaria

Plexus venosus vesicalis

M. levator ani

Crus clitoridis

M. ischiocavernosus

Urethra feminina

Labium minus pudendi

Ostium urethrae externum

Fig. 1180 Pelvic diaphragm, Diaphragma pelvis, and
pelvic organs, Organa pelvis, of the female;
frontal section (on the right) combined with a median section;
ventral view.

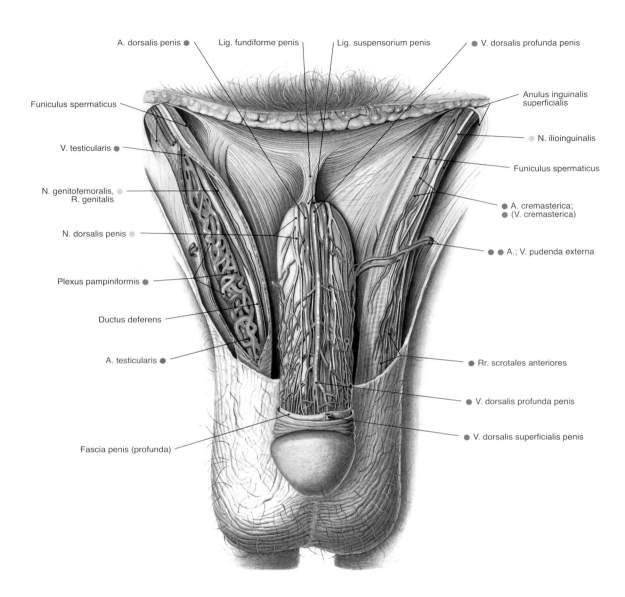

A. dorsalis penis ●

Lig. fundiforme penis

Lig. suspensorium penis

● V. dorsalis profunda penis

Funiculus spermaticus

Anulus inguinalis superficialis

V. testicularis ●

● N. ilioinguinalis

N. genitofemoralis, ●
R. genitalis

Funiculus spermaticus

N. dorsalis penis ●

● A. cremasterica;
● (V. cremasterica)

Plexus pampiniformis ●

● ● A.; V. pudenda externa

Ductus deferens

A. testicularis ●

● Rr. scrotales anteriores

● V. dorsalis profunda penis

Fascia penis (profunda)

● V. dorsalis superficialis penis

Fig. 1181   Male external genitalia,
Organa genitalia masculina externa.

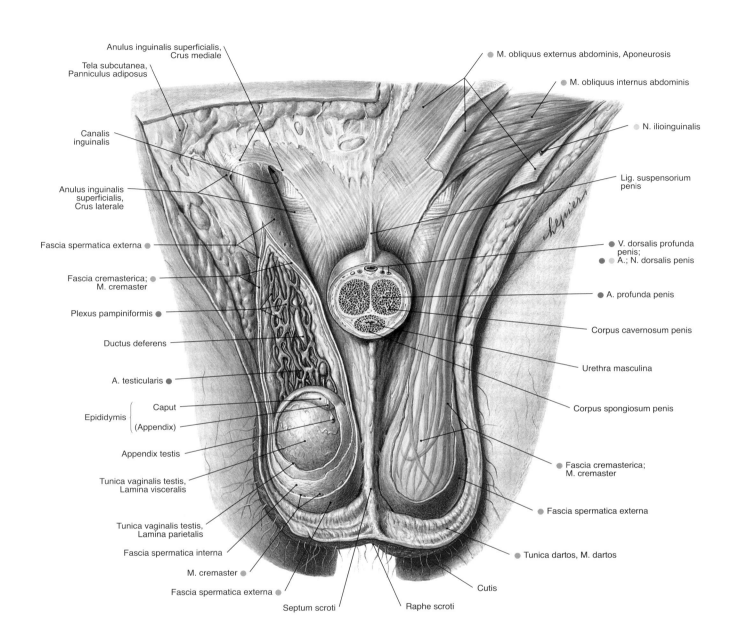

Anulus inguinalis superficialis, Crus mediale

Tela subcutanea, Panniculus adiposus

Canalis inguinalis

Anulus inguinalis superficialis, Crus laterale

Fascia spermatica externa

Fascia cremasterica; M. cremaster

Plexus pampiniformis

Ductus deferens

A. testicularis

Epididymis — Caput — (Appendix)

Appendix testis

Tunica vaginalis testis, Lamina visceralis

Tunica vaginalis testis, Lamina parietalis

Fascia spermatica interna

M. cremaster

Fascia spermatica externa

Septum scroti

Raphe scroti

M. obliquus externus abdominis, Aponeurosis

M. obliquus internus abdominis

N. ilioinguinalis

Lig. suspensorium penis

V. dorsalis profunda penis;
A.; N. dorsalis penis

A. profunda penis

Corpus cavernosum penis

Urethra masculina

Corpus spongiosum penis

Fascia cremasterica; M. cremaster

Fascia spermatica externa

Tunica dartos, M. dartos

Cutis

Fig. 1182 Male genitalia, Organa genitalia masculina.

→ 1105, 1117

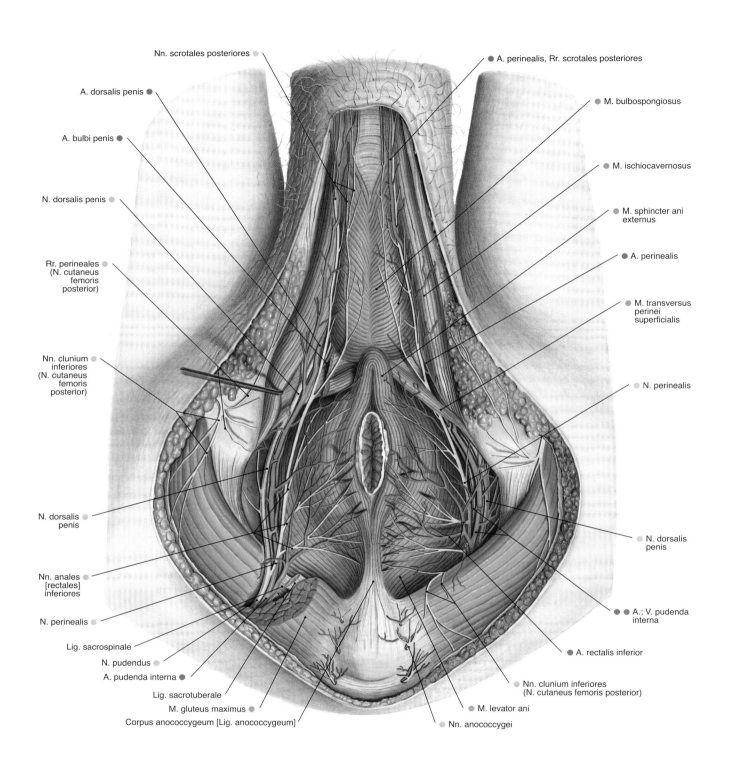

Nn. scrotales posteriores ●

A. dorsalis penis ●

A. bulbi penis ●

N. dorsalis penis ●

Rr. perineales ●
(N. cutaneus
femoris
posterior)

Nn. clunium ●
inferiores
(N. cutaneus
femoris
posterior)

N. dorsalis ●
penis

Nn. anales ●
[rectales]
inferiores

N. perinealis ●

Lig. sacrospinale

N. pudendus ●

A. pudenda interna ●

Lig. sacrotuberale

M. gluteus maximus ●

Corpus anococcygeum [Lig. anococcygeum]

● A. perinealis, Rr. scrotales posteriores

● M. bulbospongiosus

● M. ischiocavernosus

● M. sphincter ani externus

● A. perinealis

● M. transversus perinei superficialis

● N. perinealis

● N. dorsalis penis

● ● A.; V. pudenda interna

● A. rectalis inferior

● Nn. clunium inferiores (N. cutaneus femoris posterior)

● M. levator ani

● Nn. anococcygei

Fig. 1183 Vessels and nerves of the perineum, Regio perinealis, and the male external genitalia, Organa genitalia masculina externa.

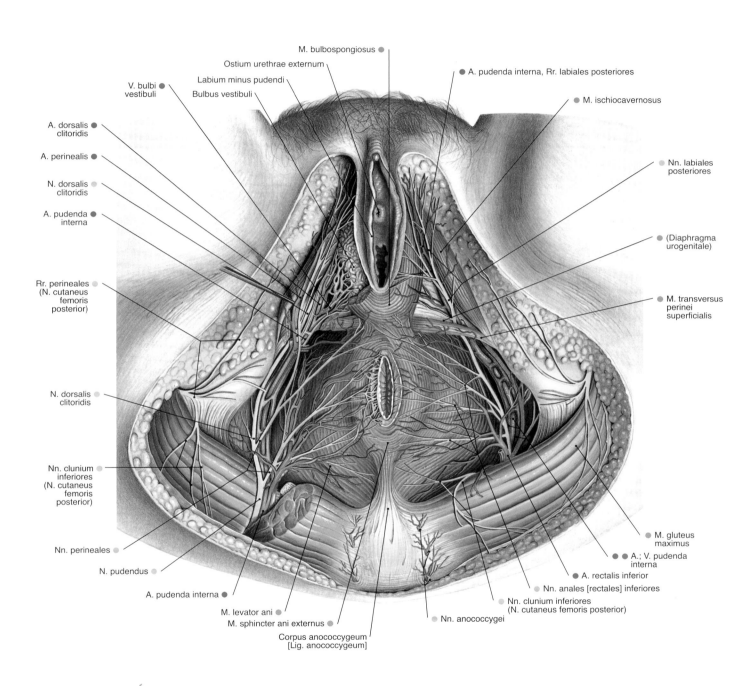

M. bulbospongiosus ●

Ostium urethrae externum

● A. pudenda interna, Rr. labiales posteriores

V. bulbi ●
vestibuli

Labium minus pudendi

Bulbus vestibuli

● M. ischiocavernosus

A. dorsalis ●
clitoridis

A. perinealis ●

N. dorsalis ●
clitoridis

A. pudenda ●
interna

● Nn. labiales
posteriores

● (Diaphragma
urogenitale)

Rr. perineales ●
(N. cutaneus
femoris
posterior)

● M. transversus
perinei
superficialis

N. dorsalis ●
clitoridis

Nn. clunium ●
inferiores
(N. cutaneus
femoris
posterior)

● M. gluteus
maximus

● ● A.; V. pudenda
interna

Nn. perineales ●

N. pudendus ●

● A. rectalis inferior

● Nn. anales [rectales] inferiores

A. pudenda interna ●

Nn. clunium inferiores
(N. cutaneus femoris posterior)

M. levator ani ●

M. sphincter ani externus ●

Nn. anococcygei ●

Corpus anococcygeum
[Lig. anococcygeum]

Fig. 1184 Vessels and nerves of the perineum,
Regio perinealis, and the female external genitalia,
Organa genitalia feminina externa.

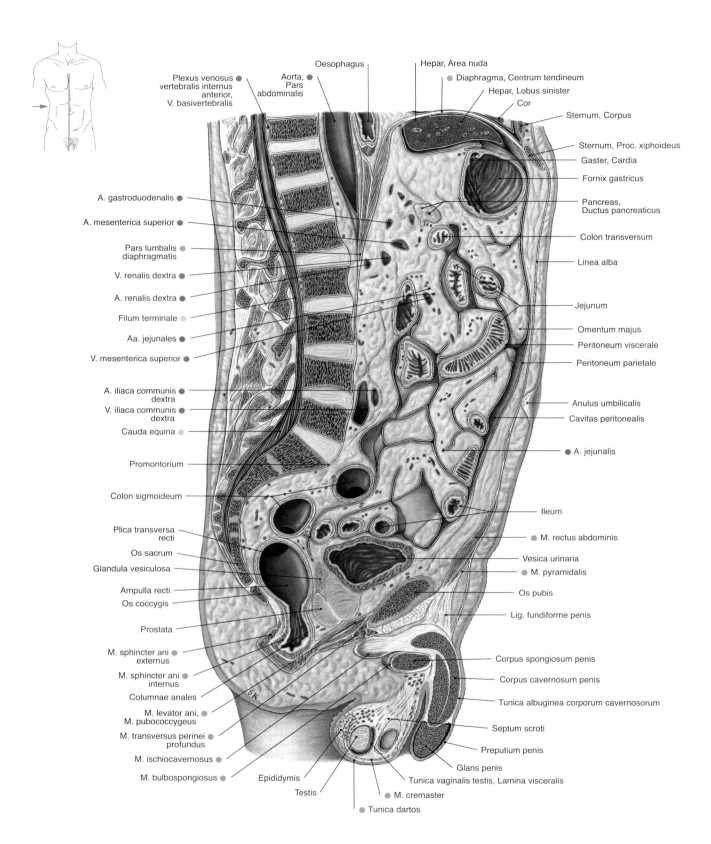

Oesophagus

Plexus venosus
vertebralis internus
anterior,
V. basivertebralis

Aorta,
Pars
abdominalis

Hepar, Area nuda

Diaphragma, Centrum tendineum

Hepar, Lobus sinister

Cor

Sternum, Corpus

Sternum, Proc. xiphoideus

Gaster, Cardia

Fornix gastricus

A. gastroduodenalis

A. mesenterica superior

Pars lumbalis
diaphragmatis

V. renalis dextra

A. renalis dextra

Filum terminale

Aa. jejunales

V. mesenterica superior

A. iliaca communis
dextra

V. iliaca communis
dextra

Cauda equina

Promontorium

Colon sigmoideum

Plica transversa
recti

Os sacrum

Glandula vesiculosa

Ampulla recti

Os coccygis

Prostata

M. sphincter ani
externus

M. sphincter ani
internus

Columnae anales

M. levator ani,
M. pubococcygeus

M. transversus perinei
profundus

M. ischiocavernosus

M. bulbospongiosus

Epididymis

Testis

Pancreas,
Ductus pancreaticus

Colon transversum

Linea alba

Jejunum

Omentum majus

Peritoneum viscerale

Peritoneum parietale

Anulus umbilicalis

Cavitas peritonealis

A. jejunalis

Ileum

M. rectus abdominis

Vesica urinaria

M. pyramidalis

Os pubis

Lig. fundiforme penis

Corpus spongiosum penis

Corpus cavernosum penis

Tunica albuginea corporum cavernosorum

Septum scroti

Preputium penis

Glans penis

Tunica vaginalis testis, Lamina visceralis

M. cremaster

Tunica dartos

Fig. 1185   Abdomen, Abdomen, and pelvis, Pelvis,
of the male;
median section.

Abdomen, sagittal section

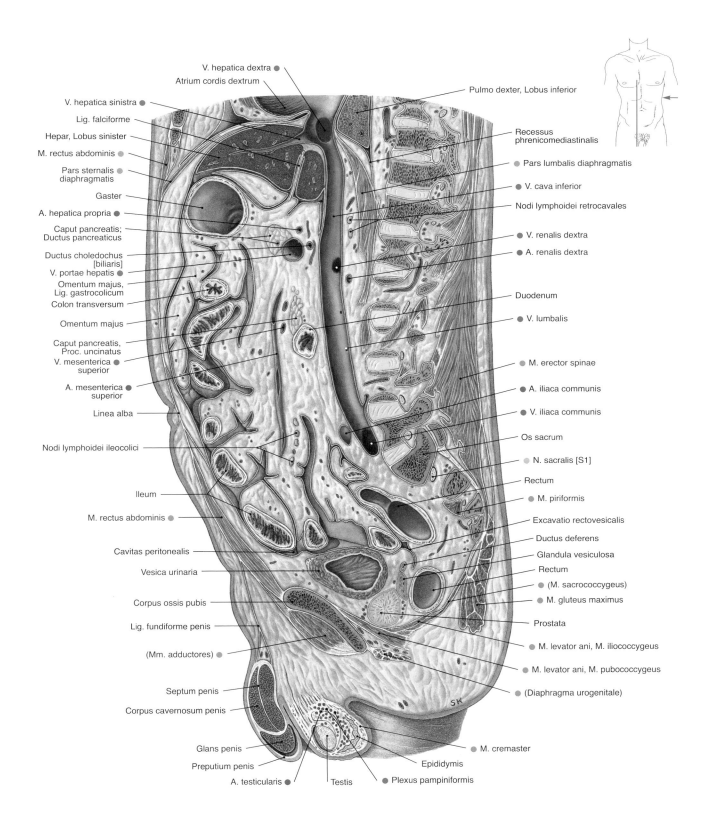

V. hepatica dextra ●
Atrium cordis dextrum
V. hepatica sinistra ●
Lig. falciforme
Hepar, Lobus sinister
M. rectus abdominis ●
Pars sternalis ● diaphragmatis
Gaster
A. hepatica propria ●
Caput pancreatis; Ductus pancreaticus
Ductus choledochus [biliaris]
V. portae hepatis ●
Omentum majus, Lig. gastrocolicum
Colon transversum
Omentum majus
Caput pancreatis, Proc. uncinatus
V. mesenterica ● superior
A. mesenterica ● superior
Linea alba
Nodi lymphoidei ileocolici
Ileum
M. rectus abdominis ●
Cavitas peritonealis
Vesica urinaria
Corpus ossis pubis
Lig. fundiforme penis
(Mm. adductores) ●
Septum penis
Corpus cavernosum penis
Glans penis
Preputium penis
A. testicularis ●
Testis

Pulmo dexter, Lobus inferior
Recessus phrenicomediastinalis
● Pars lumbalis diaphragmatis
● V. cava inferior
Nodi lymphoidei retrocavales
● V. renalis dextra
● A. renalis dextra
Duodenum
● V. lumbalis
● M. erector spinae
● A. iliaca communis
● V. iliaca communis
Os sacrum
● N. sacralis [S1]
Rectum
● M. piriformis
Excavatio rectovesicalis
Ductus deferens
Glandula vesiculosa
Rectum
● (M. sacrococcygeus)
● M. gluteus maximus
Prostata
● M. levator ani, M. iliococcygeus
● M. levator ani, M. pubococcygeus
● (Diaphragma urogenitale)
● M. cremaster
Epididymis
● Plexus pampiniformis

Fig. 1186 Abdomen, Abdomen, and pelvis, Pelvis, of the male; sagittal section to the right of the median plane.

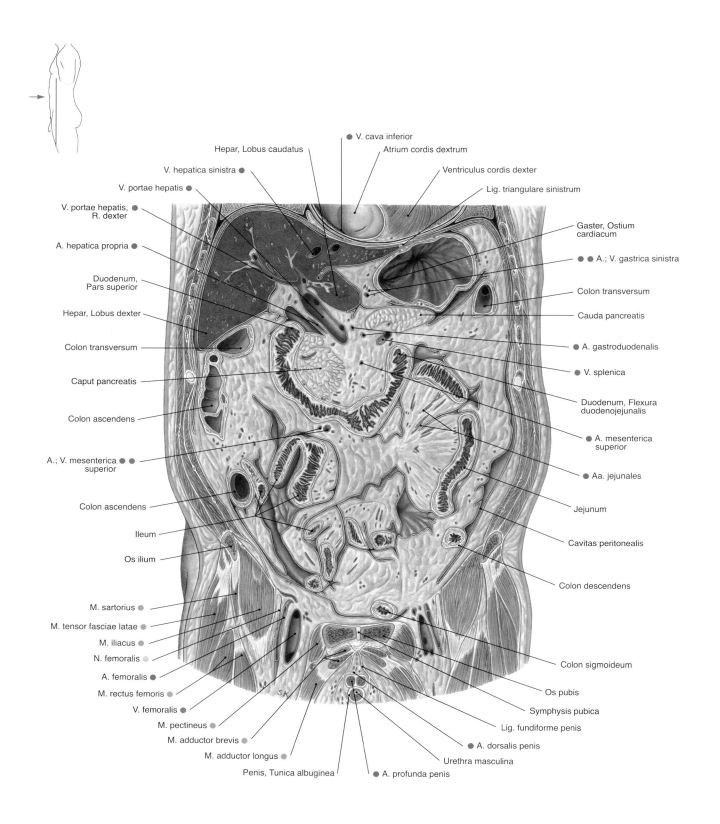

V. cava inferior

Hepar, Lobus caudatus

Atrium cordis dextrum

V. hepatica sinistra

Ventriculus cordis dexter

V. portae hepatis

Lig. triangulare sinistrum

V. portae hepatis, R. dexter

Gaster, Ostium cardiacum

A. hepatica propria

A.; V. gastrica sinistra

Duodenum, Pars superior

Colon transversum

Hepar, Lobus dexter

Cauda pancreatis

Colon transversum

A. gastroduodenalis

Caput pancreatis

V. splenica

Colon ascendens

Duodenum, Flexura duodenojejunalis

A.; V. mesenterica superior

A. mesenterica superior

Aa. jejunales

Colon ascendens

Jejunum

Ileum

Cavitas peritonealis

Os ilium

Colon descendens

M. sartorius

M. tensor fasciae latae

M. iliacus

N. femoralis

Colon sigmoideum

A. femoralis

M. rectus femoris

Os pubis

V. femoralis

Symphysis pubica

M. pectineus

Lig. fundiforme penis

M. adductor brevis

A. dorsalis penis

M. adductor longus

Urethra masculina

Penis, Tunica albuginea

A. profunda penis

→ 870

Fig. 1187 Abdomen, Abdomen;
frontal section through the most anterior part of the abdominal cavity.

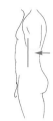

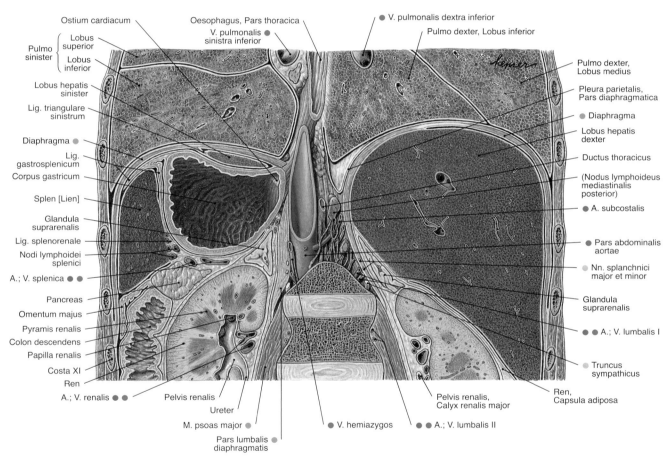

Ostium cardiacum

Oesophagus, Pars thoracica

V. pulmonalis
sinistra inferior

● V. pulmonalis dextra inferior

Pulmo dexter, Lobus inferior

Pulmo sinister — Lobus superior
Lobus inferior

Lobus hepatis sinister

Lig. triangulare sinistrum

Diaphragma ●

Lig. gastrosplenicum

Corpus gastricum

Splen [Lien]

Glandula suprarenalis

Lig. splenorenale

Nodi lymphoidei splenici

A.; V. splenica ● ●

Pancreas

Omentum majus

Pyramis renalis

Colon descendens

Papilla renalis

Costa XI

Ren

A.; V. renalis ● ●

Pelvis renalis

Ureter

M. psoas major ●

Pars lumbalis diaphragmatis

● V. hemiazygos

● ● A.; V. lumbalis II

Pelvis renalis, Calyx renalis major

Pulmo dexter, Lobus medius

Pleura parietalis, Pars diaphragmatica

● Diaphragma

Lobus hepatis dexter

Ductus thoracicus

(Nodus lymphoideus mediastinalis posterior)

● A. subcostalis

● Pars abdominalis aortae

Nn. splanchnici major et minor

Glandula suprarenalis

● ● A.; V. lumbalis I

Truncus sympathicus

Ren, Capsula adiposa

Fig. 1188 Abdomen, Abdomen;
frontal section demonstrating the diaphragm,
the organs of the upper abdomen and the kidneys;
dorsal view.

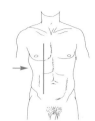

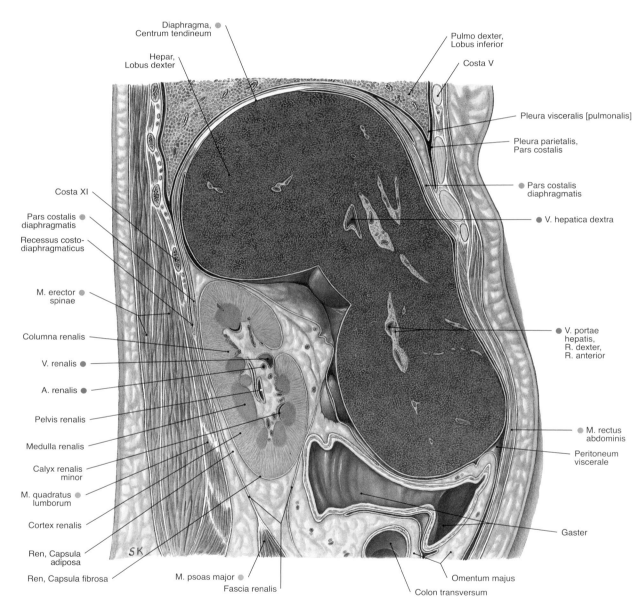

Diaphragma, ●
Centrum tendineum

Hepar,
Lobus dexter

Pulmo dexter,
Lobus inferior

Costa V

Pleura visceralis [pulmonalis]

Pleura parietalis,
Pars costalis

Pars costalis
diaphragmatis

Costa XI

Pars costalis ●
diaphragmatis

Recessus costo-
diaphragmaticus

M. erector ●
spinae

Columna renalis

V. renalis ●

A. renalis ●

Pelvis renalis

Medulla renalis

Calyx renalis
minor

M. quadratus ●
lumborum

Cortex renalis

Ren, Capsula
adiposa

Ren, Capsula fibrosa

M. psoas major ●

Fascia renalis

● V. hepatica dextra

● V. portae
hepatis,
R. dexter,
R. anterior

● M. rectus
abdominis

Peritoneum
viscerale

Gaster

Omentum majus

Colon transversum

SK

Fig. 1189   Abdomen, Abdomen;
sagittal section through the upper abdomen
at the level of the right kidney;
viewed from the right.

Upper abdomen, sagittal section

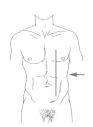

Gaster, Cardia, Ostium cardiacum

Gaster, Fornix gastricus

Lig. phrenicosplenicum

Omentum minus, Lig. hepatogastricum

Pericardium

Pulmo sinister, Lobus inferior

Costa VI

Pars costalis diaphragmatis

Hepar, Lobus sinister

A. gastrica sinistra ●

R. intercostalis anterior; ●
V. intercostalis anterior; ●
N. intercostalis ●

Costa IX

Gaster, Pars pylorica, Antrum pyloricum

A. gastroomentalis ●
sinistra

Omentum majus, Lig. gastrocolicum

M. rectus abdominis ●

Omentum majus

Colon transversum

Pleura visceralis [pulmonalis]

Pleura parietalis, Pars costalis

Splen [Lien]

Lig. gastrosplenicum

Bursa omentalis

Recessus costodiaphragmaticus

● M. erector spinae

Costa XII

Medulla renalis

Cortex renalis   Ren

Capsula fibrosa

Capsula adiposa

● M. quadratus lumborum

Fascia renalis

S K

● M. psoas major

Cavitas peritonealis

Jejunum

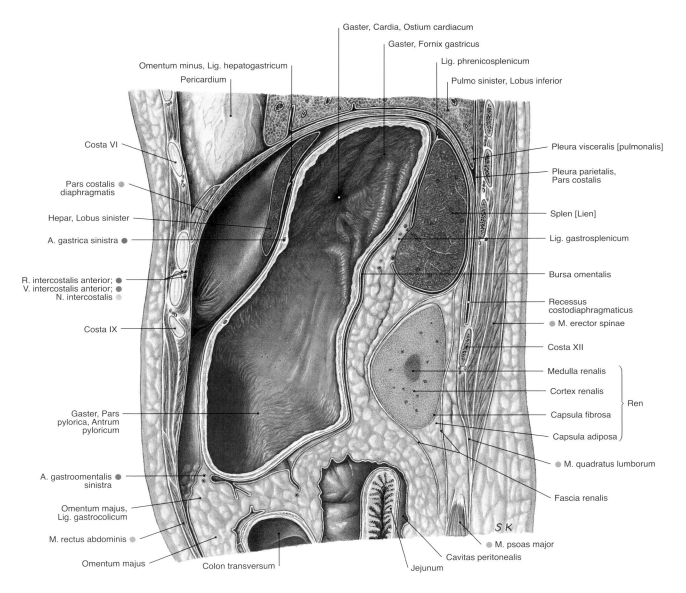

Fig. 1190   Abdomen, Abdomen;
sagittal section through the upper abdomen at the level of the spleen;
viewed from the left.

Upper abdomen, transverse sections

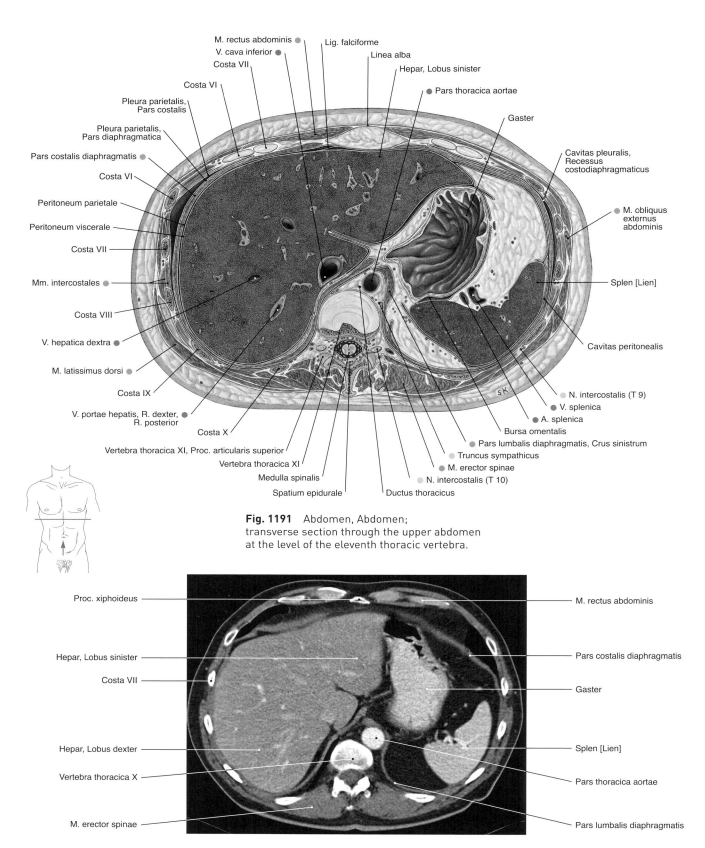

M. rectus abdominis
V. cava inferior
Costa VII
Costa VI
Pleura parietalis, Pars costalis
Pleura parietalis, Pars diaphragmatica
Pars costalis diaphragmatis
Costa VI
Peritoneum parietale
Peritoneum viscerale
Costa VII
Mm. intercostales
Costa VIII
V. hepatica dextra
M. latissimus dorsi
Costa IX
V. portae hepatis, R. dexter, R. posterior
Vertebra thoracica XI, Proc. articularis superior
Vertebra thoracica XI
Medulla spinalis
Spatium epidurale
Costa X

Lig. falciforme
Linea alba
Hepar, Lobus sinister
Pars thoracica aortae
Gaster
Cavitas pleuralis, Recessus costodiaphragmaticus
M. obliquus externus abdominis
Splen [Lien]
Cavitas peritonealis
N. intercostalis (T 9)
V. splenica
A. splenica
Bursa omentalis
Pars lumbalis diaphragmatis, Crus sinistrum
Truncus sympathicus
M. erector spinae
N. intercostalis (T 10)
Ductus thoracicus

Fig. 1191 Abdomen, Abdomen; transverse section through the upper abdomen at the level of the eleventh thoracic vertebra.

Proc. xiphoideus
Hepar, Lobus sinister
Costa VII
Hepar, Lobus dexter
Vertebra thoracica X
M. erector spinae

M. rectus abdominis
Pars costalis diaphragmatis
Gaster
Splen [Lien]
Pars thoracica aortae
Pars lumbalis diaphragmatis

Fig. 1192 Abdomen, Abdomen; computed tomographic cross-section (CT) at the level of the tenth thoracic vertebra; inferior view.

Upper abdomen, transverse sections

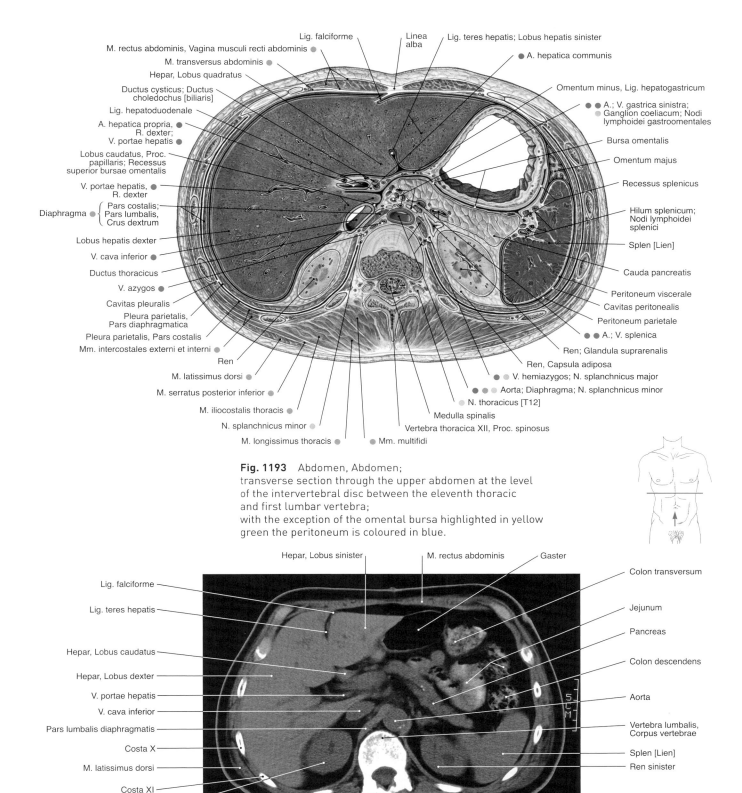

Lig. falciforme
Linea alba
Lig. teres hepatis; Lobus hepatis sinister

M. rectus abdominis, Vagina musculi recti abdominis
M. transversus abdominis
Hepar, Lobus quadratus
Ductus cysticus; Ductus choledochus [biliaris]
Lig. hepatoduodenale
A. hepatica propria, R. dexter; V. portae hepatis
Lobus caudatus, Proc. papillaris; Recessus superior bursae omentalis
V. portae hepatis, R. dexter
Diaphragma — Pars costalis; Pars lumbalis, Crus dextrum
Lobus hepatis dexter
V. cava inferior
Ductus thoracicus
V. azygos
Cavitas pleuralis
Pleura parietalis, Pars diaphragmatica
Pleura parietalis, Pars costalis
Mm. intercostales externi et interni
Ren
M. latissimus dorsi
M. serratus posterior inferior
M. iliocostalis thoracis
N. splanchnicus minor
M. longissimus thoracis

A. hepatica communis
Omentum minus, Lig. hepatogastricum
A.; V. gastrica sinistra; Ganglion coeliacum; Nodi lymphoidei gastroomentales
Bursa omentalis
Omentum majus
Recessus splenicus
Hilum splenicum; Nodi lymphoidei splenici
Splen [Lien]
Cauda pancreatis
Peritoneum viscerale
Cavitas peritonealis
Peritoneum parietale
A.; V. splenica
Ren; Glandula suprarenalis
Ren, Capsula adiposa
V. hemiazygos; N. splanchnicus major
Aorta; Diaphragma; N. splanchnicus minor
N. thoracicus [T12]
Medulla spinalis
Vertebra thoracica XII, Proc. spinosus
Mm. multifidi

Fig. 1193 Abdomen, Abdomen;
transverse section through the upper abdomen at the level
of the intervertebral disc between the eleventh thoracic
and first lumbar vertebra;
with the exception of the omental bursa highlighted in yellow
green the peritoneum is coloured in blue.

Hepar, Lobus sinister
M. rectus abdominis
Gaster
Colon transversum

Lig. falciforme
Lig. teres hepatis
Hepar, Lobus caudatus
Hepar, Lobus dexter
V. portae hepatis
V. cava inferior
Pars lumbalis diaphragmatis
Costa X
M. latissimus dorsi
Costa XI
Ren dexter
Costa XII

Jejunum
Pancreas
Colon descendens
Aorta
Vertebra lumbalis, Corpus vertebrae
Splen [Lien]
Ren sinister
M. erector spinae

Fig. 1194 Abdomen, Abdomen;
computed tomographic section (CT)
at the level of the first lumbar vertebra.
The intestine is partially filled with a contrast medium.

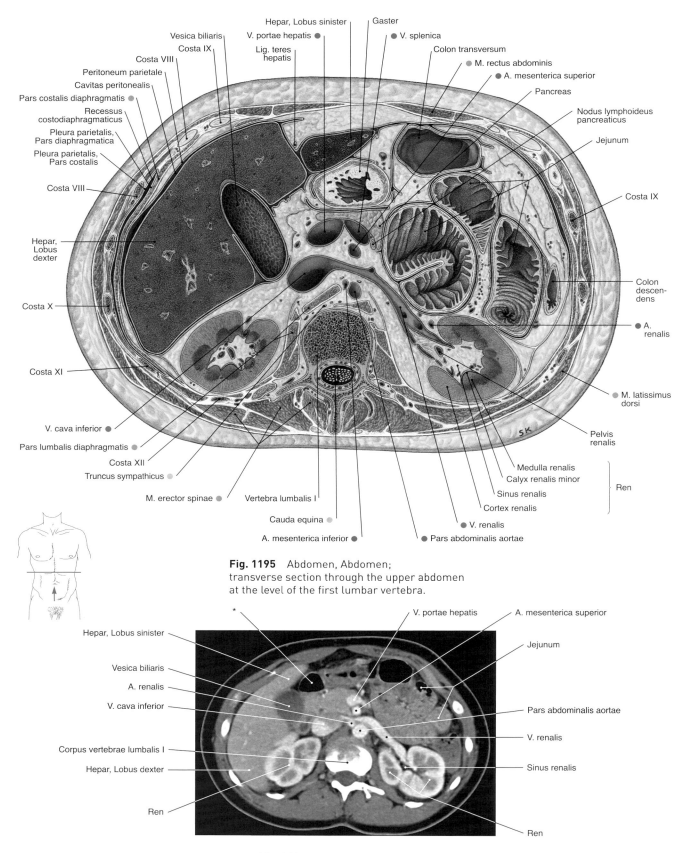

Hepar, Lobus sinister
Gaster
V. portae hepatis ●
● V. splenica
Vesica biliaris
Costa IX
Lig. teres hepatis
Colon transversum
Costa VIII
● M. rectus abdominis
Peritoneum parietale
● A. mesenterica superior
Cavitas peritonealis
Pancreas
Pars costalis diaphragmatis ●
Nodus lymphoideus pancreaticus
Recessus costodiaphragmaticus
Jejunum
Pleura parietalis, Pars diaphragmatica
Pleura parietalis, Pars costalis
Costa VIII
Costa IX
Hepar, Lobus dexter
Colon descendens
Costa X
● A. renalis
Costa XI
● M. latissimus dorsi
V. cava inferior ●
Pelvis renalis
Pars lumbalis diaphragmatis ●
Medulla renalis
Costa XII
Calyx renalis minor
Truncus sympathicus ●
Sinus renalis
Ren
M. erector spinae ●
Vertebra lumbalis I
Cortex renalis
Cauda equina ●
● V. renalis
A. mesenterica inferior ●
● Pars abdominalis aortae

Fig. 1195 Abdomen, Abdomen;
transverse section through the upper abdomen
at the level of the first lumbar vertebra.

*
V. portae hepatis
A. mesenterica superior
Hepar, Lobus sinister
Jejunum
Vesica biliaris
A. renalis
Pars abdominalis aortae
V. cava inferior
V. renalis
Corpus vertebrae lumbalis I
Hepar, Lobus dexter
Sinus renalis
Ren
Ren

Fig. 1196 Abdomen, Abdomen;
computed tomographic section (CT)
at the level of the first lumbar vertebra;
inferior view.
* Intestinal gas

Lower abdomen, transverse sections

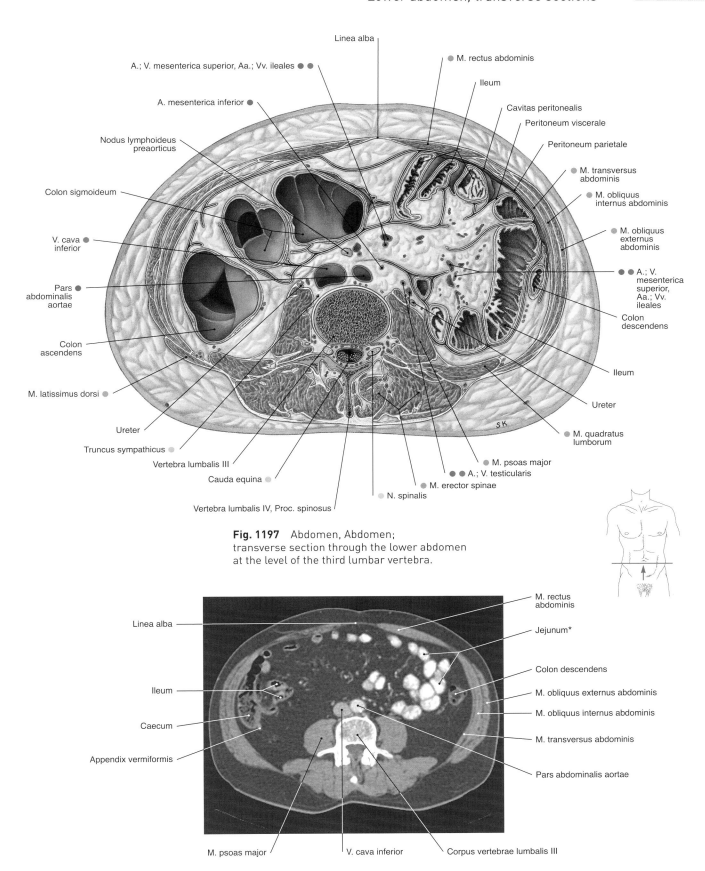

Linea alba

A.; V. mesenterica superior, Aa.; Vv. ileales ● ●

A. mesenterica inferior ●

Nodus lymphoideus preaorticus

Colon sigmoideum

V. cava ● inferior

Pars ● abdominalis aortae

Colon ascendens

M. latissimus dorsi ●

Ureter

Truncus sympathicus ●

Vertebra lumbalis III

Cauda equina ●

Vertebra lumbalis IV, Proc. spinosus

M. rectus abdominis ●

Ileum

Cavitas peritonealis

Peritoneum viscerale

Peritoneum parietale

● M. transversus abdominis

● M. obliquus internus abdominis

● M. obliquus externus abdominis

● ● A.; V. mesenterica superior, Aa.; Vv. ileales

Colon descendens

Ileum

Ureter

● M. quadratus lumborum

● M. psoas major

● ● A.; V. testicularis

● M. erector spinae

● N. spinalis

Fig. 1197   Abdomen, Abdomen;
transverse section through the lower abdomen
at the level of the third lumbar vertebra.

Linea alba

Ileum

Caecum

Appendix vermiformis

M. rectus abdominis

Jejunum*

Colon descendens

M. obliquus externus abdominis

M. obliquus internus abdominis

M. transversus abdominis

Pars abdominalis aortae

M. psoas major

V. cava inferior

Corpus vertebrae lumbalis III

Fig. 1198   Abdomen, Abdomen;
computed tomographic section (CT)
at the level of the third lumbar vertebra;
inferior view.
* Jejunum filled with a contrast medium

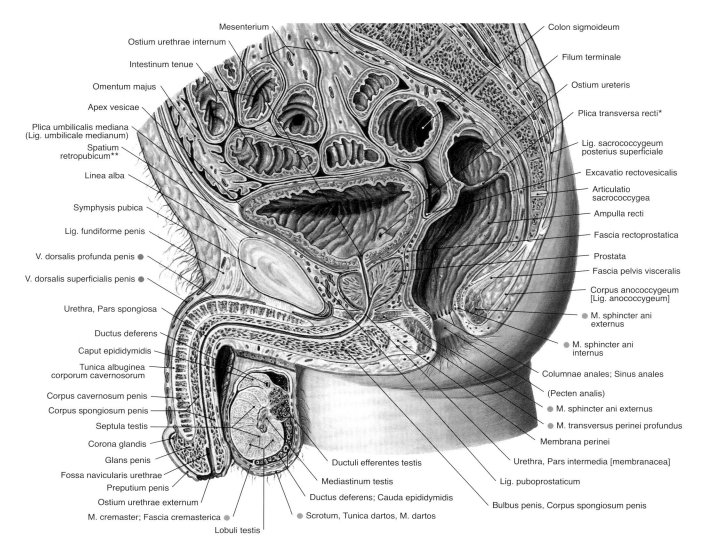

Mesenterium

Ostium urethrae internum

Intestinum tenue

Omentum majus

Apex vesicae

Plica umbilicalis mediana
(Lig. umbilicale medianum)

Spatium
retropubicum**

Linea alba

Symphysis pubica

Lig. fundiforme penis

V. dorsalis profunda penis ●

V. dorsalis superficialis penis ●

Urethra, Pars spongiosa

Ductus deferens

Caput epididymidis

Tunica albuginea
corporum cavernosorum

Corpus cavernosum penis

Corpus spongiosum penis

Septula testis

Corona glandis

Glans penis

Fossa navicularis urethrae

Preputium penis

Ostium urethrae externum

M. cremaster; Fascia cremasterica ●

Lobuli testis

Colon sigmoideum

Filum terminale

Ostium ureteris

Plica transversa recti*

Lig. sacrococcygeum
posterius superficiale

Excavatio rectovesicalis

Articulatio
sacrococcygea

Ampulla recti

Fascia rectoprostatica

Prostata

Fascia pelvis visceralis

Corpus anococcygeum
[Lig. anococcygeum]

● M. sphincter ani
externus

● M. sphincter ani
internus

Columnae anales; Sinus anales

(Pecten analis)

● M. sphincter ani externus

● M. transversus perinei profundus

Urethra, Pars intermedia [membranacea]

Lig. puboprostaticum

Bulbus penis, Corpus spongiosum penis

Ductuli efferentes testis

Mediastinum testis

Ductus deferens; Cauda epididymidis

● Scrotum, Tunica dartos, M. dartos

Fig. 1199 Pelvis, Pelvis, of the male;
median section;
viewed from the left.

* Clinical term: KOHLRAUSCH's fold
** Clinical term: cave of RETZIUS

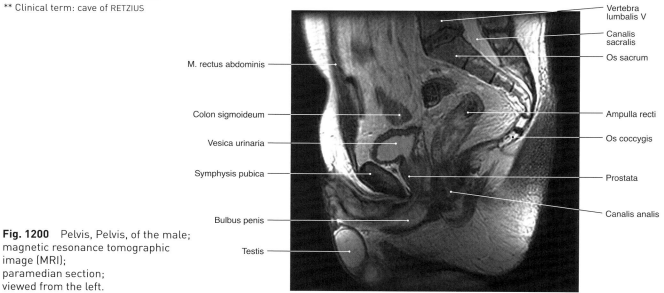

Vertebra
lumbalis V

Canalis
sacralis

Os sacrum

M. rectus abdominis

Colon sigmoideum

Vesica urinaria

Symphysis pubica

Bulbus penis

Testis

Ampulla recti

Os coccygis

Prostata

Canalis analis

Fig. 1200 Pelvis, Pelvis, of the male;
magnetic resonance tomographic
image (MRI);
paramedian section;
viewed from the left.

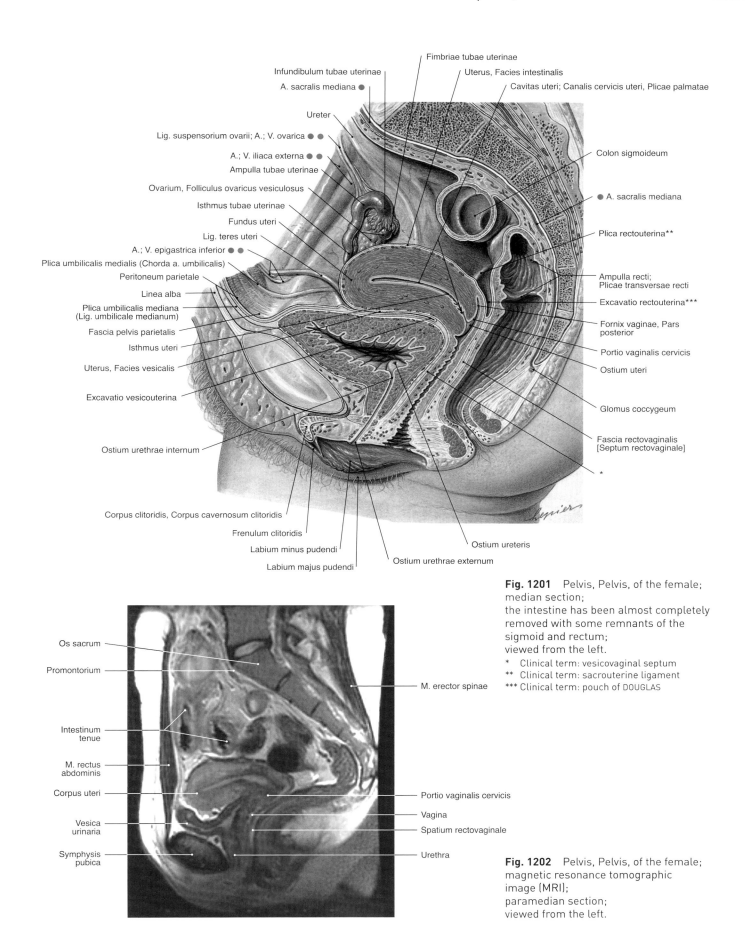

Fimbriae tubae uterinae

Infundibulum tubae uterinae

A. sacralis mediana ●

Uterus, Facies intestinalis

Cavitas uteri; Canalis cervicis uteri, Plicae palmatae

Ureter

Lig. suspensorium ovarii; A.; V. ovarica ● ●

A.; V. iliaca externa ● ●

Ampulla tubae uterinae

Ovarium, Folliculus ovaricus vesiculosus

Isthmus tubae uterinae

Fundus uteri

Lig. teres uteri

A.; V. epigastrica inferior ● ●

Plica umbilicalis medialis (Chorda a. umbilicalis)

Peritoneum parietale

Linea alba

Plica umbilicalis mediana
(Lig. umbilicale medianum)

Fascia pelvis parietalis

Isthmus uteri

Uterus, Facies vesicalis

Excavatio vesicouterina

Ostium urethrae internum

Corpus clitoridis, Corpus cavernosum clitoridis

Frenulum clitoridis

Labium minus pudendi

Labium majus pudendi

Colon sigmoideum

● A. sacralis mediana

Plica rectouterina**

Ampulla recti;
Plicae transversae recti

Excavatio rectouterina***

Fornix vaginae, Pars posterior

Portio vaginalis cervicis

Ostium uteri

Glomus coccygeum

Fascia rectovaginalis
[Septum rectovaginale]

*

Ostium ureteris

Ostium urethrae externum

Fig. 1201 Pelvis, Pelvis, of the female;
median section;
the intestine has been almost completely
removed with some remnants of the
sigmoid and rectum;
viewed from the left.

* Clinical term: vesicovaginal septum
** Clinical term: sacrouterine ligament
*** Clinical term: pouch of DOUGLAS

Os sacrum

Promontorium

Intestinum
tenue

M. rectus
abdominis

Corpus uteri

Vesica
urinaria

Symphysis
pubica

M. erector spinae

Portio vaginalis cervicis

Vagina

Spatium rectovaginale

Urethra

Fig. 1202 Pelvis, Pelvis, of the female;
magnetic resonance tomographic
image (MRI);
paramedian section;
viewed from the left.

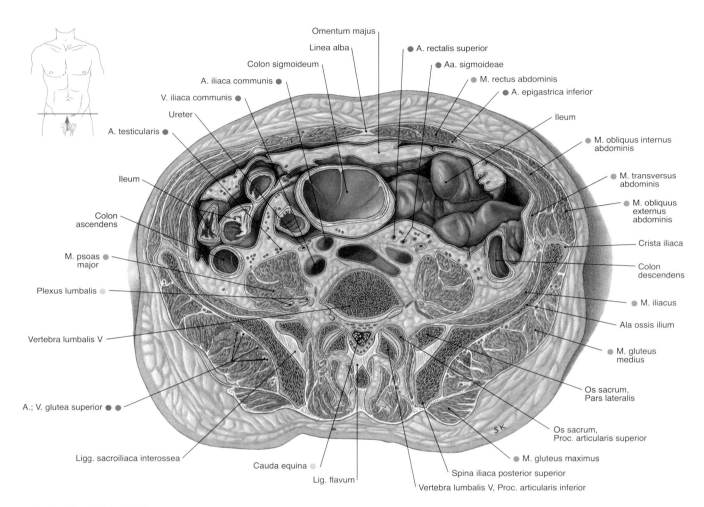

Omentum majus
Linea alba
Colon sigmoideum
A. iliaca communis ●
V. iliaca communis ●
Ureter
A. testicularis ●
Ileum
Colon ascendens
M. psoas major ●
Plexus lumbalis ●
Vertebra lumbalis V
A.; V. glutea superior ● ●
Ligg. sacroiliaca interossea
Cauda equina ●
Lig. flavum

● A. rectalis superior
● Aa. sigmoideae
● M. rectus abdominis
● A. epigastrica inferior
Ileum
● M. obliquus internus abdominis
● M. transversus abdominis
● M. obliquus externus abdominis
Crista iliaca
Colon descendens
● M. iliacus
Ala ossis ilium
● M. gluteus medius
Os sacrum, Pars lateralis
Os sacrum, Proc. articularis superior
● M. gluteus maximus
Spina iliaca posterior superior
Vertebra lumbalis V, Proc. articularis inferior

Fig. 1203   Pelvis, Pelvis;
transverse section at the level of the fifth lumbar vertebra.
This male specimen is different from Fig. 1191, 1193, 1195
and 1197.

As the sigmoid reaches far into the upper abdomen the figure
also displays the dome of colonic flexure. The thickness of the
adipose tissue layer on the gluteus medius muscle must be
taken into consideration when injecting intramuscularly.

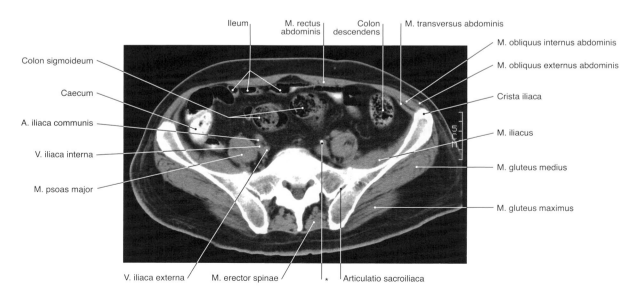

Ileum
M. rectus abdominis
Colon descendens
M. transversus abdominis
Colon sigmoideum
Caecum
A. iliaca communis
V. iliaca interna
M. psoas major
V. iliaca externa
M. erector spinae
*
Articulatio sacroiliaca
M. obliquus internus abdominis
M. obliquus externus abdominis
Crista iliaca
M. iliacus
M. gluteus medius
M. gluteus maximus

Fig. 1204   Pelvis, Pelvis;
computed tomographic cross-section (CT) at the level
of the first sacral vertebra after administration

of a contrast medium into the colon; supine position;
inferior view.

* Calcification in the wall of the iliac artery.

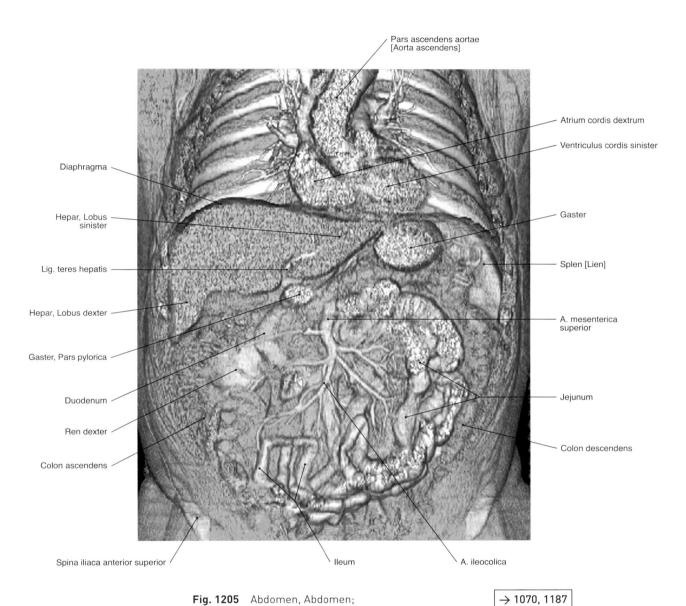

Pars ascendens aortae
[Aorta ascendens]

Atrium cordis dextrum

Ventriculus cordis sinister

Diaphragma

Hepar, Lobus
sinister

Gaster

Lig. teres hepatis

Splen [Lien]

Hepar, Lobus dexter

A. mesenterica
superior

Gaster, Pars pylorica

Duodenum

Ren dexter

Jejunum

Colon ascendens

Colon descendens

Spina iliaca anterior superior

Ileum

A. ileocolica

Fig. 1205 Abdomen, Abdomen;
volume-guided reconstruction in the frontal plane
based on horizontal computed tomographic sections (CT).
The section planes of organs such as the heart,
the stomach, the liver and parts of the small intestine,
appear granulated.

→ 1070, 1187

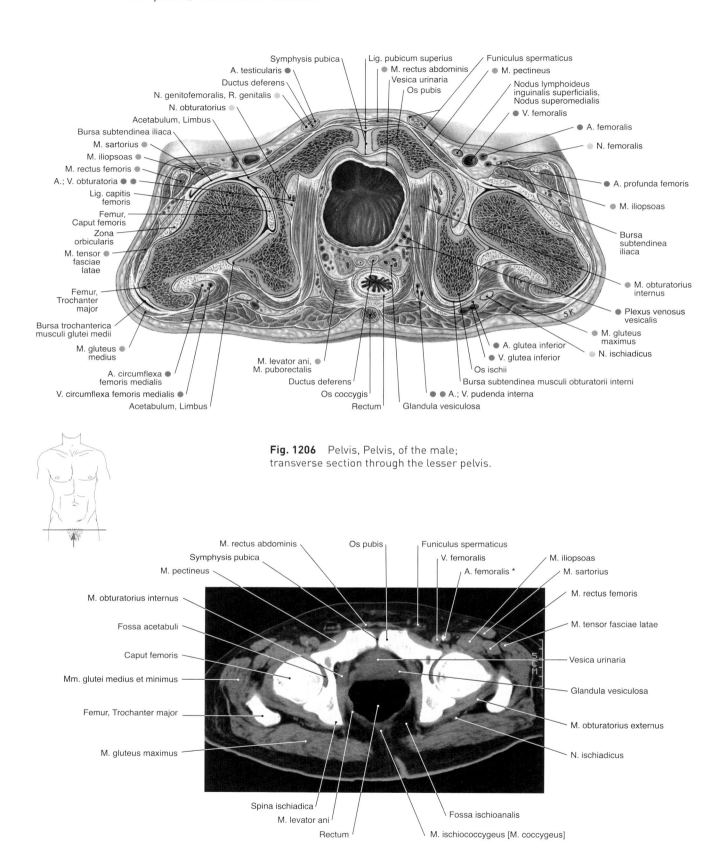

Symphysis pubica
A. testicularis ●
Ductus deferens
N. genitofemoralis, R. genitalis ●
N. obturatorius ●
Acetabulum, Limbus
Bursa subtendinea iliaca
M. sartorius ●
M. iliopsoas ●
M. rectus femoris ●
A.; V. obturatoria ● ●
Lig. capitis femoris
Femur, Caput femoris
Zona orbicularis
M. tensor fasciae latae ●
Femur, Trochanter major
Bursa trochanterica musculi glutei medii
M. gluteus medius ●
A. circumflexa femoris medialis ●
V. circumflexa femoris medialis ●
Acetabulum, Limbus

Lig. pubicum superius
● M. rectus abdominis
Vesica urinaria
Os pubis

Funiculus spermaticus
● M. pectineus
Nodus lymphoideus inguinalis superficialis, Nodus superomedialis
● V. femoralis
● A. femoralis
○ N. femoralis
● A. profunda femoris
● M. iliopsoas
Bursa subtendinea iliaca
● M. obturatorius internus
● Plexus venosus vesicalis
● M. gluteus maximus
● N. ischiadicus

M. levator ani, ●
M. puborectalis
Ductus deferens
Os coccygis
Rectum

● A. glutea inferior
● V. glutea inferior
Os ischii
Bursa subtendinea musculi obturatorii interni
● ● A.; V. pudenda interna
Glandula vesiculosa

Fig. 1206 Pelvis, Pelvis, of the male;
transverse section through the lesser pelvis.

M. rectus abdominis
Symphysis pubica
M. pectineus
M. obturatorius internus
Fossa acetabuli
Caput femoris
Mm. glutei medius et minimus
Femur, Trochanter major
M. gluteus maximus

Os pubis
Funiculus spermaticus
V. femoralis
A. femoralis *
M. iliopsoas
M. sartorius
M. rectus femoris
M. tensor fasciae latae
Vesica urinaria
Glandula vesiculosa
M. obturatorius externus
N. ischiadicus

Spina ischiadica
M. levator ani
Rectum
Fossa ischioanalis
M. ischiococcygeus [M. coccygeus]

Fig. 1207 Pelvis, Pelvis, of the male;
computed tomographic cross-section (CT) through
the lesser pelvis with the subject in supine position.
* Calcification in the medial part of the femoral artery

Female pelvis, transverse sections

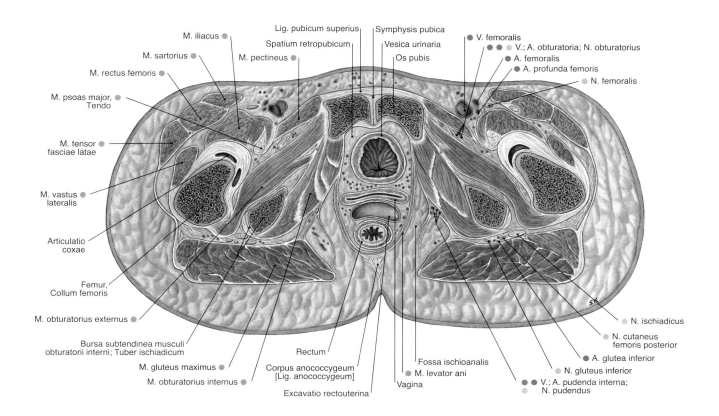

M. iliacus
M. sartorius
M. rectus femoris
M. psoas major, Tendo
M. tensor fasciae latae
M. vastus lateralis
Articulatio coxae
Femur, Collum femoris
M. obturatorius externus
Bursa subtendinea musculi obturatorii interni; Tuber ischiadicum
M. gluteus maximus
M. obturatorius internus

Lig. pubicum superius
Spatium retropubicum
M. pectineus

Symphysis pubica
Vesica urinaria
Os pubis

V. femoralis
V.; A. obturatoria; N. obturatorius
A. femoralis
A. profunda femoris
N. femoralis

Rectum
Corpus anococcygeum [Lig. anococcygeum]
Excavatio rectouterina

Fossa ischioanalis
M. levator ani
Vagina

N. ischiadicus
N. cutaneus femoris posterior
A. glutea inferior
N. gluteus inferior
V.; A. pudenda interna; N. pudendus

Fig. 1208   Pelvis, Pelvis, of the female; transverse section through the lesser pelvis at the level of the symphysis.

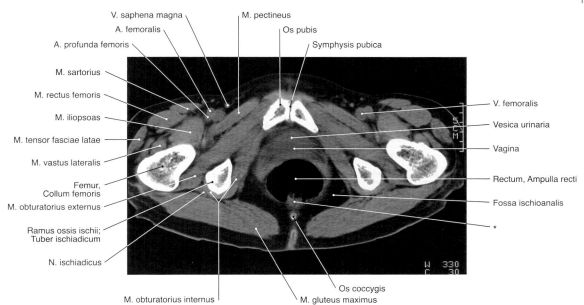

V. saphena magna
A. femoralis
A. profunda femoris
M. sartorius
M. rectus femoris
M. iliopsoas
M. tensor fasciae latae
M. vastus lateralis
Femur, Collum femoris
M. obturatorius externus
Ramus ossis ischii; Tuber ischiadicum
N. ischiadicus

M. pectineus
Os pubis
Symphysis pubica

V. femoralis
Vesica urinaria
Vagina
Rectum, Ampulla recti
Fossa ischioanalis
*

M. obturatorius internus
M. gluteus maximus
Os coccygis

Fig. 1209   Pelvis, Pelvis, of the female; computed tomographic cross-section (CT) through the lesser pelvis with the subject in supine position.
* Remnants of contrasting intestinal contents

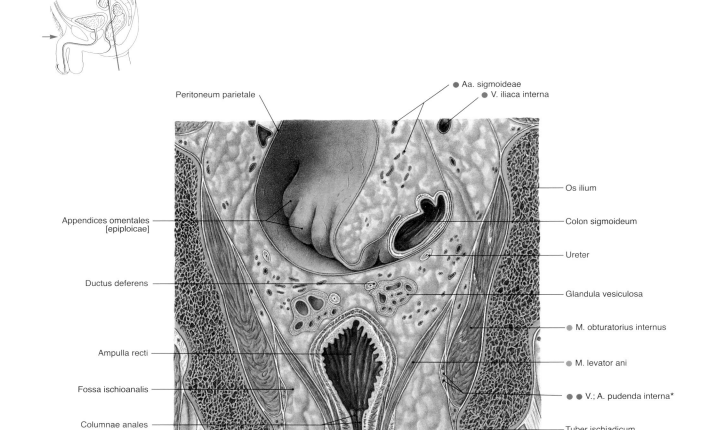

Peritoneum parietale

● Aa. sigmoideae
● V. iliaca interna

Os ilium

Appendices omentales [epiploicae]

Colon sigmoideum

Ureter

Ductus deferens

Glandula vesiculosa

● M. obturatorius internus

Ampulla recti

● M. levator ani

Fossa ischioanalis

● ● V.; A. pudenda interna*

Columnae anales

Tuber ischiadicum

● M. biceps femoris;
M. semitendinosus;
M. semimembranosus

Cutis

● M. levator ani, M. puborectalis

M. sphincter ani internus ●

● M. sphincter ani externus

Fig. 1210 Pelvis, Pelvis, of the male;
oblique frontal section through the lesser pelvis.
* Clinical term: ALCOCK's canal

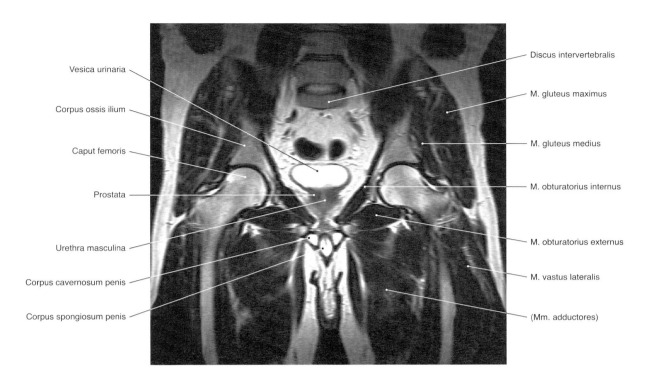

Vesica urinaria

Corpus ossis ilium

Caput femoris

Prostata

Urethra masculina

Corpus cavernosum penis

Corpus spongiosum penis

Discus intervertebralis

M. gluteus maximus

M. gluteus medius

M. obturatorius internus

M. obturatorius externus

M. vastus lateralis

(Mm. adductores)

Fig. 1211   Pelvis, Pelvis, of the male;
magnetic resonance tomographic image (MRI);
frontal section at the level of the hip joints;
ventral view.

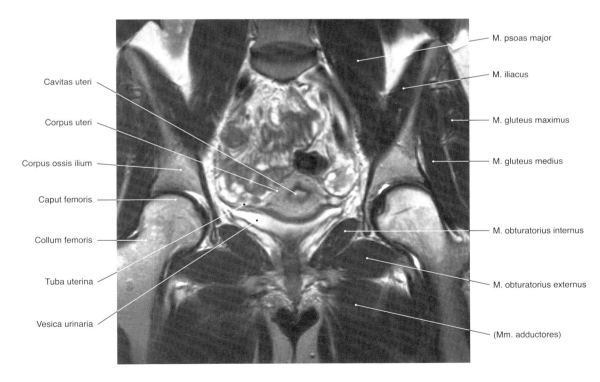

Cavitas uteri

Corpus uteri

Corpus ossis ilium

Caput femoris

Collum femoris

Tuba uterina

Vesica urinaria

M. psoas major

M. iliacus

M. gluteus maximus

M. gluteus medius

M. obturatorius internus

M. obturatorius externus

(Mm. adductores)

Fig. 1212   Pelvis, Pelvis, of the female;
magnetic resonance tomographic image (MRI);
frontal section at the level of the hip joints;
ventral view.

When the urinary bladder is empty, the uterus lies on the apex
of the bladder due to its anteflexion.

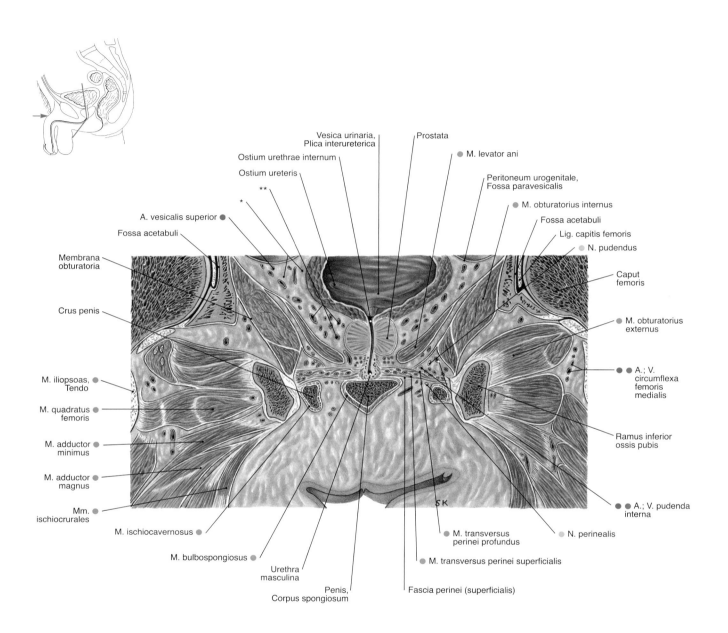

Vesica urinaria, Plica interureterica

Prostata

Ostium urethrae internum

● M. levator ani

Ostium ureteris

Peritoneum urogenitale, Fossa paravesicalis

**

*

● M. obturatorius internus

A. vesicalis superior ●

Fossa acetabuli

Fossa acetabuli

Lig. capitis femoris

Membrana obturatoria

● N. pudendus

Caput femoris

Crus penis

● M. obturatorius externus

M. iliopsoas, Tendo ●

●● A.; V. circumflexa femoris medialis

M. quadratus femoris ●

M. adductor minimus ●

Ramus inferior ossis pubis

M. adductor magnus ●

Mm. ● ischiocrurales

SK

●● A.; V. pudenda interna

M. ischiocavernosus ●

● M. transversus perinei profundus

● N. perinealis

M. bulbospongiosus ●

● M. transversus perinei superficialis

Urethra masculina

Penis, Corpus spongiosum

Fascia perinei (superficialis)

Fig. 1213 Pelvis, Pelvis, of the male; angled-frontal section through the urinary bladder.
* Clinical term: paracystium
** Clinical term: prostatic venous plexus

Female pelvic diaphragm, angled-frontal section

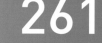

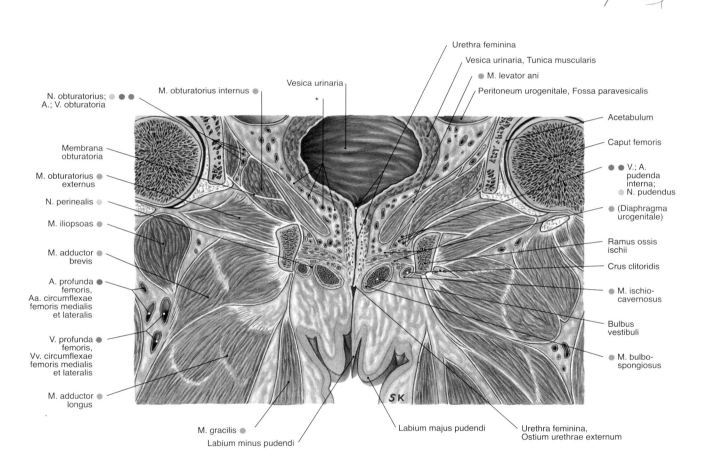

N. obturatorius; ●● ●
A.; V. obturatoria

Membrana
obturatoria

M. obturatorius ●
externus

N. perinealis ●

M. iliopsoas ●

M. adductor ●
brevis

A. profunda ●
femoris,
Aa. circumflexae
femoris medialis
et lateralis

V. profunda ●
femoris,
Vv. circumflexae
femoris medialis
et lateralis

M. adductor ●
longus

M. obturatorius internus ●

Vesica urinaria

*

M. gracilis ●

Labium minus pudendi

Urethra feminina

Vesica urinaria, Tunica muscularis

● M. levator ani

Peritoneum urogenitale, Fossa paravesicalis

Acetabulum

Caput femoris

●● V.; A.
pudenda
interna;
● N. pudendus

● (Diaphragma
urogenitale)

Ramus ossis
ischii

Crus clitoridis

● M. ischio-
cavernosus

Bulbus
vestibuli

● M. bulbo-
spongiosus

Labium majus pudendi

Urethra feminina,
Ostium urethrae externum

S K

Fig. 1214 Pelvis, Pelvis, of the female;
angled-frontal section through the urinary bladder.
* Paracystium with venous plexus

Surface anatomy

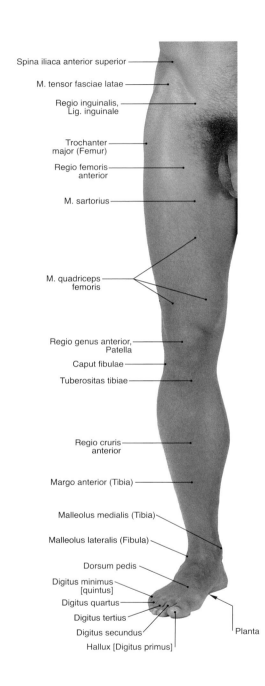

Spina iliaca anterior superior
M. tensor fasciae latae
Regio inguinalis, Lig. inguinale
Trochanter major (Femur)
Regio femoris anterior
M. sartorius
M. quadriceps femoris
Regio genus anterior, Patella
Caput fibulae
Tuberositas tibiae
Regio cruris anterior
Margo anterior (Tibia)
Malleolus medialis (Tibia)
Malleolus lateralis (Fibula)
Dorsum pedis
Digitus minimus [quintus]
Digitus quartus
Digitus tertius
Digitus secundus
Hallux [Digitus primus]
Planta

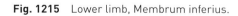

Fig. 1215 Lower limb, Membrum inferius.

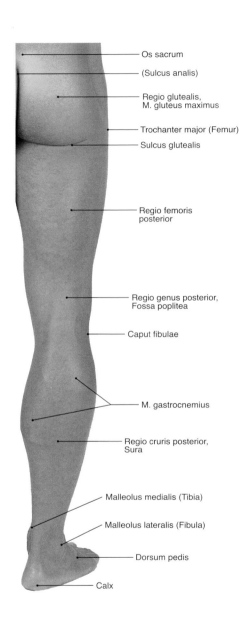

Os sacrum
(Sulcus analis)
Regio glutealis, M. gluteus maximus
Trochanter major (Femur)
Sulcus glutealis
Regio femoris posterior
Regio genus posterior, Fossa poplitea
Caput fibulae
M. gastrocnemius
Regio cruris posterior, Sura
Malleolus medialis (Tibia)
Malleolus lateralis (Fibula)
Dorsum pedis
Calx

Fig. 1216 Lower limb, Membrum inferius.

Skeleton of the lower limb, overview

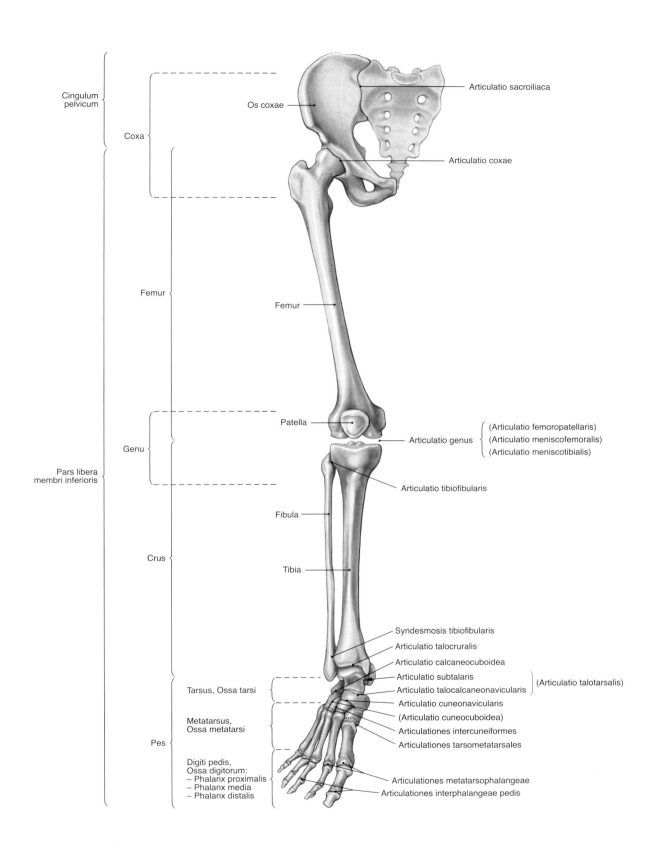

Cingulum
pelvicum

Coxa

Os coxae

Articulatio sacroiliaca

Articulatio coxae

Femur

Femur

Genu

Patella

Articulatio genus

{ (Articulatio femoropatellaris)
(Articulatio meniscofemoralis)
(Articulatio meniscotibialis) }

Articulatio tibiofibularis

Pars libera
membri inferioris

Crus

Fibula

Tibia

Syndesmosis tibiofibularis
Articulatio talocruralis
Articulatio calcaneocuboidea
Articulatio subtalaris
Articulatio talocalcaneonavicularis
} (Articulatio talotarsalis)

Tarsus, Ossa tarsi

Articulatio cuneonavicularis
(Articulatio cuneocuboidea)
Articulationes intercuneiformes
Articulationes tarsometatarsales

Metatarsus,
Ossa metatarsi

Pes

Digiti pedis,
Ossa digitorum:
– Phalanx proximalis
– Phalanx media
– Phalanx distalis

Articulationes metatarsophalangeae
Articulationes interphalangeae pedis

Fig. 1217   Lower limb, Membrum inferius;
skeleton and joints.

Pelvis

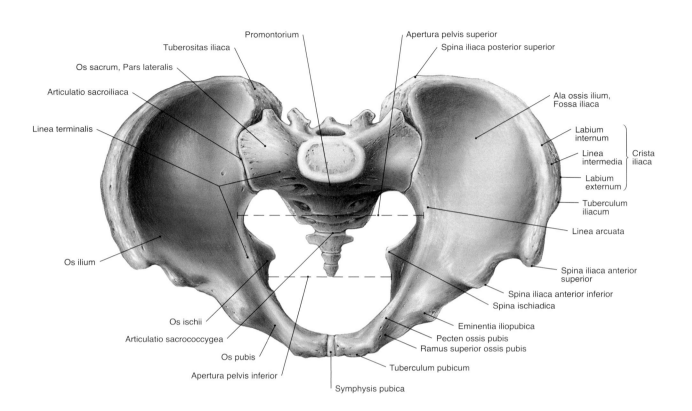

Promontorium

Tuberositas iliaca

Os sacrum, Pars lateralis

Articulatio sacroiliaca

Linea terminalis

Apertura pelvis superior

Spina iliaca posterior superior

Ala ossis ilium, Fossa iliaca

Labium internum

Linea intermedia } Crista iliaca

Labium externum

Tuberculum iliacum

Linea arcuata

Os ilium

Spina iliaca anterior superior

Spina iliaca anterior inferior

Spina ischiadica

Eminentia iliopubica

Pecten ossis pubis

Ramus superior ossis pubis

Os ischii

Articulatio sacrococcygea

Os pubis

Apertura pelvis inferior

Tuberculum pubicum

Symphysis pubica

Fig. 1218 Sacrum, Os sacrum, and pelvic girdle, Cingulum pelvicum.
The region cranial to the linea terminalis is referred to as the greater pelvis, Pelvis major, and the region caudal to it is known as lesser pelvis, Pelvis minor.

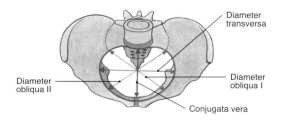

Diameter transversa

Diameter obliqua II

Diameter obliqua I

Conjugata vera

Fig. 1219 Pelvis, Pelvis; shape and dimensions of the pelvic inlet of the female.

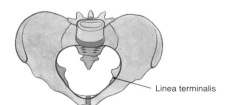

Linea terminalis

Fig. 1220 Pelvis, Pelvis; shape of the pelvic inlet of the male.

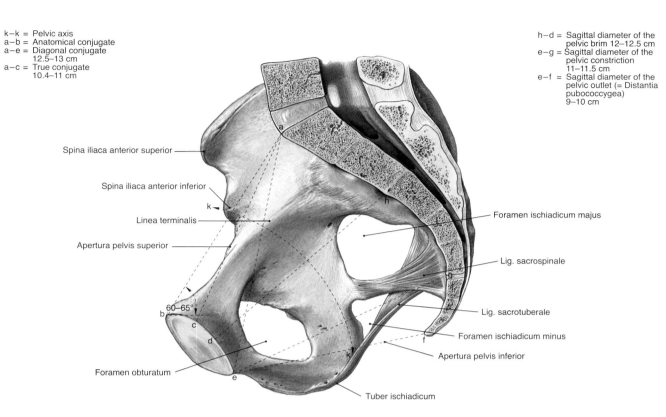

k−k = Pelvic axis
a−b = Anatomical conjugate
a−e = Diagonal conjugate
     12.5–13 cm
a−c = True conjugate
     10.4–11 cm

h−d = Sagittal diameter of the
     pelvic brim 12–12.5 cm
e−g = Sagittal diameter of the
     pelvic constriction
     11–11.5 cm
e−f = Sagittal diameter of the
     pelvic outlet (= Distantia
     pubococcygea)
     9–10 cm

Spina iliaca anterior superior

Spina iliaca anterior inferior

Linea terminalis

Apertura pelvis superior

60–65°

Foramen obturatum

Tuber ischiadicum

Foramen ischiadicum majus

Lig. sacrospinale

Lig. sacrotuberale

Foramen ischiadicum minus

Apertura pelvis inferior

Fig. 1221 Pelvis, Pelvis;
dimensions in the female;
median section.

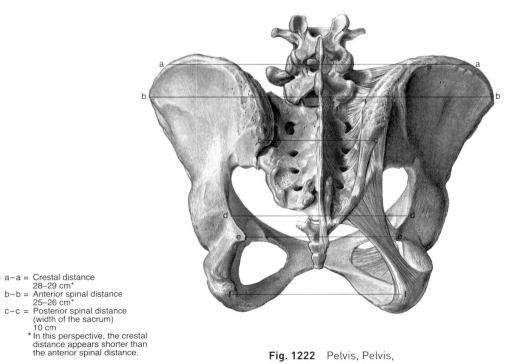

a−a = Crestal distance
     28–29 cm*
b−b = Anterior spinal distance
     25–26 cm*
c−c = Posterior spinal distance
     (width of the sacrum)
     10 cm
     * In this perspective, the crestal
     distance appears shorter than
     the anterior spinal distance.

d−d = Transverse diameter
     of the pelvic brim
     (= interacetabular line)
     12–12.5 cm
e−e = Transverse diameter of
     the pelvic constriction
     (= interspinal line)
     10.5 cm
f−f = Transverse diameter of
     the pelvic outlet
     (= tuberal diameter)
     11–12 cm)

Fig. 1222 Pelvis, Pelvis,
dimensions in the female.

Hip bone

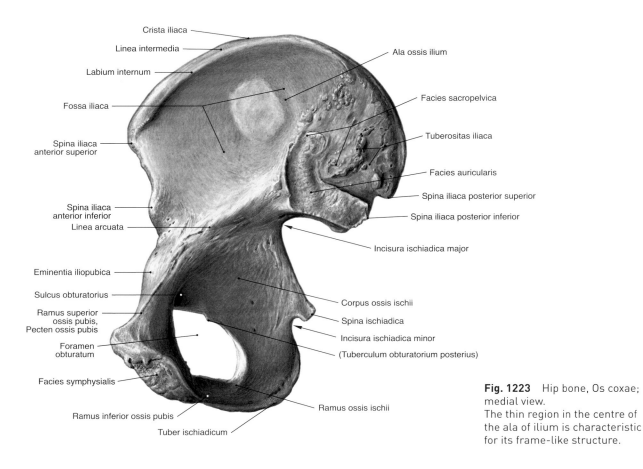

Crista iliaca
Linea intermedia
Labium internum
Fossa iliaca
Spina iliaca anterior superior
Spina iliaca anterior inferior
Linea arcuata
Eminentia iliopubica
Sulcus obturatorius
Ramus superior ossis pubis, Pecten ossis pubis
Foramen obturatum
Facies symphysialis
Ramus inferior ossis pubis
Tuber ischiadicum

Ala ossis ilium
Facies sacropelvica
Tuberositas iliaca
Facies auricularis
Spina iliaca posterior superior
Spina iliaca posterior inferior
Incisura ischiadica major
Corpus ossis ischii
Spina ischiadica
Incisura ischiadica minor
(Tuberculum obturatorium posterius)
Ramus ossis ischii

Fig. 1223 Hip bone, Os coxae; medial view.
The thin region in the centre of the ala of ilium is characteristic for its frame-like structure.

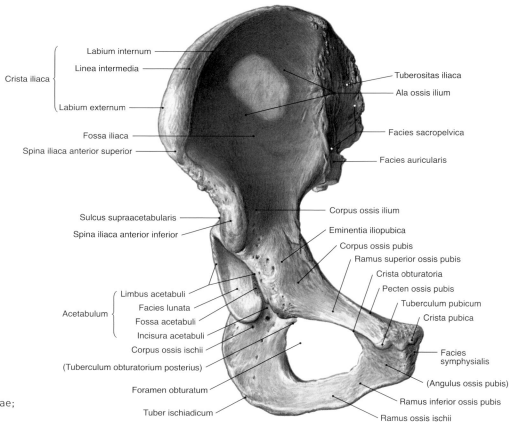

Crista iliaca
Labium internum
Linea intermedia
Labium externum
Fossa iliaca
Spina iliaca anterior superior
Sulcus supraacetabularis
Spina iliaca anterior inferior
Acetabulum
Limbus acetabuli
Facies lunata
Fossa acetabuli
Incisura acetabuli
Corpus ossis ischii
(Tuberculum obturatorium posterius)
Foramen obturatum
Tuber ischiadicum

Tuberositas iliaca
Ala ossis ilium
Facies sacropelvica
Facies auricularis
Corpus ossis ilium
Eminentia iliopubica
Corpus ossis pubis
Ramus superior ossis pubis
Crista obturatoria
Pecten ossis pubis
Tuberculum pubicum
Crista pubica
Facies symphysialis
(Angulus ossis pubis)
Ramus inferior ossis pubis
Ramus ossis ischii

Fig. 1224 Hip bone, Os coxae; ventral view.

Hip bone

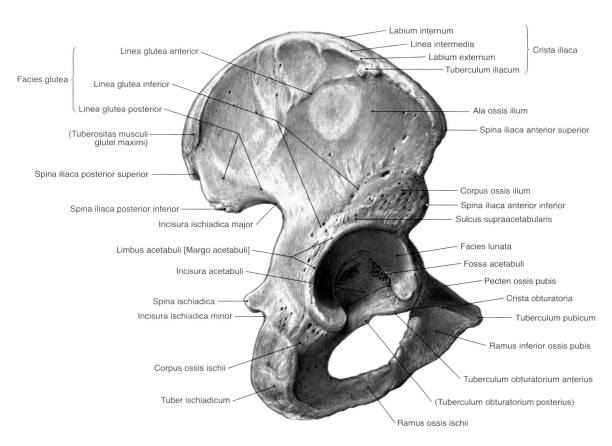

Labium internum
Linea intermedia
Labium externum
Tuberculum iliacum
Crista iliaca

Linea glutea anterior

Facies glutea
Linea glutea inferior

Linea glutea posterior

(Tuberositas musculi glutei maximi)

Spina iliaca posterior superior

Spina iliaca posterior inferior

Incisura ischiadica major

Limbus acetabuli [Margo acetabuli]

Incisura acetabuli

Spina ischiadica
Incisura ischiadica minor

Corpus ossis ischii

Tuber ischiadicum

Ala ossis ilium

Spina iliaca anterior superior

Corpus ossis ilium
Spina iliaca anterior inferior
Sulcus supraacetabularis

Facies lunata
Fossa acetabuli

Pecten ossis pubis
Crista obturatoria

Tuberculum pubicum

Ramus inferior ossis pubis

Tuberculum obturatorium anterius

(Tuberculum obturatorium posterius)

Ramus ossis ischii

Fig. 1225   Hip bone, Os coxae;
dorsolateral view.

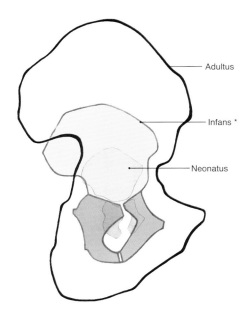

Adultus

Infans *

Neonatus

Fig. 1226   Hip bone, Os coxae;
development.
* Approximately sixth year of life

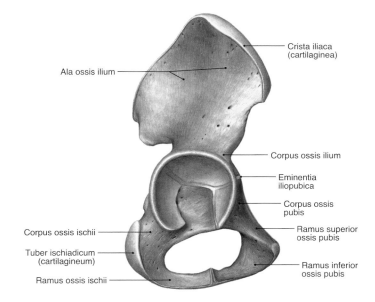

Ala ossis ilium

Crista iliaca
(cartilaginea)

Corpus ossis ilium

Eminentia
iliopubica

Corpus ossis
pubis

Ramus superior
ossis pubis

Corpus ossis ischii

Tuber ischiadicum
(cartilagineum)

Ramus ossis ischii

Ramus inferior
ossis pubis

Fig. 1227   Hip bone, Os coxae;
stage of development in a 6-year-old child.
In the acetabulum, the three parts of the hip bone are fused
to a Y-shaped cartilaginous junction. This junction ossifies at
the age of 13–18 years.

Joints of the pelvic girdle

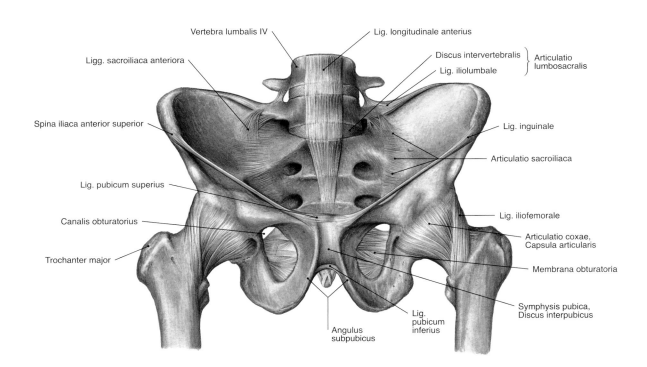

Vertebra lumbalis IV
Lig. longitudinale anterius
Ligg. sacroiliaca anteriora
Discus intervertebralis ⎱ Articulatio
Lig. iliolumbale ⎰ lumbosacralis
Spina iliaca anterior superior
Lig. inguinale
Articulatio sacroiliaca
Lig. pubicum superius
Lig. iliofemorale
Canalis obturatorius
Articulatio coxae, Capsula articularis
Trochanter major
Membrana obturatoria
Symphysis pubica, Discus interpubicus
Angulus subpubicus
Lig. pubicum inferius

Fig. 1228 Joints of the pelvic girdle,
Juncturae cinguli pelvici, and the lumbosacral joint,
Articulatio lumbosacralis, of the male.

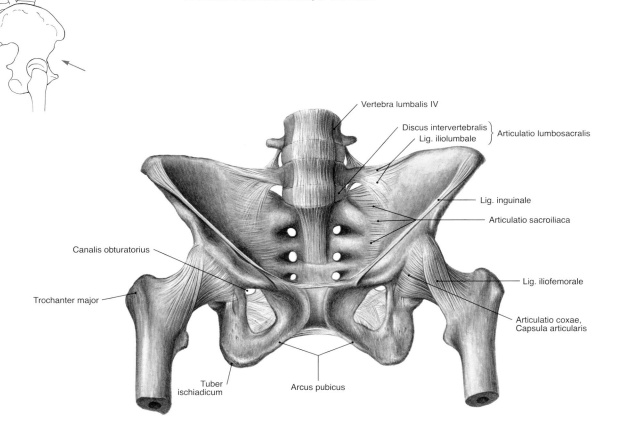

Vertebra lumbalis IV
Discus intervertebralis ⎱ Articulatio lumbosacralis
Lig. iliolumbale ⎰
Lig. inguinale
Articulatio sacroiliaca
Canalis obturatorius
Lig. iliofemorale
Trochanter major
Articulatio coxae, Capsula articularis
Tuber ischiadicum
Arcus pubicus

Fig. 1229 Joints of the pelvic girdle,
Juncturae cinguli pelvici, and the lumbosacral joint,
Articulatio lumbosacralis, of the female.

Joints of the pelvic girdle

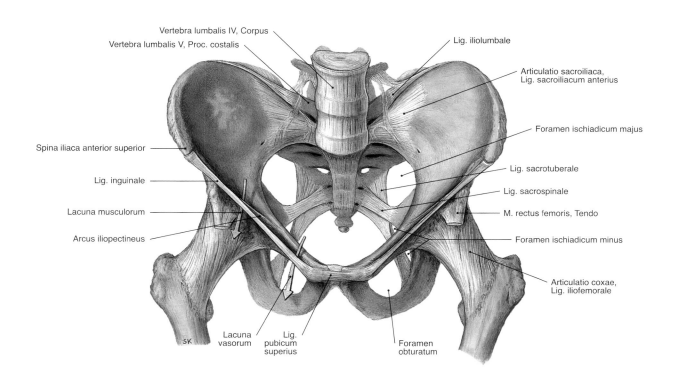

Vertebra lumbalis IV, Corpus
Vertebra lumbalis V, Proc. costalis
Lig. iliolumbale
Articulatio sacroiliaca, Lig. sacroiliacum anterius
Foramen ischiadicum majus
Spina iliaca anterior superior
Lig. inguinale
Lacuna musculorum
Arcus iliopectineus
Lig. sacrotuberale
Lig. sacrospinale
M. rectus femoris, Tendo
Foramen ischiadicum minus
Articulatio coxae, Lig. iliofemorale
Lacuna vasorum
Lig. pubicum superius
Foramen obturatum

Fig. 1230 Joints of the pelvic girdle, Juncturae cinguli pelvici, and the lumbosacral joint, Articulatio lumbosacralis, of the male.

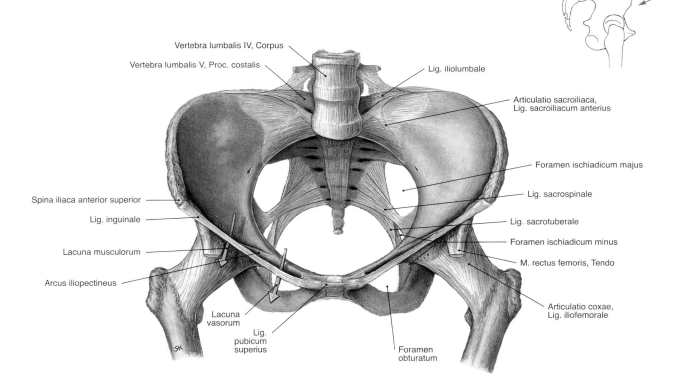

Vertebra lumbalis IV, Corpus
Vertebra lumbalis V, Proc. costalis
Lig. iliolumbale
Articulatio sacroiliaca, Lig. sacroiliacum anterius
Foramen ischiadicum majus
Lig. sacrospinale
Spina iliaca anterior superior
Lig. inguinale
Lig. sacrotuberale
Foramen ischiadicum minus
Lacuna musculorum
M. rectus femoris, Tendo
Arcus iliopectineus
Articulatio coxae, Lig. iliofemorale
Lacuna vasorum
Lig. pubicum superius
Foramen obturatum

Fig. 1231 Joints of the pelvic girdle, Juncturae cinguli pelvici, and the lumbosacral joint, Articulatio lumbosacralis, of the female.

Joints of the pelvic girdle

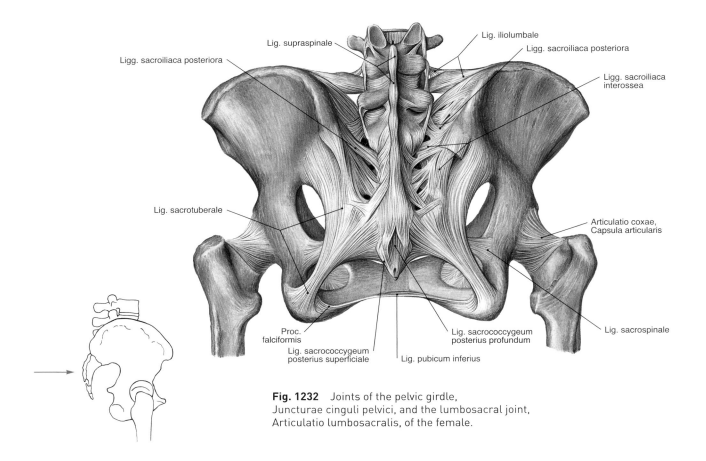

Lig. supraspinale

Ligg. sacroiliaca posteriora

Lig. iliolumbale

Ligg. sacroiliaca posteriora

Ligg. sacroiliaca interossea

Lig. sacrotuberale

Articulatio coxae, Capsula articularis

Proc. falciformis

Lig. sacrococcygeum posterius superficiale

Lig. sacrococcygeum posterius profundum

Lig. pubicum inferius

Lig. sacrospinale

Fig. 1232 Joints of the pelvic girdle, Juncturae cinguli pelvici, and the lumbosacral joint, Articulatio lumbosacralis, of the female.

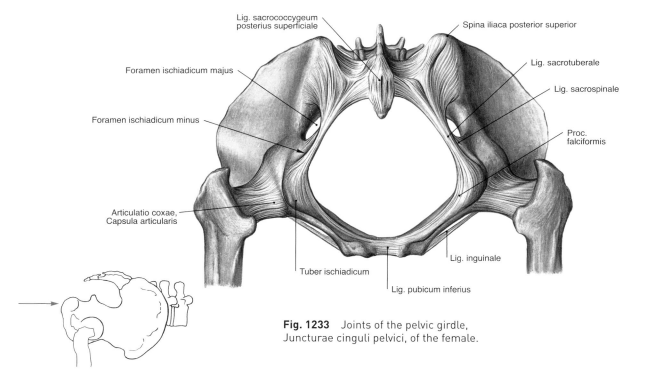

Lig. sacrococcygeum posterius superficiale

Spina iliaca posterior superior

Foramen ischiadicum majus

Lig. sacrotuberale

Lig. sacrospinale

Foramen ischiadicum minus

Proc. falciformis

Articulatio coxae, Capsula articularis

Lig. inguinale

Tuber ischiadicum

Lig. pubicum inferius

Fig. 1233 Joints of the pelvic girdle, Juncturae cinguli pelvici, of the female.

Joints of the pelvic girdle

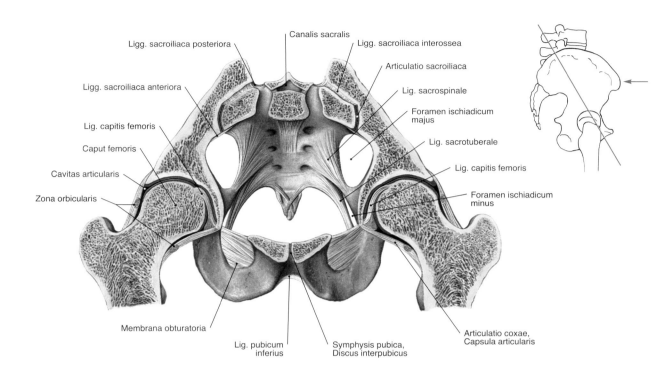

Ligg. sacroiliaca posteriora

Ligg. sacroiliaca anteriora

Lig. capitis femoris

Caput femoris

Cavitas articularis

Zona orbicularis

Canalis sacralis

Ligg. sacroiliaca interossea

Articulatio sacroiliaca

Lig. sacrospinale

Foramen ischiadicum majus

Lig. sacrotuberale

Lig. capitis femoris

Foramen ischiadicum minus

Membrana obturatoria

Lig. pubicum inferius

Symphysis pubica, Discus interpubicus

Articulatio coxae, Capsula articularis

Fig. 1234   Joints of the pelvic girdle,
Juncturae cinguli pelvici, of the female.

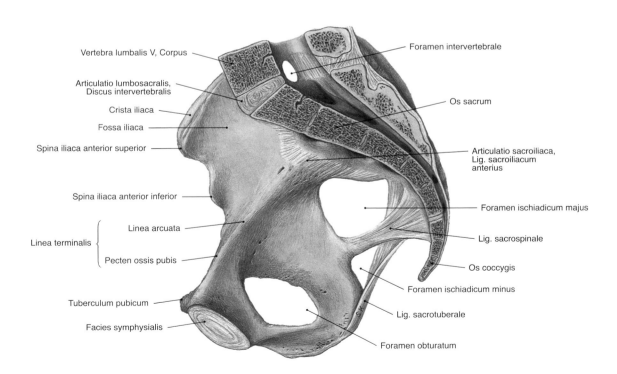

Vertebra lumbalis V, Corpus

Articulatio lumbosacralis, Discus intervertebralis

Crista iliaca

Fossa iliaca

Spina iliaca anterior superior

Spina iliaca anterior inferior

Linea arcuata

Linea terminalis

Pecten ossis pubis

Tuberculum pubicum

Facies symphysialis

Foramen intervertebrale

Os sacrum

Articulatio sacroiliaca, Lig. sacroiliacum anterius

Foramen ischiadicum majus

Lig. sacrospinale

Os coccygis

Foramen ischiadicum minus

Lig. sacrotuberale

Foramen obturatum

Fig. 1235   Joints of the pelvic girdle,
Juncturae cinguli pelvici, and the lumbosacral joint,
Articulatio lumbosacralis, of the female;
median section.

Normally, the anterior border of the lowest intervertebral disc
forms the furthest projecting point of the posterior circumference
of the pelvic inlet. Radiographically, the most anterior part of the
sacrum is referred to as promontory.

Joints of the pelvic girdle

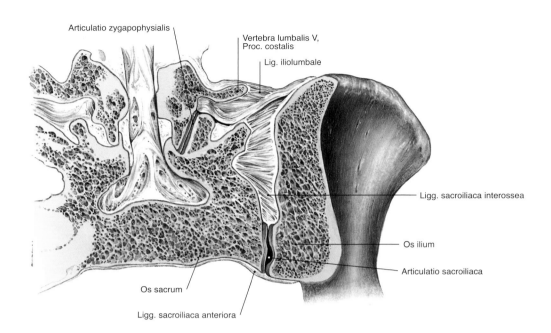

Articulatio zygapophysialis

Vertebra lumbalis V, Proc. costalis

Lig. iliolumbale

Ligg. sacroiliaca interossea

Os ilium

Articulatio sacroiliaca

Os sacrum

Ligg. sacroiliaca anteriora

Fig. 1236   Sacroiliac joint, Articulatio sacroiliaca; frontal section.

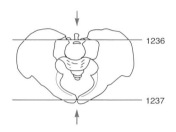

1236

1237

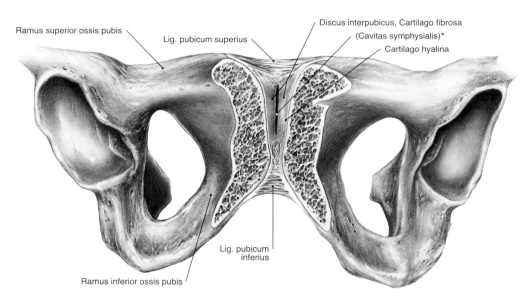

Ramus superior ossis pubis

Lig. pubicum superius

Discus interpubicus, Cartilago fibrosa

(Cavitas symphysialis)*

Cartilago hyalina

Lig. pubicum inferius

Ramus inferior ossis pubis

Fig. 1237   Pubic symphysis, Symphysis pubica; oblique section in the direction of the longitudinal axis of the symphysis.
The interpubic disc consists of fibrous cartilage, with the exception of the articular symphysial surfaces of both pubic bones that are covered with hyaline cartilage. A longitudinal flat cleft occurs after the first decade of life (*).

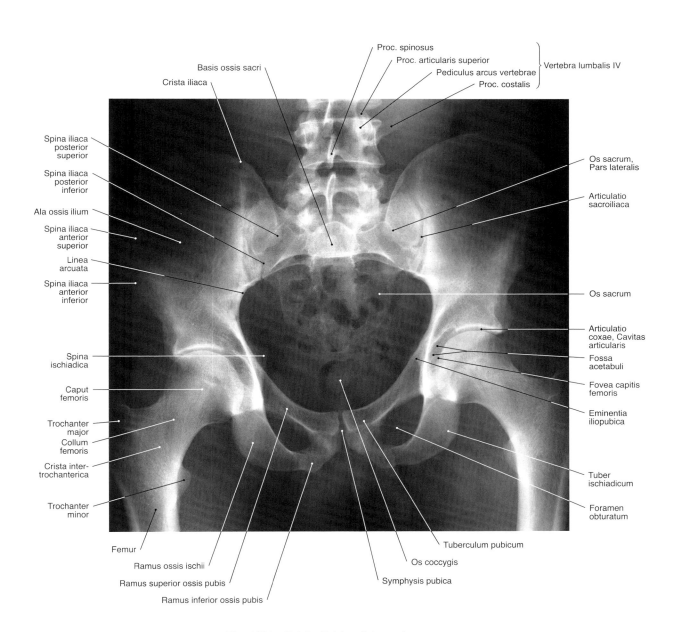

Proc. spinosus
Proc. articularis superior
Basis ossis sacri
Pediculus arcus vertebrae
Crista iliaca
Proc. costalis
Vertebra lumbalis IV

Spina iliaca posterior superior
Os sacrum, Pars lateralis

Spina iliaca posterior inferior
Articulatio sacroiliaca

Ala ossis ilium
Spina iliaca anterior superior
Linea arcuata
Spina iliaca anterior inferior
Os sacrum

Articulatio coxae, Cavitas articularis
Spina ischiadica
Fossa acetabuli
Caput femoris
Fovea capitis femoris
Trochanter major
Collum femoris
Eminentia iliopubica
Crista inter-trochanterica
Trochanter minor
Tuber ischiadicum
Femur
Foramen obturatum
Ramus ossis ischii
Tuberculum pubicum
Ramus superior ossis pubis
Os coccygis
Ramus inferior ossis pubis
Symphysis pubica

Fig. 1238 Pelvis, Pelvis, of the male;
AP-radiograph with the central beam directed
onto the third sacral segment; upright position.

Pelvis, development

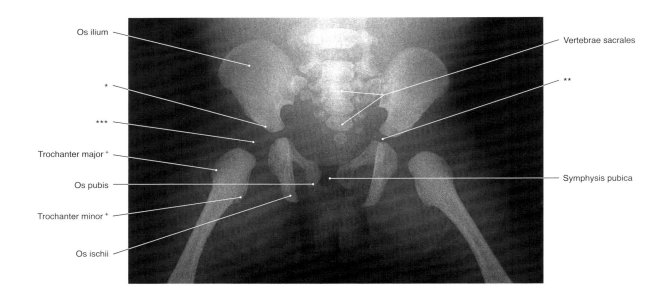

Os ilium

*

***

Trochanter major +

Os pubis

Trochanter minor +

Os ischii

Vertebrae sacrales

**

Symphysis pubica

Fig. 1239 Pelvis, Pelvis, and femur, Femur; AP-radiograph of a female, premature baby (eighth month of pregnancy).

*   Osseous roof of the acetabulum
**   Y-shaped junction in the acetabular fossa
***The ossification centre in the head of the femur does not appear before the third to fifth month of life.
\+   At this age, both greater trochanters only become apparent as small protuberances of the bone of the diaphysis.

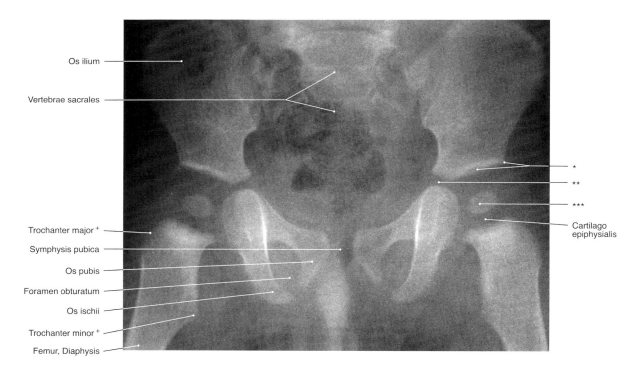

Os ilium

Vertebrae sacrales

Trochanter major +

Symphysis pubica

Os pubis

Foramen obturatum

Os ischii

Trochanter minor +

Femur, Diaphysis

*

**

***

Cartilago epiphysialis

Fig. 1240 Pelvis, Pelvis, and femur, Femur; AP-radiograph of a 12-month-old boy.

*   Osseous roof of the acetabulum
**   Y-shaped junction in the acetabular fossa
***Ossification centre in the epiphysis of the head of the femur
\+   At this age, both greater trochanters only become apparent as small protuberances of the bone of the diaphysis.

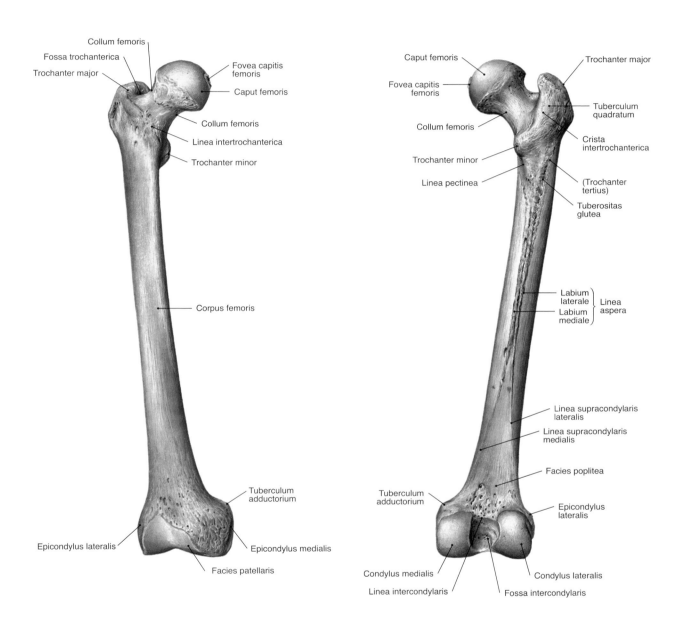

Collum femoris
Fossa trochanterica
Trochanter major
Fovea capitis femoris
Caput femoris
Collum femoris
Linea intertrochanterica
Trochanter minor
Corpus femoris
Tuberculum adductorium
Epicondylus lateralis
Epicondylus medialis
Facies patellaris

Caput femoris
Fovea capitis femoris
Collum femoris
Trochanter minor
Linea pectinea
Trochanter major
Tuberculum quadratum
Crista intertrochanterica
(Trochanter tertius)
Tuberositas glutea
Labium laterale
Labium mediale
Linea aspera
Linea supracondylaris lateralis
Linea supracondylaris medialis
Facies poplitea
Tuberculum adductorium
Epicondylus lateralis
Condylus medialis
Linea intercondylaris
Fossa intercondylaris
Condylus lateralis

Fig. 1241 Femur, Femur;
ventral view.

Fig. 1242 Femur, Femur;
dorsal view.

Femur

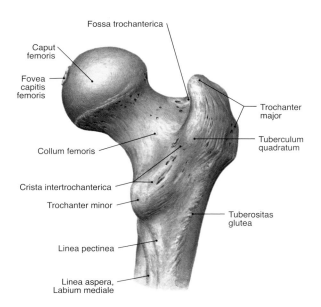

Fossa trochanterica
Caput femoris
Fovea capitis femoris
Collum femoris
Crista intertrochanterica
Trochanter minor
Linea pectinea
Linea aspera, Labium mediale
Trochanter major
Tuberculum quadratum
Tuberositas glutea

Fig. 1243   Femur, Femur;
proximal extremity;
dorsal view.

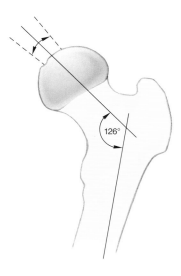

126°

Fig. 1244   Femur, Femur;
variability of the angle of the neck of the femur;
dorsal view.
The angle between the neck and the shaft of the femur is
referred to as neck-shaft angle. It is 150° in infants and about
126° in the adult.

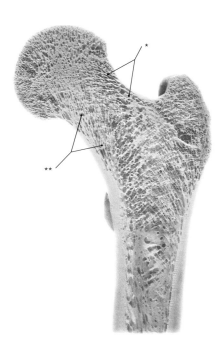

*

**

Fig. 1245   Femur, Femur;
trabecular structure of the femoral bone with a large
neck-shaft angle (coxa valga); section in the plane of the
angle of anterior torsion (60%).
The lateral plates of the trabecular bone* ("tensile system")
are only poorly developed, whereas the medial plates**
("compressive system") are much stronger.

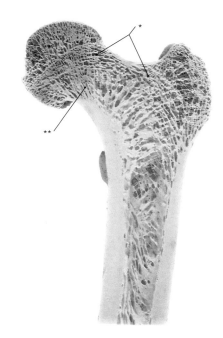

*

**

Fig. 1246   Femur, Femur;
trabecular structure of the femoral bone with a small
neck-shaft angle (coxa vara); section in the plane of the
angle of anterior torsion (60%).
The lateral plates of the trabecular bone * ("tensile system")
are well developed, while the medial plates **
("compressive system") are developed less strong. As a
result of the high demand of flexion, the cortex on the inner
side of the femoral neck is particularly thick.

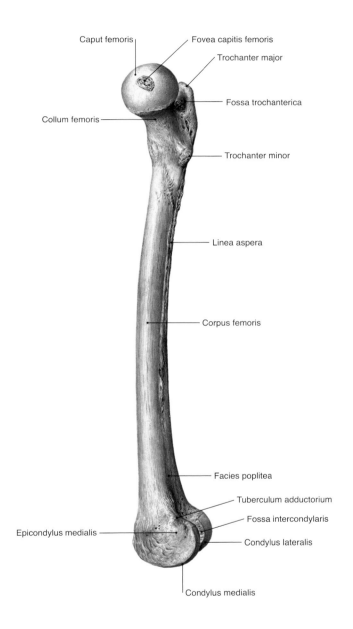

Caput femoris
Fovea capitis femoris
Trochanter major
Fossa trochanterica
Collum femoris
Trochanter minor
Linea aspera
Corpus femoris
Facies poplitea
Tuberculum adductorium
Fossa intercondylaris
Epicondylus medialis
Condylus lateralis
Condylus medialis

Fig. 1247 Femur, Femur;
medial view.

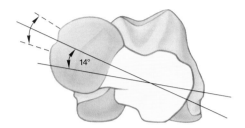

14°

Fig. 1248 Femur, Femur;
variability of the angle of anterior torsion; the proximal
end of the femur has been projected over the distal end;
proximal view.
The angle of anterior torsion is about 30° in infants
and about 14° in adults.

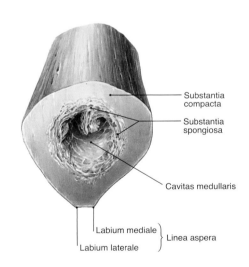

Substantia
compacta
Substantia
spongiosa
Cavitas medullaris
Labium mediale
Labium laterale
Linea aspera

Fig. 1249 Femur, Femur;
cross-section through the middle of the shaft;
distal view.

Hip joint

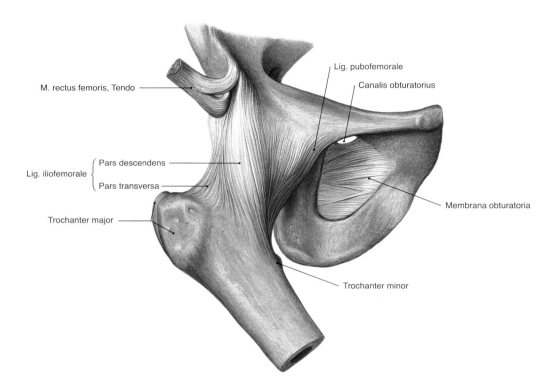

M. rectus femoris, Tendo

Lig. pubofemorale
Canalis obturatorius

Lig. iliofemorale {
Pars descendens
Pars transversa

Trochanter major

Membrana obturatoria

Trochanter minor

Fig. 1250 Hip joint, Articulatio coxae; ventrodistal view.

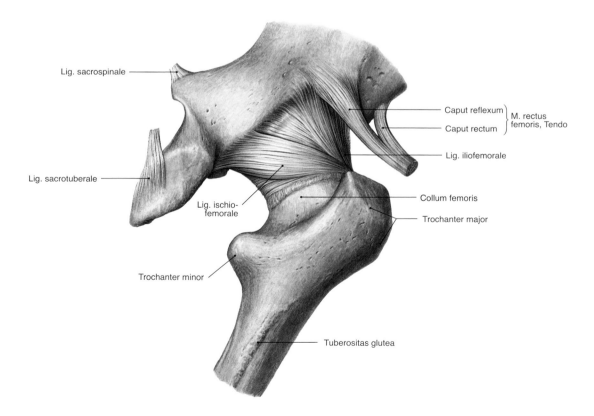

Lig. sacrospinale

Caput reflexum
Caput rectum
} M. rectus femoris, Tendo

Lig. iliofemorale

Lig. sacrotuberale

Lig. ischio-femorale

Collum femoris

Trochanter major

Trochanter minor

Tuberositas glutea

Fig. 1251 Hip joint, Articulatio coxae; dorsal view.

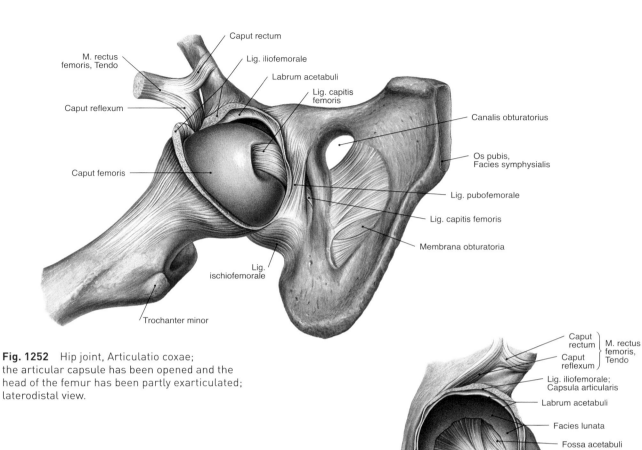

Fig. 1252 Hip joint, Articulatio coxae;
the articular capsule has been opened and the
head of the femur has been partly exarticulated;
laterodistal view.

Fig. 1253 Hip joint, Articulatio coxae;
aspect of the acetabulum after removal of the articular
capsule and exarticulation of the head of the femur;
laterodistal view.

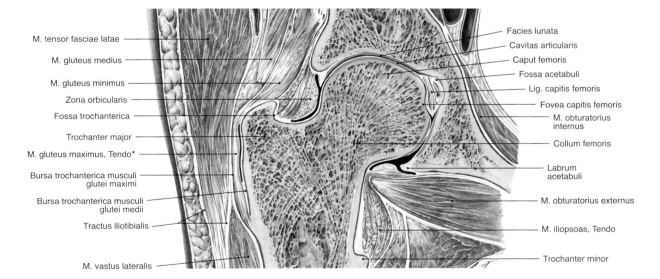

Fig. 1254 Hip joint, Articulatio coxae;
vertical section at the plane of the angle of antetorsion.
* Radiations into the iliotibial tract

Hip joint, radiography

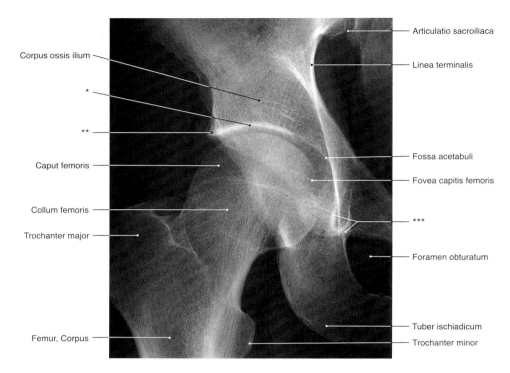

Fig. 1255 Hip joint, Articulatio coxae;
AP-radiograph; upright position on both legs.

* Clinical term: acetabular roof = tangential projection of the lunate surface
** Clinical term: edge of the acetabular roof = the most lateral projection
of the acetabulum
*** Clinical term: KÖHLER's teardrop = projection of the acetabular fossa

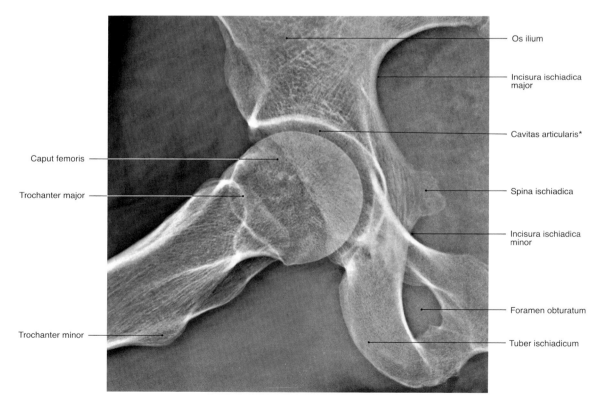

Fig. 1256 Hip joint, Articulatio coxae;
AP-radiograph; supine position with the thigh abducted
and flexed (so-called LAUENSTEIN projection).

* Due to minimal absorption of X-rays by cartilage, the articular cleft
appears abnormally broad.

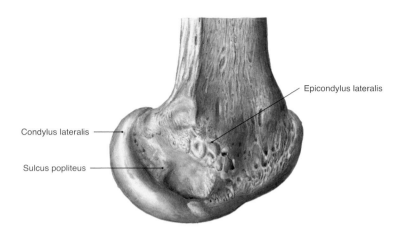

Fig. 1257 Femur, Femur;
distal extremity;
lateral view.

Epicondylus lateralis

Condylus lateralis

Sulcus popliteus

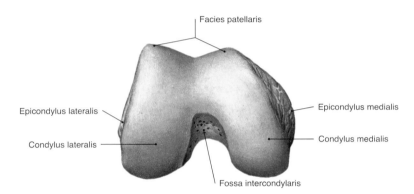

Facies patellaris

Epicondylus lateralis

Condylus lateralis

Epicondylus medialis

Condylus medialis

Fossa intercondylaris

Fig. 1258 Femur, Femur;
distal extremity;
distal view.

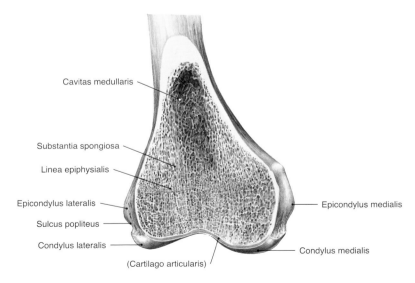

Cavitas medullaris

Substantia spongiosa

Linea epiphysialis

Epicondylus lateralis

Sulcus popliteus

Condylus lateralis

(Cartilago articularis)

Epicondylus medialis

Condylus medialis

Fig. 1259 Femur, Femur;
frontal section through the distal part;
ventral view.

Tibia

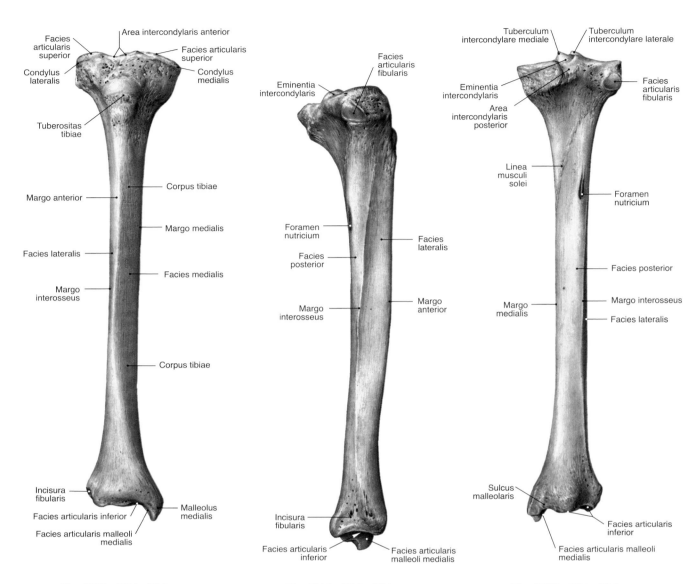

Fig. 1260 Tibia, Tibia; ventral view.

Fig. 1261 Tibia, Tibia; lateral view.

Fig. 1262 Tibia, Tibia; dorsal view.

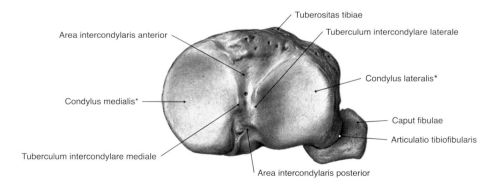

Fig. 1263 Tibia, Tibia, and fibula, Fibula; proximal view.

* The articular surfaces of the condyles together are referred to as superior articular surface.

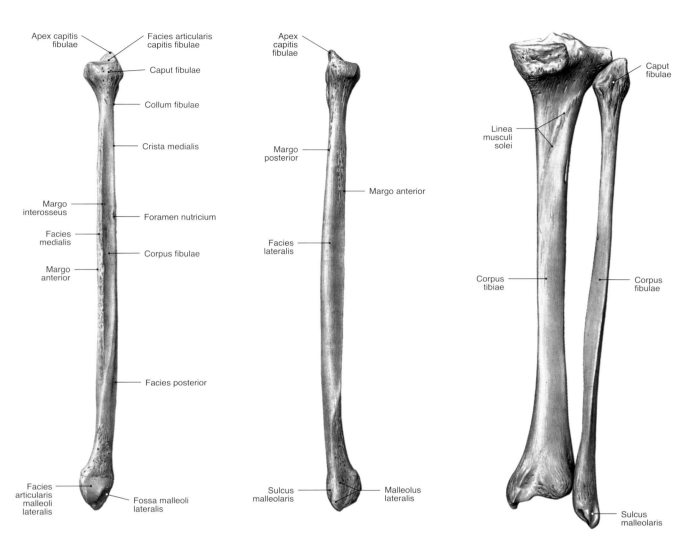

Apex capitis
fibulae

Facies articularis
capitis fibulae

Caput fibulae

Collum fibulae

Crista medialis

Margo
interosseus

Facies
medialis

Margo
anterior

Facies posterior

Facies
articularis
malleoli
lateralis

Foramen nutricium

Corpus fibulae

Fossa malleoli
lateralis

Fig. 1264   Fibula, Fibula;
medial view.

Apex
capitis
fibulae

Margo
posterior

Margo anterior

Facies
lateralis

Sulcus
malleolaris

Malleolus
lateralis

Fig. 1265   Fibula, Fibula;
lateral view.

Caput
fibulae

Linea
musculi
solei

Corpus
tibiae

Corpus
fibulae

Sulcus
malleolaris

Fig. 1266   Tibia, Tibia, and
fibula, Fibula;
dorsal view.

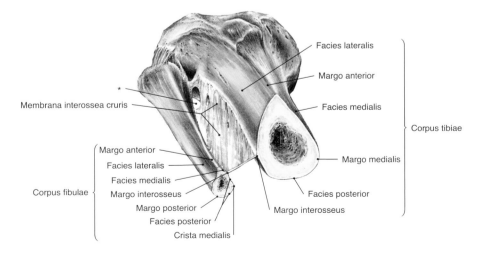

Facies lateralis

Margo anterior

Facies medialis

*

Membrana interossea cruris

Corpus tibiae

Margo anterior

Facies lateralis

Facies medialis

Margo interosseus

Margo posterior

Facies posterior

Crista medialis

Corpus fibulae

Margo medialis

Facies posterior

Margo interosseus

Fig. 1267   Tibia, Tibia, and fibula, Fibula;
cross-section with the interosseous membrane of leg;
distal view.
* Opening for the anterior tibial artery

Patella and knee joint

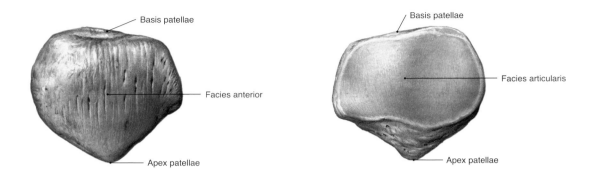

Fig. 1268 Patella, Patella;
ventral view.

Fig. 1269 Patella, Patella;
dorsal view.

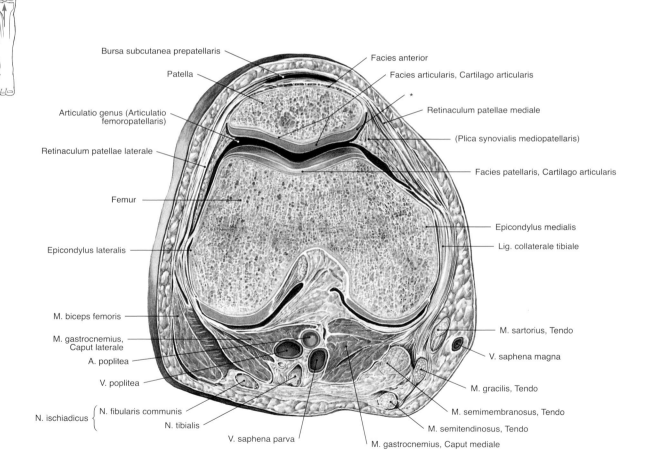

Fig. 1270 Knee joint, Articulatio genus;
cross-section.
* Medial border facet

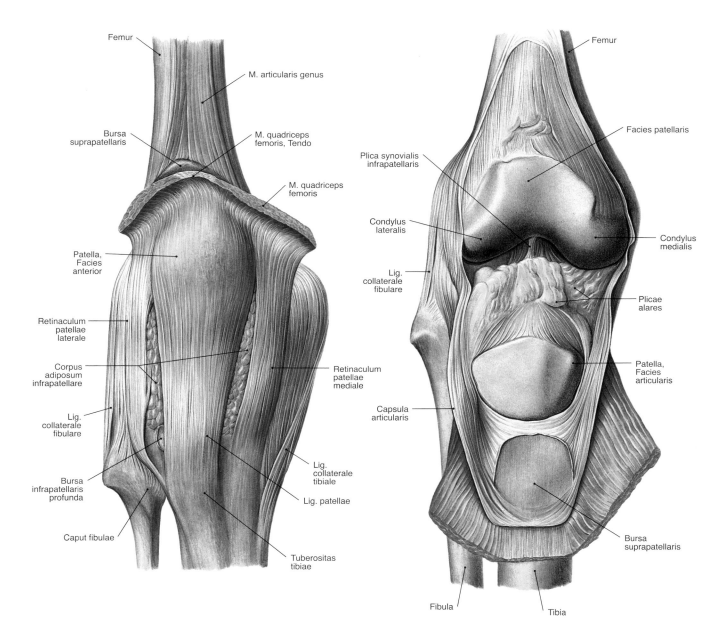

Femur

M. articularis genus

Bursa
suprapatellaris

M. quadriceps
femoris, Tendo

M. quadriceps
femoris

Patella,
Facies
anterior

Retinaculum
patellae
laterale

Corpus
adiposum
infrapatellare

Retinaculum
patellae
mediale

Lig.
collaterale
fibulare

Bursa
infrapatellaris
profunda

Lig.
collaterale
tibiale

Lig. patellae

Caput fibulae

Tuberositas
tibiae

Femur

Plica synovialis
infrapatellaris

Facies patellaris

Condylus
lateralis

Condylus
medialis

Lig.
collaterale
fibulare

Plicae
alares

Patella,
Facies
articularis

Capsula
articularis

Bursa
suprapatellaris

Fibula

Tibia

Fig. 1271 Knee joint, Articulatio genus;
intact articular capsule;
ventral view.

Fig. 1272 Knee joint, Articulatio genus;
the anterior part of the articular capsule has
been reflected downwards after dissection of
the quadriceps muscle;
the suprapatellar bursa has been opened;
ventral view.

Knee joint

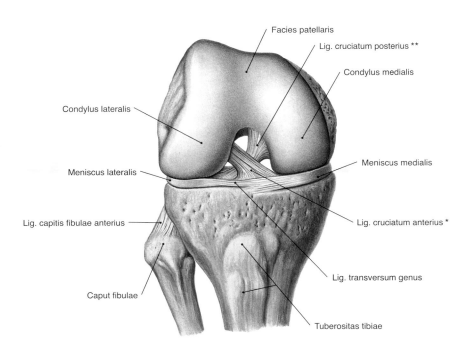

Facies patellaris

Lig. cruciatum posterius **

Condylus medialis

Condylus lateralis

Meniscus medialis

Meniscus lateralis

Lig. capitis fibulae anterius

Lig. cruciatum anterius *

Lig. transversum genus

Caput fibulae

Tuberositas tibiae

Fig. 1273   Knee joint, Articulatio genus;
in 90° flexion; the articular capsule and the lateral
ligaments have been removed;
ventral view.

* Clinical term: ACL (= anterior cruciate ligament)
** Clinical term: PCL (= posterior cruciate ligament)

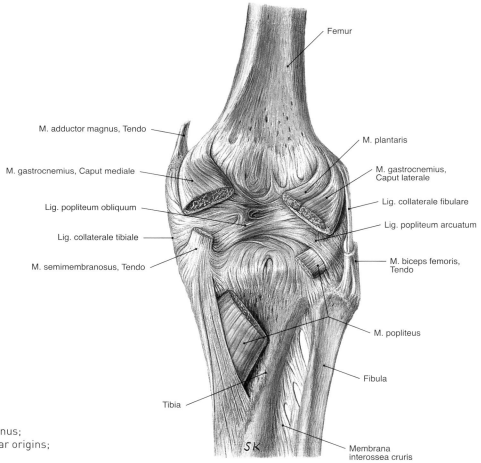

Femur

M. adductor magnus, Tendo

M. plantaris

M. gastrocnemius, Caput mediale

M. gastrocnemius,
Caput laterale

Lig. popliteum obliquum

Lig. collaterale fibulare

Lig. popliteum arcuatum

Lig. collaterale tibiale

M. semimembranosus, Tendo

M. biceps femoris,
Tendo

M. popliteus

Fibula

Tibia

Membrana
interossea cruris

Fig. 1274   Knee joint, Articulatio genus;
intact articular capsule with muscular origins;
dorsal view.

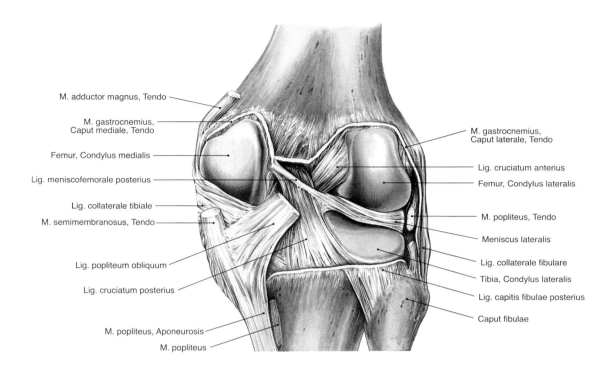

M. adductor magnus, Tendo

M. gastrocnemius,
Caput mediale, Tendo

Femur, Condylus medialis

Lig. meniscofemorale posterius

Lig. collaterale tibiale

M. semimembranosus, Tendo

Lig. popliteum obliquum

Lig. cruciatum posterius

M. popliteus, Aponeurosis

M. popliteus

M. gastrocnemius,
Caput laterale, Tendo

Lig. cruciatum anterius

Femur, Condylus lateralis

M. popliteus, Tendo

Meniscus lateralis

Lig. collaterale fibulare

Tibia, Condylus lateralis

Lig. capitis fibulae posterius

Caput fibulae

Fig. 1275 Knee joint, Articulatio genus;
exposure of the cruciate ligaments and the menisci;
dorsal view.

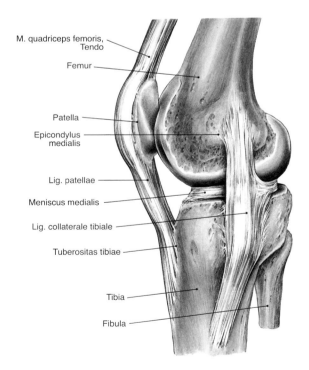

M. quadriceps femoris, Tendo

Femur

Patella

Epicondylus medialis

Lig. patellae

Meniscus medialis

Lig. collaterale tibiale

Tuberositas tibiae

Tibia

Fibula

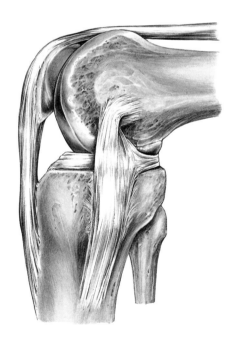

Fig. 1276 Tibial collateral ligament, Lig. collaterale tibiale;
knee in extended position;
medial view.
Only the posterior fibres of the tibial collateral ligament are
attached to the medial meniscus.

Fig. 1277 Tibial collateral ligament, Lig. collaterale tibiale;
knee in flexed position (90°);
medial view.
In the course of flexion, the posterior and proximal fibres of the
tibial collateral ligament become twisted, thereby stabilizing
the medial meniscus.

Knee joint

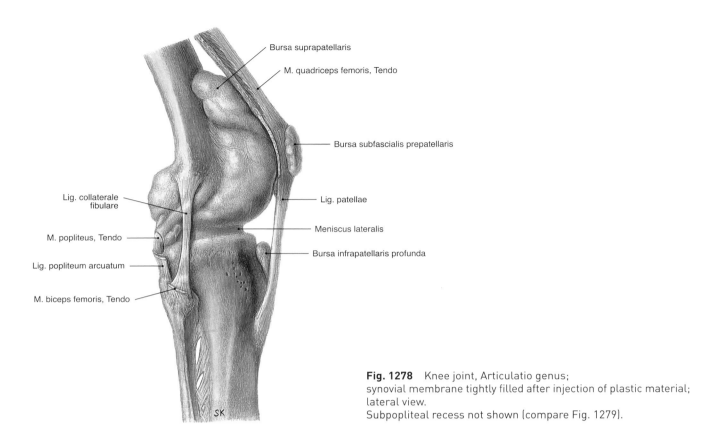

Bursa suprapatellaris

M. quadriceps femoris, Tendo

Bursa subfascialis prepatellaris

Lig. collaterale fibulare

Lig. patellae

M. popliteus, Tendo

Meniscus lateralis

Lig. popliteum arcuatum

Bursa infrapatellaris profunda

M. biceps femoris, Tendo

Fig. 1278 Knee joint, Articulatio genus;
synovial membrane tightly filled after injection of plastic material;
lateral view.
Subpopliteal recess not shown (compare Fig. 1279).

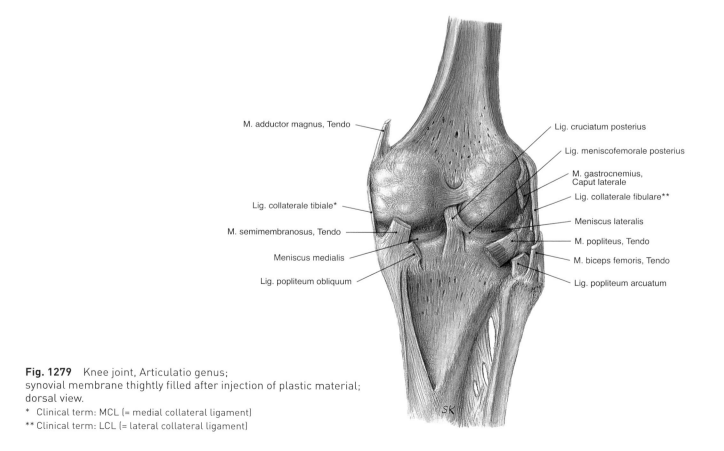

M. adductor magnus, Tendo

Lig. cruciatum posterius

Lig. meniscofemorale posterius

M. gastrocnemius, Caput laterale

Lig. collaterale tibiale*

Lig. collaterale fibulare**

M. semimembranosus, Tendo

Meniscus lateralis

Meniscus medialis

M. popliteus, Tendo

Lig. popliteum obliquum

M. biceps femoris, Tendo

Lig. popliteum arcuatum

Fig. 1279 Knee joint, Articulatio genus;
synovial membrane thightly filled after injection of plastic material;
dorsal view.
* Clinical term: MCL (= medial collateral ligament)
** Clinical term: LCL (= lateral collateral ligament)

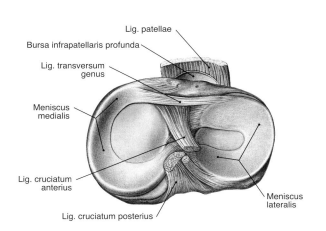

Lig. patellae

Bursa infrapatellaris profunda

Lig. transversum genus

Meniscus medialis

Lig. cruciatum anterius

Lig. cruciatum posterius

Meniscus lateralis

Fig. 1280 Menisci of the knee joint, Articulatio genus, and cruciate ligaments, Ligg. cruciata; proximal view.

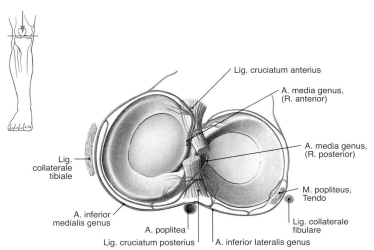

Lig. cruciatum anterius

A. media genus, (R. anterior)

A. media genus, (R. posterior)

M. popliteus, Tendo

Lig. collaterale fibulare

A. inferior lateralis genus

Lig. cruciatum posterius

A. poplitea

A. inferior medialis genus

Lig. collaterale tibiale

Fig. 1281 Menisci of the knee joint, Articulatio genus; arterial supply; proximal view.

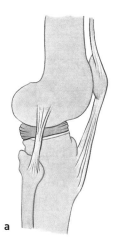

a

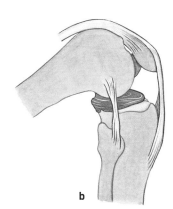

b

Fig. 1282 a, b Displacement of the menisci during flexion; lateral view.

a Extended position
b Flexed position

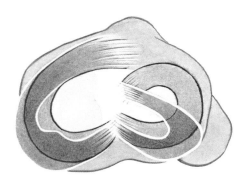

Fig. 1283 Displacement of the menisci during flexion; proximal view.
In flexion, both menisci are displaced posteriorly over the edges of the tibial condyles. The greater mobility of the lateral meniscus accounts for its lesser risk of damage.

Knee joint, sections

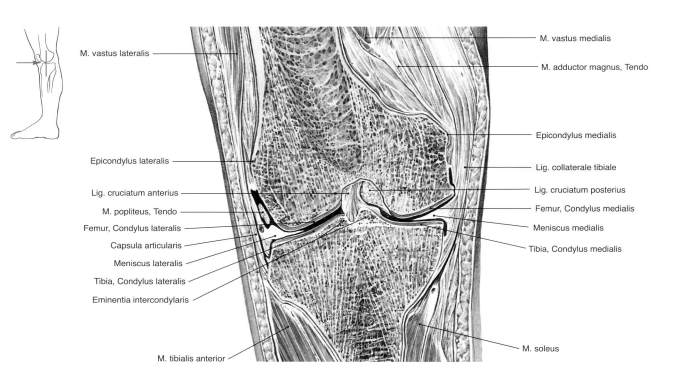

M. vastus lateralis

M. vastus medialis

M. adductor magnus, Tendo

Epicondylus medialis

Epicondylus lateralis

Lig. collaterale tibiale

Lig. cruciatum anterius

Lig. cruciatum posterius

M. popliteus, Tendo

Femur, Condylus medialis

Femur, Condylus lateralis

Meniscus medialis

Capsula articularis

Tibia, Condylus medialis

Meniscus lateralis

Tibia, Condylus lateralis

Eminentia intercondylaris

M. soleus

M. tibialis anterior

Fig. 1284 Knee joint, Articulatio genus;
frontal section.

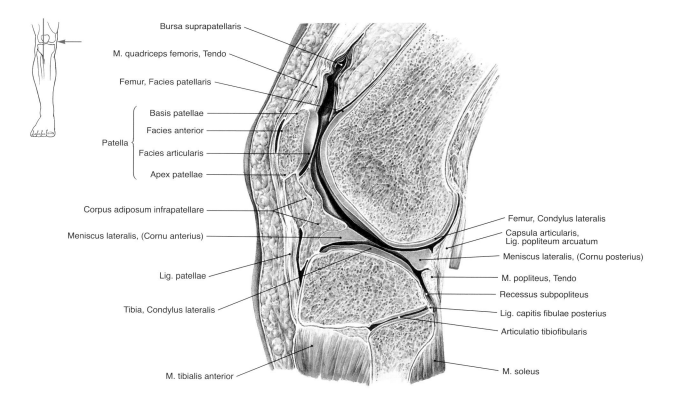

Bursa suprapatellaris

M. quadriceps femoris, Tendo

Femur, Facies patellaris

Basis patellae

Facies anterior

Patella

Facies articularis

Apex patellae

Corpus adiposum infrapatellare

Femur, Condylus lateralis

Capsula articularis,
Lig. popliteum arcuatum

Meniscus lateralis, (Cornu anterius)

Meniscus lateralis, (Cornu posterius)

M. popliteus, Tendo

Lig. patellae

Recessus subpopliteus

Lig. capitis fibulae posterius

Tibia, Condylus lateralis

Articulatio tibiofibularis

M. tibialis anterior

M. soleus

Fig. 1285 Knee joint, Articulatio genus;
sagittal section through the lateral part of the joint.

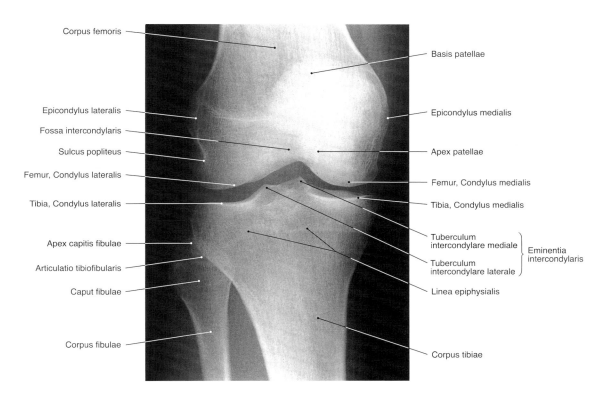

Corpus femoris

Basis patellae

Epicondylus lateralis

Epicondylus medialis

Fossa intercondylaris

Sulcus popliteus

Apex patellae

Femur, Condylus lateralis

Femur, Condylus medialis

Tibia, Condylus lateralis

Tibia, Condylus medialis

Apex capitis fibulae

Tuberculum intercondylare mediale

Tuberculum intercondylare laterale

} Eminentia intercondylaris

Articulatio tibiofibularis

Caput fibulae

Linea epiphysialis

Corpus fibulae

Corpus tibiae

Fig. 1286   Knee joint, Articulatio genus;
AP-radiograph with the central beam directed onto
the middle of the joint; subject reclined.

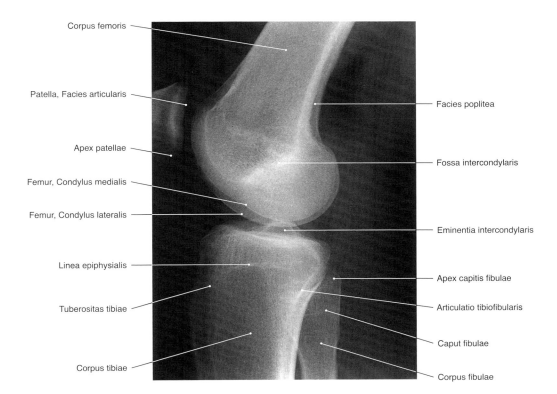

Corpus femoris

Patella, Facies articularis

Facies poplitea

Apex patellae

Fossa intercondylaris

Femur, Condylus medialis

Femur, Condylus lateralis

Eminentia intercondylaris

Linea epiphysialis

Apex capitis fibulae

Tuberositas tibiae

Articulatio tibiofibularis

Caput fibulae

Corpus tibiae

Corpus fibulae

Fig. 1287   Knee joint, Articulatio genus;
lateral radiograph with the central beam directed onto
the middle of the joint; subject reclined.

Knee joint, arthroscopy

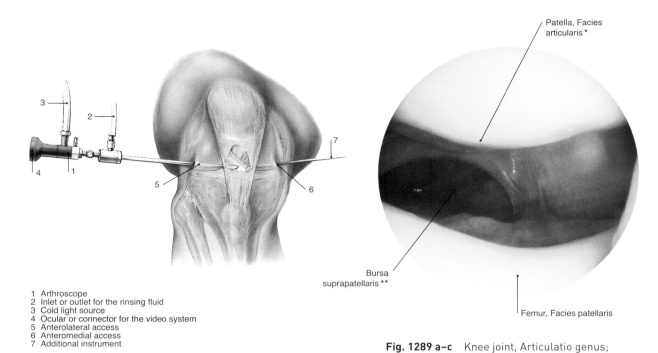

1 Arthroscope
2 Inlet or outlet for the rinsing fluid
3 Cold light source
4 Ocular or connector for the video system
5 Anterolateral access
6 Anteromedial access
7 Additional instrument

Fig. 1288 Accesses for arthroscopy.

Fig. 1289 a–c Knee joint, Articulatio genus; arthroscopy.
a Distal view into the femoropatellar joint
* Patellar roof ridge: ridge between the medial and lateral articular surfaces
** Clinical term: suprapatellar recess

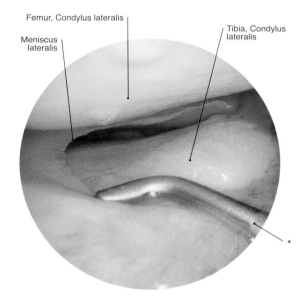

b Medial view of the free inner edge of the lateral meniscus;
retractor (*) slightly depressing the anterior part of the meniscus

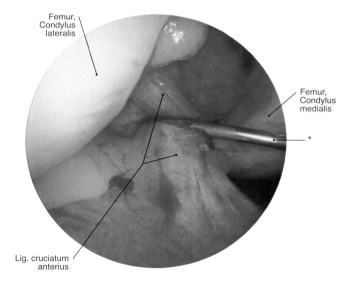

c Anterolateral view of the distal part of the anterior cruciate ligament, Lig. cruciatum anterius.
The ligament is covered by a richly vascularized synovial membrane. It is drawn medially by a retractor (*).

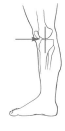

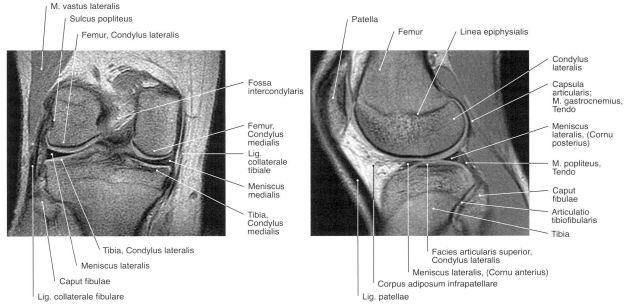

M. vastus lateralis
Sulcus popliteus
Femur, Condylus lateralis

Fossa intercondylaris

Femur, Condylus medialis

Lig. collaterale tibiale

Meniscus medialis

Tibia, Condylus medialis

Tibia, Condylus lateralis

Meniscus lateralis

Caput fibulae

Lig. collaterale fibulare

Patella
Femur
Linea epiphysialis

Condylus lateralis

Capsula articularis; M. gastrocnemius, Tendo

Meniscus lateralis, (Cornu posterius)

M. popliteus, Tendo

Caput fibulae

Articulatio tibiofibularis

Tibia

Facies articularis superior, Condylus lateralis

Meniscus lateralis, (Cornu anterius)

Corpus adiposum infrapatellare

Lig. patellae

Fig. 1290   Knee joint, Articulatio genus;
magnetic resonance tomographic image (MRI);
frontal section;
knee in the extended position.
In this imaging technique, compact bone appears black.

Fig. 1291   Knee joint, Articulatio genus;
magnetic resonance tomographic image (MRI);
sagittal section through the lateral part of the joint;
knee in the extended position.

1291
1292a
1292b

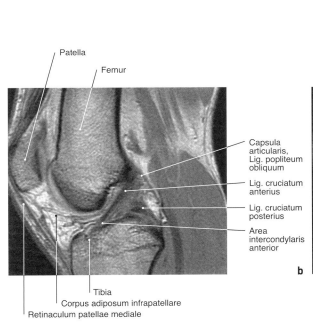

Patella
Femur

Capsula articularis, Lig. popliteum obliquum

Lig. cruciatum anterius

Lig. cruciatum posterius

Area intercondylaris anterior

a

Tibia
Corpus adiposum infrapatellare
Retinaculum patellae mediale

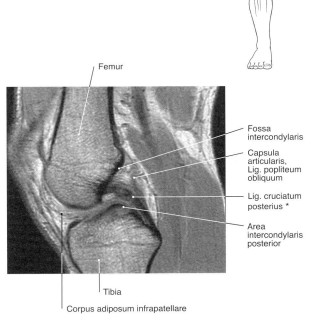

Femur

Fossa intercondylaris

Capsula articularis, Lig. popliteum obliquum

Lig. cruciatum posterius *

Area intercondylaris posterior

b

Tibia

Corpus adiposum infrapatellare

Fig. 1292 a, b   Knee joint, Articulatio genus;
magnetic resonance tomographic image (MRI);
sagittal sections to demonstrate the cruciate
ligaments;
knee in the extended position.

a Anterior cruciate ligament, Lig. cruciatum anterius, (ACL)
b Posterior cruciate ligament, Lig. cruciatum posterius, (PCL)
*   The inhomogeneity is due to oblique sectioning of the fibre bundles.

Joints of the bones of the leg

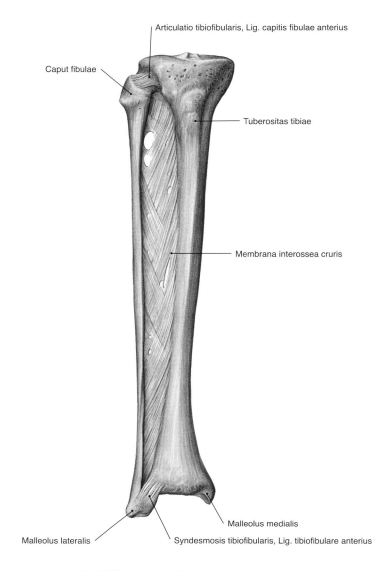

Articulatio tibiofibularis, Lig. capitis fibulae anterius

Caput fibulae

Tuberositas tibiae

Membrana interossea cruris

Malleolus medialis

Malleolus lateralis

Syndesmosis tibiofibularis, Lig. tibiofibulare anterius

Fig. 1293   Joints of the bones of the leg;
ventral view.

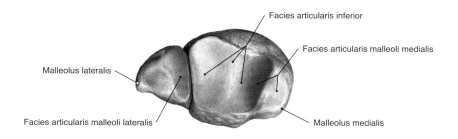

Facies articularis inferior

Facies articularis malleoli medialis

Malleolus lateralis

Facies articularis malleoli lateralis

Malleolus medialis

Fig. 1294   Tibia, Tibia, and fibula, Fibula;
distal view.

Skeleton of the foot

Fig. 1295   Skeleton of the foot, Ossa pedis; proximal view.

I   Hallux [Digitus primus]
II   Digitus secundus
III   Digitus tertius
IV   Digitus quartus
V   Digitus minimus [quintus]

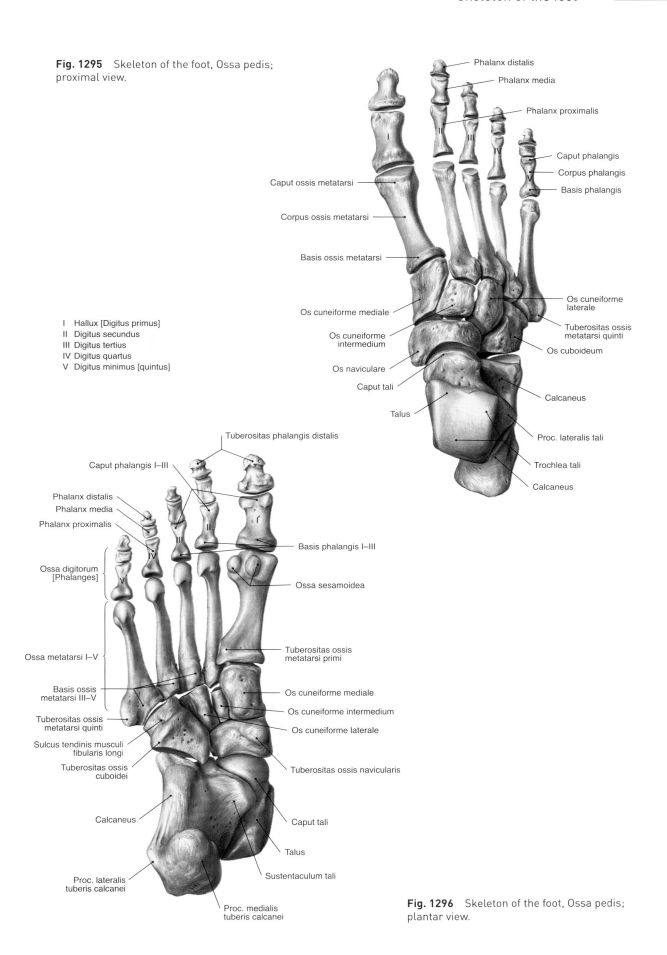

Phalanx distalis
Phalanx media
Phalanx proximalis
Caput phalangis
Corpus phalangis
Basis phalangis
Caput ossis metatarsi
Corpus ossis metatarsi
Basis ossis metatarsi
Os cuneiforme laterale
Os cuneiforme mediale
Tuberositas ossis metatarsi quinti
Os cuneiforme intermedium
Os cuboideum
Os naviculare
Caput tali
Calcaneus
Talus
Proc. lateralis tali
Trochlea tali
Calcaneus

Tuberositas phalangis distalis
Caput phalangis I–III
Phalanx distalis
Phalanx media
Phalanx proximalis
Basis phalangis I–III
Ossa digitorum [Phalanges]
Ossa sesamoidea
Ossa metatarsi I–V
Tuberositas ossis metatarsi primi
Basis ossis metatarsi III–V
Os cuneiforme mediale
Os cuneiforme intermedium
Tuberositas ossis metatarsi quinti
Os cuneiforme laterale
Sulcus tendinis musculi fibularis longi
Tuberositas ossis cuboidei
Tuberositas ossis navicularis
Calcaneus
Caput tali
Talus
Proc. lateralis tuberis calcanei
Sustentaculum tali
Proc. medialis tuberis calcanei

Fig. 1296   Skeleton of the foot, Ossa pedis; plantar view.

Skeleton of the foot

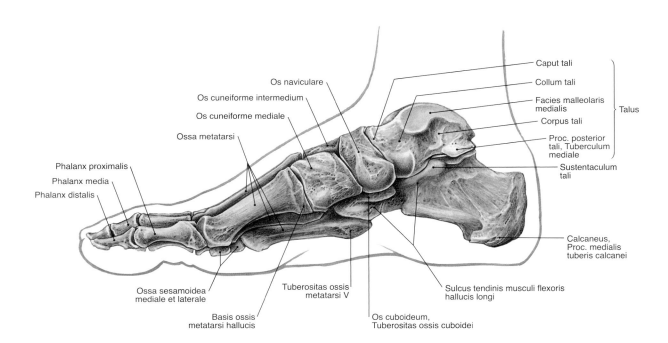

Os naviculare

Os cuneiforme intermedium

Os cuneiforme mediale

Ossa metatarsi

Phalanx proximalis

Phalanx media

Phalanx distalis

Caput tali

Collum tali

Facies malleolaris medialis

Corpus tali

Proc. posterior tali, Tuberculum mediale

Talus

Sustentaculum tali

Calcaneus, Proc. medialis tuberis calcanei

Ossa sesamoidea mediale et laterale

Basis ossis metatarsi hallucis

Tuberositas ossis metatarsi V

Sulcus tendinis musculi flexoris hallucis longi

Os cuboideum, Tuberositas ossis cuboidei

Fig. 1297   Skeleton of the foot, Ossa pedis; medial view.

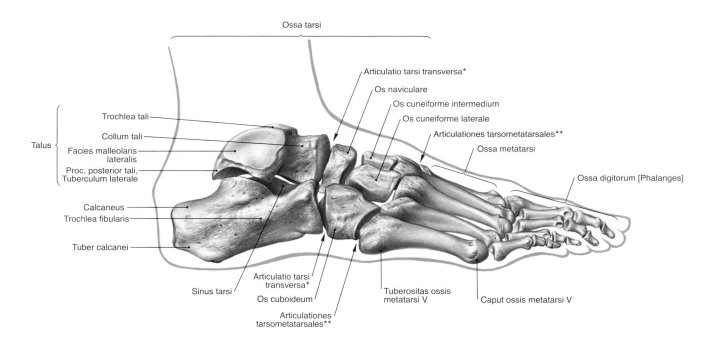

Ossa tarsi

Articulatio tarsi transversa*

Os naviculare

Os cuneiforme intermedium

Os cuneiforme laterale

Articulationes tarsometatarsales**

Ossa metatarsi

Trochlea tali

Collum tali

Facies malleolaris lateralis

Proc. posterior tali, Tuberculum laterale

Talus

Calcaneus

Trochlea fibularis

Tuber calcanei

Ossa digitorum [Phalanges]

Articulatio tarsi transversa*

Os cuboideum

Articulationes tarsometatarsales**

Sinus tarsi

Tuberositas ossis metatarsi V

Caput ossis metatarsi V

Fig. 1298   Skeleton of the foot, Ossa pedis; lateral view.

* Also: CHOPART's joint

** Also: LISFRANC's joint

Talus and calcaneus

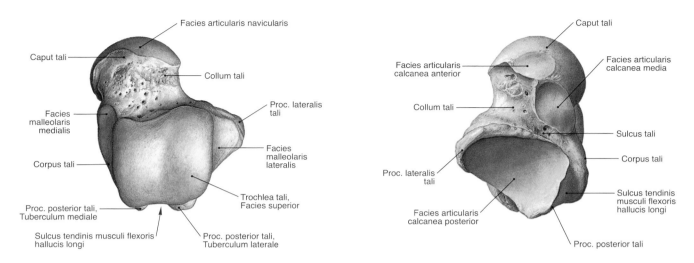

Fig. 1299 Talus, Talus; proximal view.

Facies articularis navicularis

Caput tali

Collum tali

Facies malleolaris medialis

Proc. lateralis tali

Corpus tali

Facies malleolaris lateralis

Trochlea tali, Facies superior

Proc. posterior tali, Tuberculum mediale

Sulcus tendinis musculi flexoris hallucis longi

Proc. posterior tali, Tuberculum laterale

Fig. 1300 Talus, Talus; plantar view.

Caput tali

Facies articularis calcanea anterior

Facies articularis calcanea media

Collum tali

Sulcus tali

Corpus tali

Proc. lateralis tali

Sulcus tendinis musculi flexoris hallucis longi

Facies articularis calcanea posterior

Proc. posterior tali

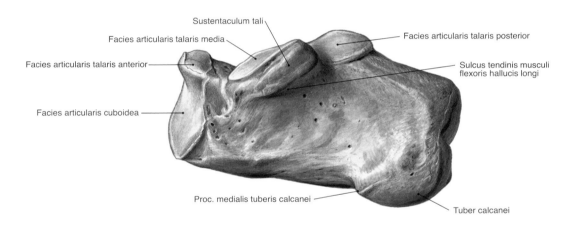

Fig. 1301 Calcaneus, Calcaneus; medial view.

Sustentaculum tali

Facies articularis talaris media

Facies articularis talaris posterior

Facies articularis talaris anterior

Sulcus tendinis musculi flexoris hallucis longi

Facies articularis cuboidea

Proc. medialis tuberis calcanei

Tuber calcanei

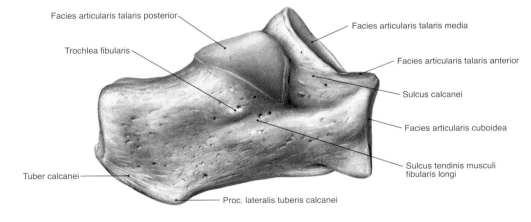

Fig. 1302 Calcaneus, Calcaneus; lateral view.

Facies articularis talaris posterior

Facies articularis talaris media

Trochlea fibularis

Facies articularis talaris anterior

Sulcus calcanei

Facies articularis cuboidea

Sulcus tendinis musculi fibularis longi

Tuber calcanei

Proc. lateralis tuberis calcanei

Tarsal bones

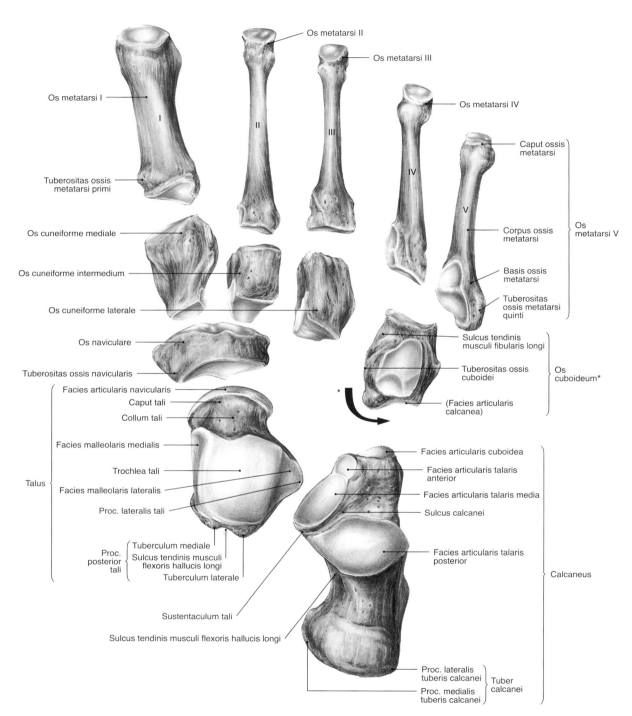

Os metatarsi II

Os metatarsi III

Os metatarsi I

Os metatarsi IV

Caput ossis metatarsi

Tuberositas ossis metatarsi primi

I

II

III

IV

V

Os cuneiforme mediale

Corpus ossis metatarsi

Os metatarsi V

Os cuneiforme intermedium

Os cuneiforme laterale

Basis ossis metatarsi

Tuberositas ossis metatarsi quinti

Os naviculare

Sulcus tendinis musculi fibularis longi

Tuberositas ossis navicularis

Tuberositas ossis cuboidei

Os cuboideum*

Facies articularis navicularis

(Facies articularis calcanea)

Caput tali

Collum tali

*

Facies malleolaris medialis

Facies articularis cuboidea

Facies articularis talaris anterior

Talus

Trochlea tali

Facies articularis talaris media

Facies malleolaris lateralis

Sulcus calcanei

Proc. lateralis tali

Facies articularis talaris posterior

Proc. posterior tali

Tuberculum mediale

Sulcus tendinis musculi flexoris hallucis longi

Tuberculum laterale

Calcaneus

Sustentaculum tali

Sulcus tendinis musculi flexoris hallucis longi

Proc. lateralis tuberis calcanei

Tuber calcanei

Proc. medialis tuberis calcanei

Fig. 1303   Tarsal bones, Ossa tarsi, and metatarsal bones, Ossa metatarsi; proximal view.

* The cuboid bone is shown in a medial view.

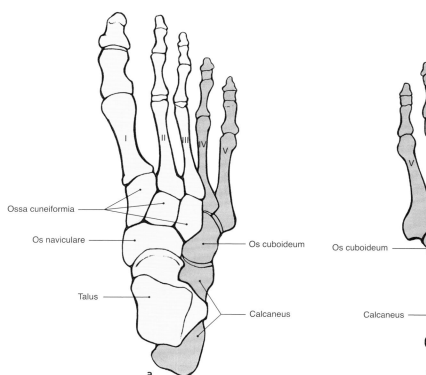

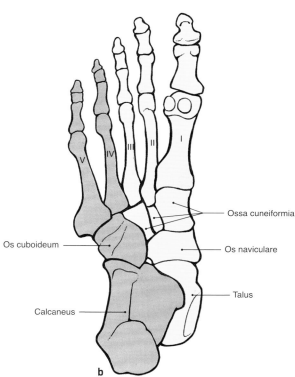

Fig. 1304 a, b Skeleton of the foot, Ossa pedis; structural organisation.
a Proximal view
b Plantar view

The heads of all metatarsal bones lie in the plantar plane. The cuneiform bones, the navicular bone and the talus rest upon the lateral parts of the skeleton, especially in the posterior part of the foot. The talus is therefore situated above the calcaneus and the longitudinal arch is formed.

The wedge-shaped cross-section of the cuneiform bones and the bases of the metatarsal bones contribute to the formation of the transverse vault.

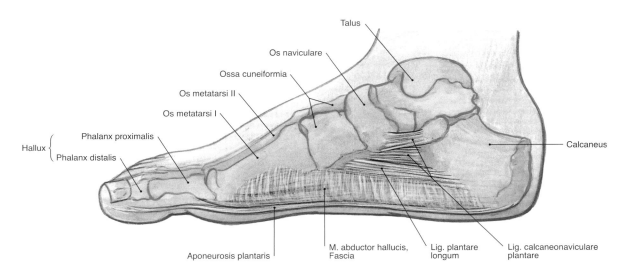

Fig. 1305 Supporting structures of the medial arch of the longitudinal vault of the foot; medial view.

The ligaments shown in this illustration are mostly directed in the longitudinal axis of the foot and support passively the longitudinal vault of the foot. The short muscles of the foot primarily support this construction.

Joints of the foot

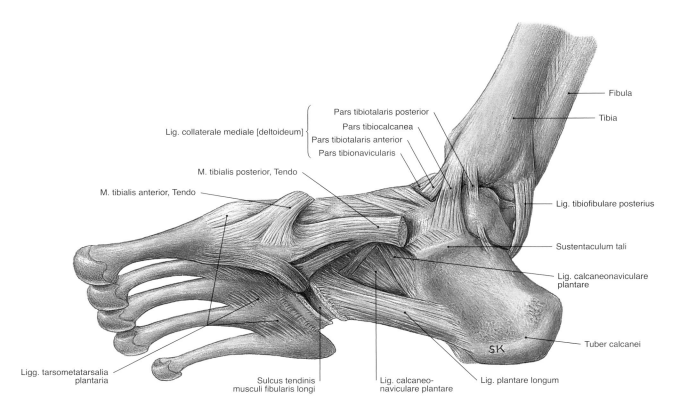

Fig. 1306   Joints of the foot, Articulationes pedis;
ligaments and tendons;
medial view.

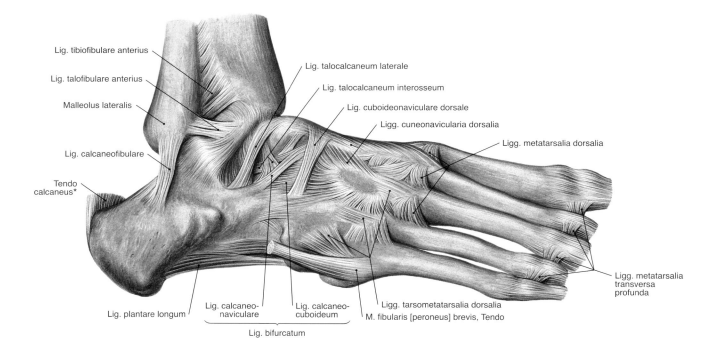

Fig. 1307   Joints of the foot, Articulationes pedis;
ligaments and tendons;
lateral view.
* Also: Achilles tendon

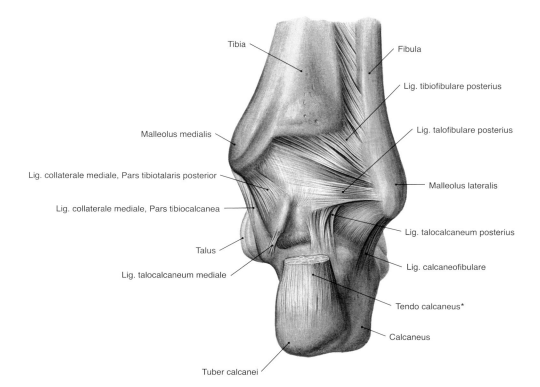

Tibia

Fibula

Lig. tibiofibulare posterius

Lig. talofibulare posterius

Malleolus medialis

Lig. collaterale mediale, Pars tibiotalaris posterior

Malleolus lateralis

Lig. collaterale mediale, Pars tibiocalcanea

Lig. talocalcaneum posterius

Talus

Lig. calcaneofibulare

Lig. talocalcaneum mediale

Tendo calcaneus*

Calcaneus

Tuber calcanei

Fig. 1308   Joints of the foot, Articulationes pedis;
ligaments and tendons of the posterior part of the foot.
* Also: Achilles tendon

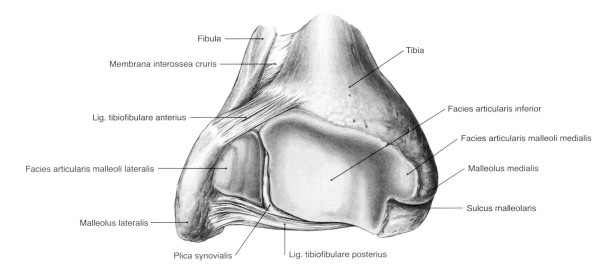

Fibula

Membrana interossea cruris

Tibia

Lig. tibiofibulare anterius

Facies articularis inferior

Facies articularis malleoli medialis

Facies articularis malleoli lateralis

Malleolus medialis

Sulcus malleolaris

Malleolus lateralis

Plica synovialis

Lig. tibiofibulare posterius

Fig. 1309   Ankle joint, Articulatio talocruralis;
proximal articular surfaces;
distal view.

Joints of the foot

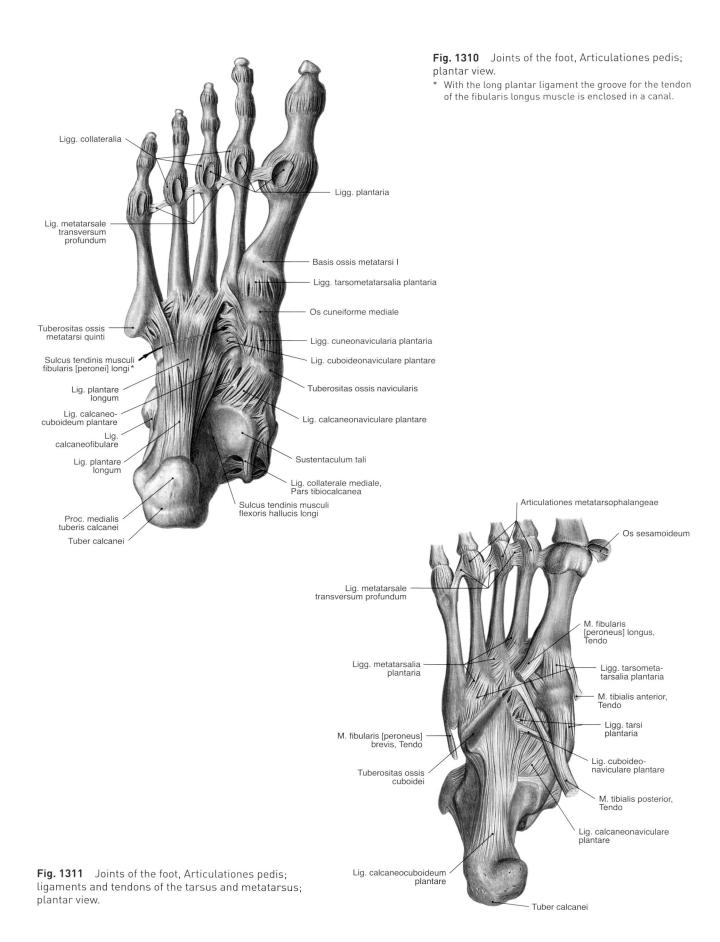

Fig. 1310 Joints of the foot, Articulationes pedis; plantar view.

* With the long plantar ligament the groove for the tendon of the fibularis longus muscle is enclosed in a canal.

Ligg. collateralia

Ligg. plantaria

Lig. metatarsale transversum profundum

Basis ossis metatarsi I

Ligg. tarsometatarsalia plantaria

Os cuneiforme mediale

Tuberositas ossis metatarsi quinti

Ligg. cuneonavicularia plantaria

Sulcus tendinis musculi fibularis [peronei] longi *

Lig. cuboideonaviculare plantare

Lig. plantare longum

Tuberositas ossis navicularis

Lig. calcaneo-cuboideum plantare

Lig. calcaneonaviculare plantare

Lig. calcaneofibulare

Lig. plantare longum

Sustentaculum tali

Proc. medialis tuberis calcanei

Lig. collaterale mediale, Pars tibiocalcanea

Tuber calcanei

Sulcus tendinis musculi flexoris hallucis longi

Articulationes metatarsophalangeae

Os sesamoideum

Lig. metatarsale transversum profundum

M. fibularis [peroneus] longus, Tendo

Ligg. metatarsalia plantaria

Ligg. tarsometa-tarsalia plantaria

M. tibialis anterior, Tendo

Ligg. tarsi plantaria

M. fibularis [peroneus] brevis, Tendo

Lig. cuboideo-naviculare plantare

Tuberositas ossis cuboidei

M. tibialis posterior, Tendo

Lig. calcaneonaviculare plantare

Lig. calcaneocuboideum plantare

Tuber calcanei

Fig. 1311 Joints of the foot, Articulationes pedis; ligaments and tendons of the tarsus and metatarsus; plantar view.

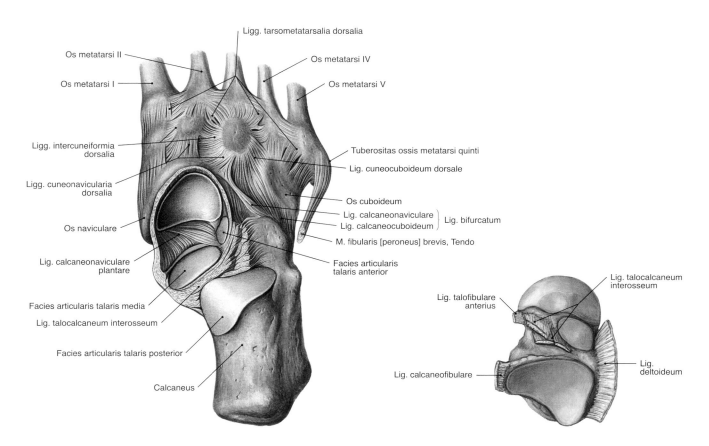

Os metatarsi II

Os metatarsi I

Ligg. intercuneiformia
dorsalia

Ligg. cuneonavicularia
dorsalia

Os naviculare

Lig. calcaneonaviculare
plantare

Facies articularis talaris media

Lig. talocalcaneum interosseum

Facies articularis talaris posterior

Calcaneus

Ligg. tarsometatarsalia dorsalia

Os metatarsi IV

Os metatarsi V

Tuberositas ossis metatarsi quinti

Lig. cuneocuboideum dorsale

Os cuboideum

Lig. calcaneonaviculare ⎫
Lig. calcaneocuboideum ⎭ Lig. bifurcatum

M. fibularis [peroneus] brevis, Tendo

Facies articularis
talaris anterior

Lig. talofibulare
anterius

Lig. calcaneofibulare

Lig. talocalcaneum
interosseum

Lig.
deltoideum

Fig. 1312 Talotarsal joint,
Articulatio talotarsalis;
distal articular surfaces;
proximal view.

Fig. 1313 Talotarsal joint,
Articulatio talotarsalis;
proximal articular surfaces;
distal view.

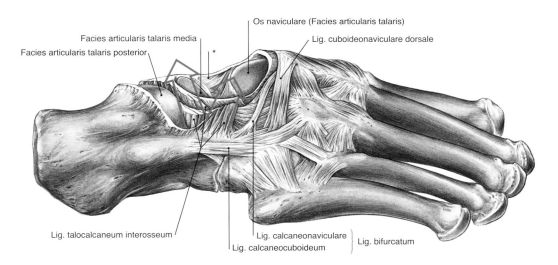

Facies articularis talaris media

Facies articularis talaris posterior

Os naviculare (Facies articularis talaris)

Lig. cuboideonaviculare dorsale

Lig. talocalcaneum interosseum

Lig. calcaneonaviculare ⎫
Lig. calcaneocuboideum ⎭ Lig. bifurcatum

Fig. 1314 Talotarsal joint, Articulatio talotarsalis;
the talus and the lateral ligaments have been removed;
lateral view.
The two arrows point out the helical distorsion of the
talocalcaneal interosseous ligament.

* Tight connective tissue layer between the plantar calcaneonavicular
ligament and the tibionavicular part of the deltoid ligament limiting
a medially directed gliding of the head of the talus; slackening of this
layer results in flattening of the longitudinal vault (flat-foot, pes valgus)

Ankle and talotarsal joint, sections

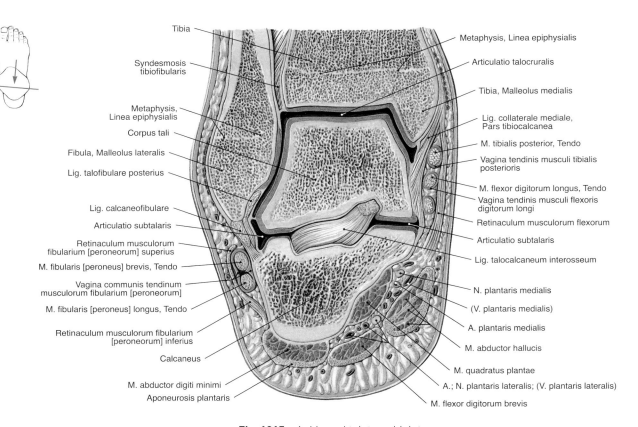

Tibia

Syndesmosis tibiofibularis

Metaphysis, Linea epiphysialis

Corpus tali

Fibula, Malleolus lateralis

Lig. talofibulare posterius

Lig. calcaneofibulare

Articulatio subtalaris

Retinaculum musculorum fibularium [peroneorum] superius

M. fibularis [peroneus] brevis, Tendo

Vagina communis tendinum musculorum fibularium [peroneorum]

M. fibularis [peroneus] longus, Tendo

Retinaculum musculorum fibularium [peroneorum] inferius

Calcaneus

M. abductor digiti minimi

Aponeurosis plantaris

Metaphysis, Linea epiphysialis

Articulatio talocruralis

Tibia, Malleolus medialis

Lig. collaterale mediale, Pars tibiocalcanea

M. tibialis posterior, Tendo

Vagina tendinis musculi tibialis posterioris

M. flexor digitorum longus, Tendo

Vagina tendinis musculi flexoris digitorum longi

Retinaculum musculorum flexorum

Articulatio subtalaris

Lig. talocalcaneum interosseum

N. plantaris medialis

(V. plantaris medialis)

A. plantaris medialis

M. abductor hallucis

M. quadratus plantae

A.; N. plantaris lateralis; (V. plantaris lateralis)

M. flexor digitorum brevis

Fig. 1315 Ankle and talotarsal joint, Articulationes talocruralis et talotarsalis; frontal section.

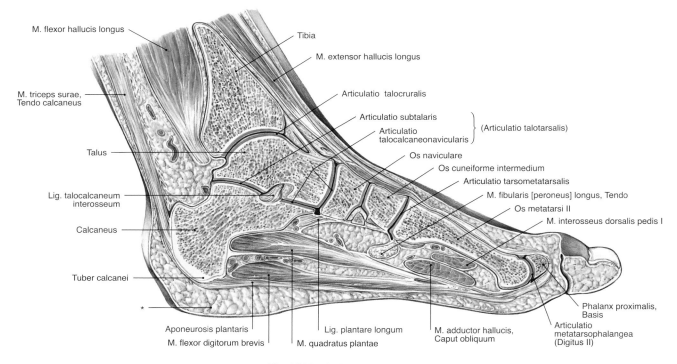

M. flexor hallucis longus

M. triceps surae, Tendo calcaneus

Talus

Lig. talocalcaneum interosseum

Calcaneus

Tuber calcanei

*

Aponeurosis plantaris

M. flexor digitorum brevis

Tibia

M. extensor hallucis longus

Articulatio talocruralis

Articulatio subtalaris

Articulatio talocalcaneonavicularis

(Articulatio talotarsalis)

Os naviculare

Os cuneiforme intermedium

Articulatio tarsometatarsalis

M. fibularis [peroneus] longus, Tendo

Os metatarsi II

M. interosseus dorsalis pedis I

Phalanx proximalis, Basis

Articulatio metatarsophalangea (Digitus II)

M. adductor hallucis, Caput obliquum

M. quadratus plantae

Lig. plantare longum

Fig. 1316 Ankle and talotarsal joint, Articulationes talocruralis et talotarsalis; sagittal section.
* Fat pad of the heel

Ankle and talotarsal joint, radiography

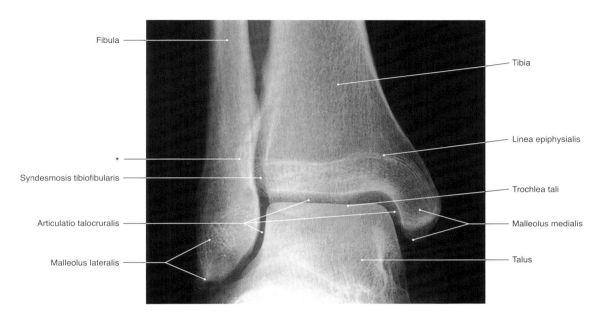

Fibula

Tibia

Linea epiphysialis

*

Syndesmosis tibiofibularis

Trochlea tali

Articulatio talocruralis

Malleolus medialis

Malleolus lateralis

Talus

Fig. 1317   Ankle joint, Articulatio talocruralis;
AP-radiograph with the subject reclined and the central beam
directed tangentially onto the trochlea of talus.

* Clinically, the posterior border of the fibular notch is also referred to
as the third malleolus.

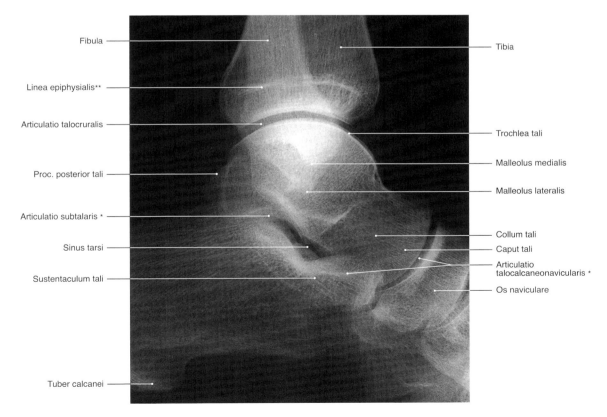

Fibula

Tibia

Linea epiphysialis**

Articulatio talocruralis

Trochlea tali

Proc. posterior tali

Malleolus medialis

Malleolus lateralis

Articulatio subtalaris *

Collum tali

Sinus tarsi

Caput tali

Articulatio
talocalcaneonavicularis *

Sustentaculum tali

Os naviculare

Tuber calcanei

Fig. 1318   Ankle and talotarsal joint,
Articulationes talocruralis et talotarsalis;
AP-radiograph with the subject reclined and the central beam
directed tangentially onto the apex of the trochlea of talus.

* Due to their helical distorsion, the joint clefts are not displayed
orthogonally.
** Overlapping epiphyseal lines of the tibia and fibula

→ 1428, 1429

Fasciae of the lower limb

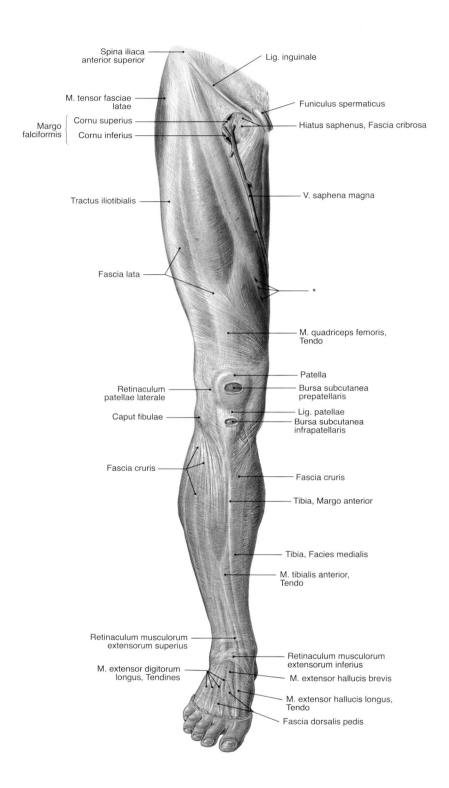

Fig. 1319 Fascia lata, Fascia lata, and deep fascia of leg, Fascia cruris.

The transition zone between the aponeurosis of the external oblique abdominal muscle and the fascia lata is known as inguinal ligament. This ligament extends laterally from the anterior superior iliac spine to its attachment on the pubic tubercle medially.

* Openings in the fascia for the perforator veins (DODD's veins)

Fasciae of the lower limb

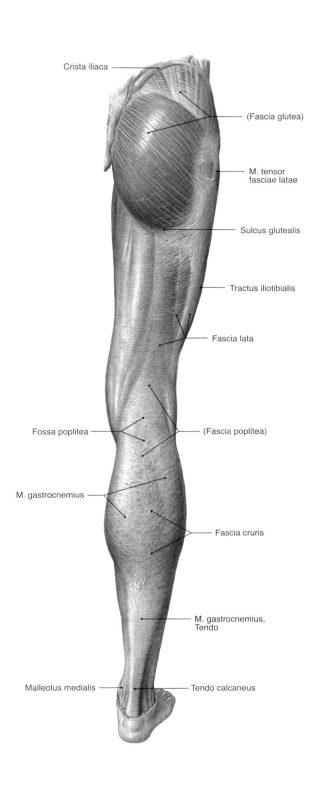

Crista iliaca

(Fascia glutea)

M. tensor fasciae latae

Sulcus glutealis

Tractus iliotibialis

Fascia lata

Fossa poplitea

(Fascia poplitea)

M. gastrocnemius

Fascia cruris

M. gastrocnemius, Tendo

Malleolus medialis

Tendo calcaneus

Fig. 1320   Fascia lata, Fascia lata, and deep fascia of leg, Fascia cruris.

Muscles of the lower limb, overview

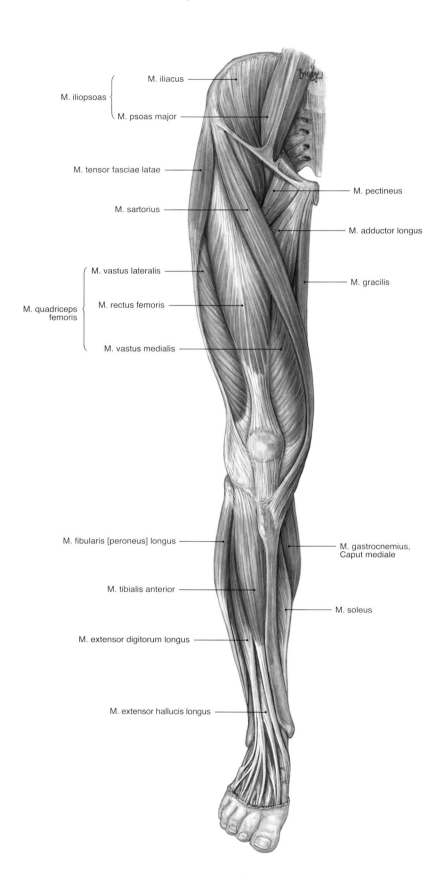

M. iliacus

M. iliopsoas

M. psoas major

M. tensor fasciae latae

M. pectineus

M. sartorius

M. adductor longus

M. vastus lateralis

M. gracilis

M. quadriceps femoris

M. rectus femoris

M. vastus medialis

M. fibularis [peroneus] longus

M. gastrocnemius, Caput mediale

M. tibialis anterior

M. soleus

M. extensor digitorum longus

M. extensor hallucis longus

→ T 42, T 44, T 45, T 47, T 48

Fig. 1321   Muscles of the lower limb, Mm. extremitatis inferioris; overview.

Muscles of the lower limb, overview

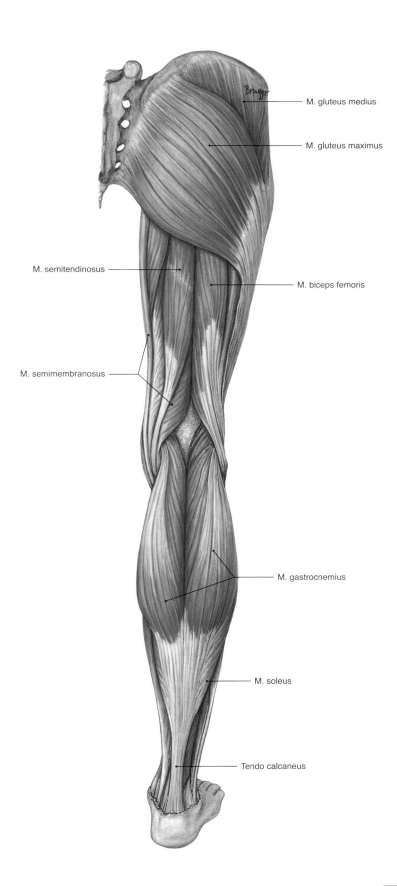

M. gluteus medius

M. gluteus maximus

M. semitendinosus

M. biceps femoris

M. semimembranosus

M. gastrocnemius

M. soleus

Tendo calcaneus

Fig. 1322   Muscles of the lower limb, Mm. extremitatis inferioris; overview.

→ T 43, T 46, T 49

Origins and insertions of the muscles of the hip, the thigh and the leg

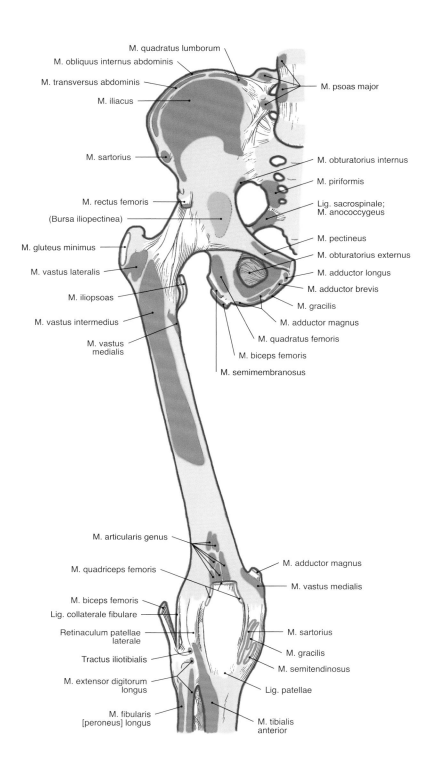

M. quadratus lumborum

M. obliquus internus abdominis

M. transversus abdominis

M. iliacus

M. psoas major

M. sartorius

M. obturatorius internus

M. piriformis

M. rectus femoris

Lig. sacrospinale;
M. anococcygeus

(Bursa iliopectinea)

M. pectineus

M. gluteus minimus

M. obturatorius externus

M. vastus lateralis

M. adductor longus

M. iliopsoas

M. adductor brevis

M. gracilis

M. vastus intermedius

M. adductor magnus

M. vastus
medialis

M. quadratus femoris

M. biceps femoris

M. semimembranosus

M. articularis genus

M. adductor magnus

M. quadriceps femoris

M. vastus medialis

M. biceps femoris

Lig. collaterale fibulare

Retinaculum patellae
laterale

M. sartorius

Tractus iliotibialis

M. gracilis

M. extensor digitorum
longus

M. semitendinosus

Lig. patellae

M. fibularis
[peroneus] longus

M. tibialis
anterior

→ T 42–T 48

Fig. 1323 Origins and insertions of the muscles at the
lower lumbar vertebrae, the pelvic bones, the femur and
the proximal extremities of the bones of the leg;
ventral view.

Origins and insertions of the muscles of the hip, the thigh and the leg

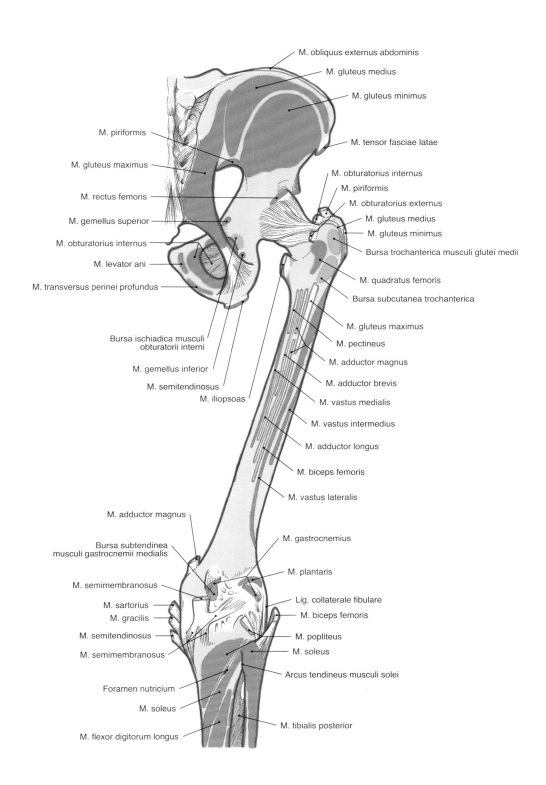

M. obliquus externus abdominis
M. gluteus medius
M. gluteus minimus
M. tensor fasciae latae
M. piriformis
M. gluteus maximus
M. rectus femoris
M. gemellus superior
M. obturatorius internus
M. levator ani
M. transversus perinei profundus
M. obturatorius internus
M. piriformis
M. obturatorius externus
M. gluteus medius
M. gluteus minimus
Bursa trochanterica musculi glutei medii
M. quadratus femoris
Bursa subcutanea trochanterica
M. gluteus maximus
M. pectineus
M. adductor magnus
M. adductor brevis
M. vastus medialis
M. vastus intermedius
M. adductor longus
M. biceps femoris
M. vastus lateralis
Bursa ischiadica musculi obturatorii interni
M. gemellus inferior
M. semitendinosus
M. iliopsoas
M. adductor magnus
Bursa subtendinea musculi gastrocnemii medialis
M. gastrocnemius
M. plantaris
M. semimembranosus
M. sartorius
M. gracilis
M. semitendinosus
M. semimembranosus
Lig. collaterale fibulare
M. biceps femoris
M. popliteus
M. soleus
Arcus tendineus musculi solei
Foramen nutricium
M. soleus
M. tibialis posterior
M. flexor digitorum longus

Fig. 1324   Origins and insertions of the muscles at the pelvic bones, the femur and the proximal extremities of the bones of the leg; dorsal view.

→ T 43–T 46, T 49, T 50

Muscles of the thigh

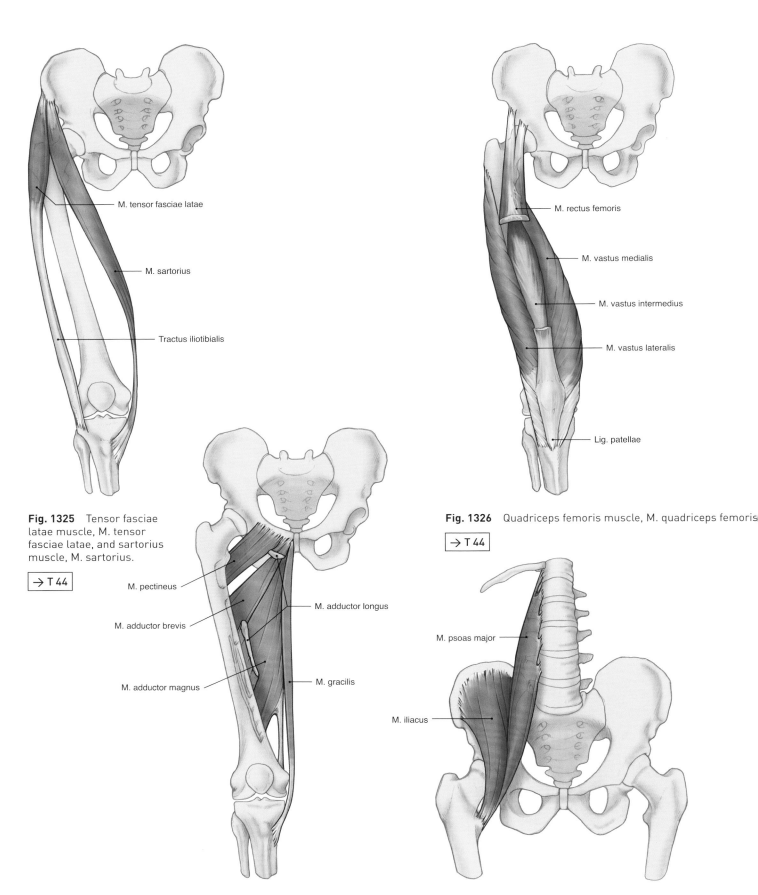

M. tensor fasciae latae

M. sartorius

Tractus iliotibialis

Fig. 1325 Tensor fasciae latae muscle, M. tensor fasciae latae, and sartorius muscle, M. sartorius.

→ T 44

M. rectus femoris

M. vastus medialis

M. vastus intermedius

M. vastus lateralis

Lig. patellae

Fig. 1326 Quadriceps femoris muscle, M. quadriceps femoris

→ T 44

M. pectineus

M. adductor brevis

M. adductor longus

M. adductor magnus

M. gracilis

Fig. 1327 Adductor muscles, Mm. adductores.

→ T 45

M. psoas major

M. iliacus

Fig. 1328 Iliopsoas muscle, M. iliopsoas.

→ T 42

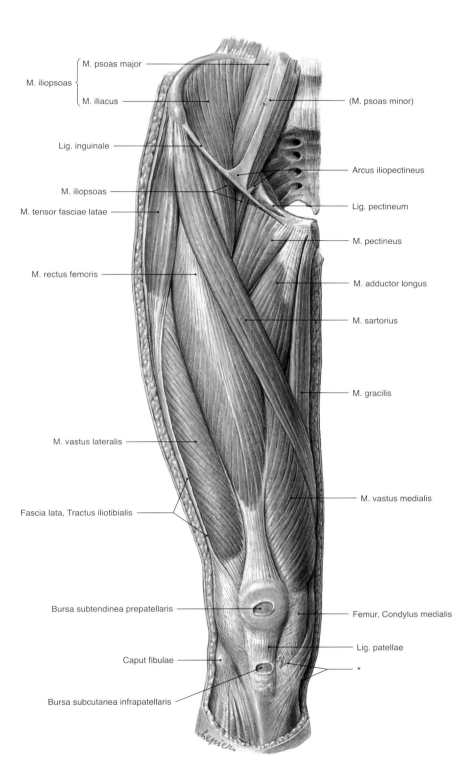

M. iliopsoas
— M. psoas major
— M. iliacus

(M. psoas minor)

Lig. inguinale

Arcus iliopectineus

M. iliopsoas

Lig. pectineum

M. tensor fasciae latae

M. pectineus

M. rectus femoris

M. adductor longus

M. sartorius

M. gracilis

M. vastus lateralis

M. vastus medialis

Fascia lata, Tractus iliotibialis

Bursa subtendinea prepatellaris

Femur, Condylus medialis

Lig. patellae

Caput fibulae

*

Bursa subcutanea infrapatellaris

Fig. 1329 Muscles of the thigh and the hip;
after removal of the fascia lata except for the iliotibial tract.
* Common insertion of the sartorius, gracilis and semitendinosus
  muscles just below the medial condyle of the tibia (formerly known
  as the superficial pes anserinus, Pes anserinus superficialis)

→ T 42, T 44, T 45

Muscles of the thigh

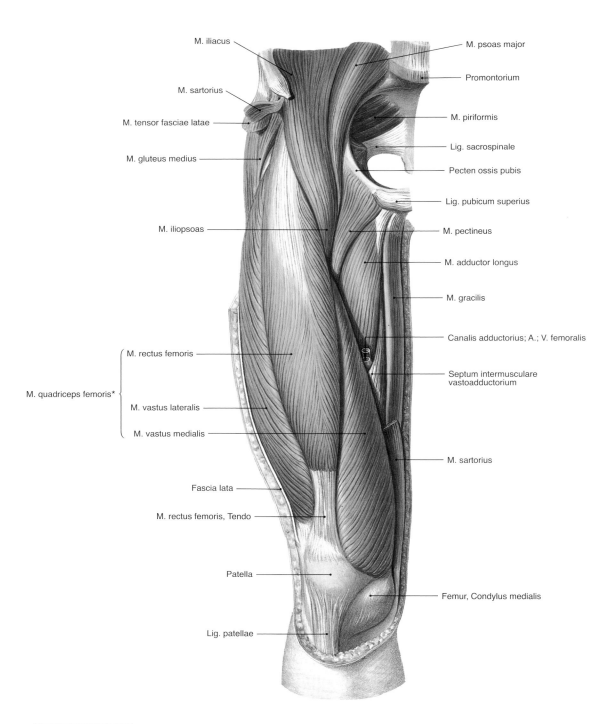

M. iliacus

M. sartorius

M. tensor fasciae latae

M. gluteus medius

M. iliopsoas

M. rectus femoris

M. quadriceps femoris*

M. vastus lateralis

M. vastus medialis

Fascia lata

M. rectus femoris, Tendo

Patella

Lig. patellae

M. psoas major

Promontorium

M. piriformis

Lig. sacrospinale

Pecten ossis pubis

Lig. pubicum superius

M. pectineus

M. adductor longus

M. gracilis

Canalis adductorius; A.; V. femoralis

Septum intermusculare vastoadductorium

M. sartorius

Femur, Condylus medialis

→ T 42, T 44, T 45

Fig. 1330 Muscles of the thigh and the hip; after removal of the fascia lata, the tensor fasciae latae muscle and the sartorius muscle.

* The fourth head of the quadriceps muscle, the vastus intermedius muscle, is covered by the rectus femoris muscle.

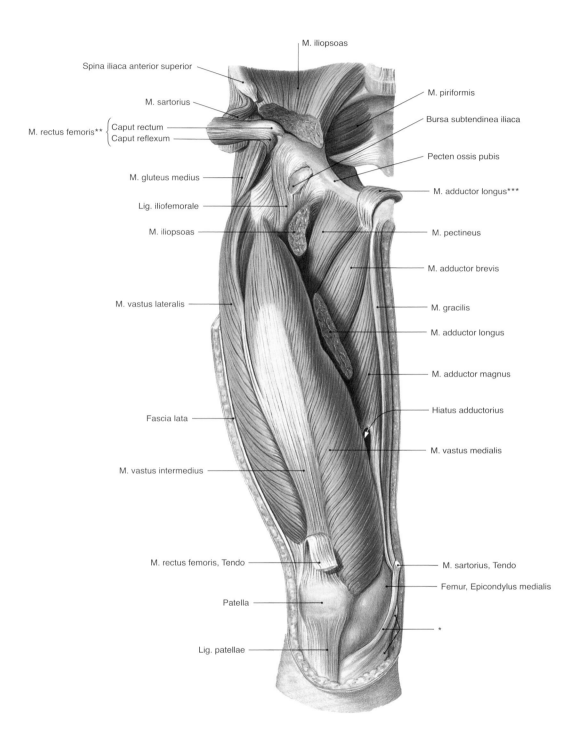

M. iliopsoas

Spina iliaca anterior superior

M. sartorius

M. rectus femoris** { Caput rectum
Caput reflexum

M. gluteus medius

Lig. iliofemorale

M. iliopsoas

M. vastus lateralis

Fascia lata

M. vastus intermedius

M. rectus femoris, Tendo

Patella

Lig. patellae

M. piriformis

Bursa subtendinea iliaca

Pecten ossis pubis

M. adductor longus***

M. pectineus

M. adductor brevis

M. gracilis

M. adductor longus

M. adductor magnus

Hiatus adductorius

M. vastus medialis

M. sartorius, Tendo

Femur, Epicondylus medialis

*

Fig. 1331 Muscles of the thigh and the hip;
deep layer after removal of the sartorius, the rectus femoris
and the adductor longus muscles as well as parts of the
iliopsoas muscle in the joint region.

* Common insertion of the sartorius, gracilis and semitendinosus
muscles just below the medial condyle of the tibia
** The origin of the rectus femoris muscle has been flapped laterally
upwards.
***A part of the adductor longus muscle has been flapped upwards.

→ T 42, T 44, T 45

Muscles of the thigh

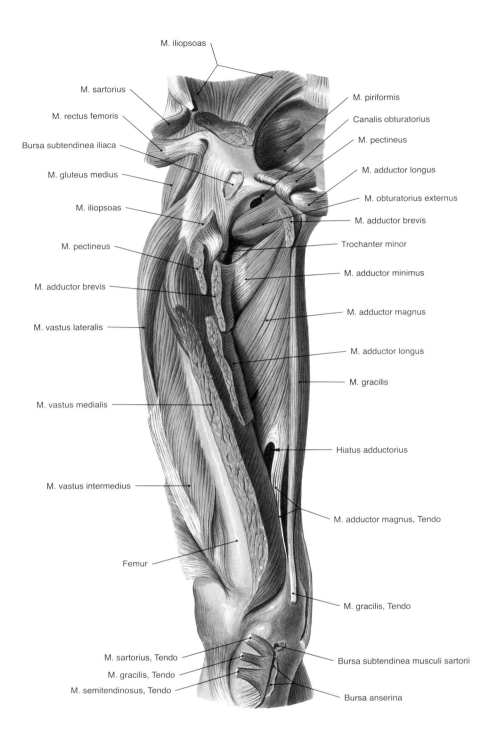

M. iliopsoas

M. sartorius

M. rectus femoris

Bursa subtendinea iliaca

M. gluteus medius

M. iliopsoas

M. pectineus

M. adductor brevis

M. vastus lateralis

M. vastus medialis

M. vastus intermedius

Femur

M. sartorius, Tendo

M. gracilis, Tendo

M. semitendinosus, Tendo

M. piriformis

Canalis obturatorius

M. pectineus

M. adductor longus

M. obturatorius externus

M. adductor brevis

Trochanter minor

M. adductor minimus

M. adductor magnus

M. adductor longus

M. gracilis

Hiatus adductorius

M. adductor magnus, Tendo

M. gracilis, Tendo

Bursa subtendinea musculi sartorii

Bursa anserina

→ T 42, T 44, T 45

Fig. 1332 Muscles of the thigh and the hip;
after almost complete removal of superficial and
several deeper muscles;
ventral view.

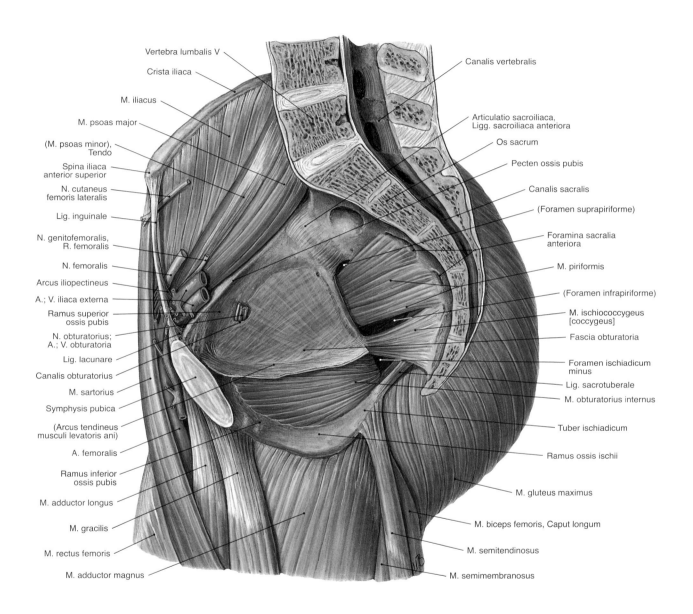

Vertebra lumbalis V

Crista iliaca

M. iliacus

M. psoas major

(M. psoas minor),
Tendo

Spina iliaca
anterior superior

N. cutaneus
femoris lateralis

Lig. inguinale

N. genitofemoralis,
R. femoralis

N. femoralis

Arcus iliopectineus

A.; V. iliaca externa

Ramus superior
ossis pubis

N. obturatorius;
A.; V. obturatoria

Lig. lacunare

Canalis obturatorius

M. sartorius

Symphysis pubica

(Arcus tendineus
musculi levatoris ani)

A. femoralis

Ramus inferior
ossis pubis

M. adductor longus

M. gracilis

M. rectus femoris

M. adductor magnus

Canalis vertebralis

Articulatio sacroiliaca,
Ligg. sacroiliaca anteriora

Os sacrum

Pecten ossis pubis

Canalis sacralis

(Foramen suprapiriforme)

Foramina sacralia
anteriora

M. piriformis

(Foramen infrapiriforme)

M. ischiococcygeus
[coccygeus]

Fascia obturatoria

Foramen ischiadicum
minus

Lig. sacrotuberale

M. obturatorius internus

Tuber ischiadicum

Ramus ossis ischii

M. gluteus maximus

M. biceps femoris, Caput longum

M. semitendinosus

M. semimembranosus

Fig. 1333   Muscles of the thigh and the hip;
medial view.

→ T 22 a, T 42–T 46

Muscles of the thigh and the hip

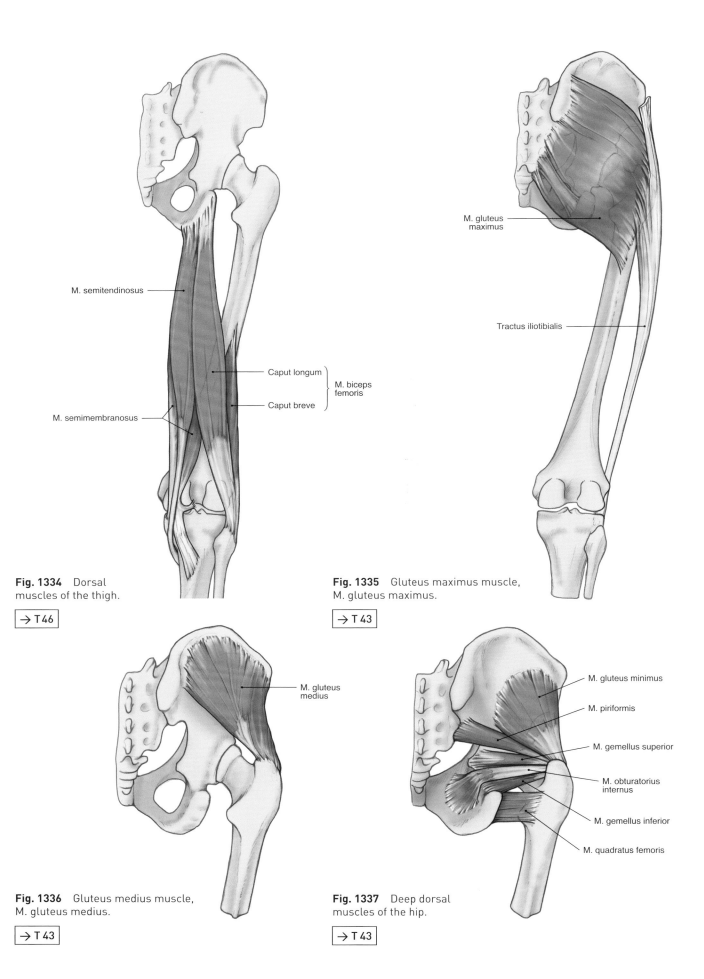

M. semitendinosus

Caput longum ⎤
            ⎥ M. biceps
Caput breve ⎦ femoris

M. semimembranosus

Fig. 1334 Dorsal
muscles of the thigh.

→ T 46

M. gluteus
maximus

Tractus iliotibialis

Fig. 1335 Gluteus maximus muscle,
M. gluteus maximus.

→ T 43

M. gluteus
medius

Fig. 1336 Gluteus medius muscle,
M. gluteus medius.

→ T 43

M. gluteus minimus

M. piriformis

M. gemellus superior

M. obturatorius
internus

M. gemellus inferior

M. quadratus femoris

Fig. 1337 Deep dorsal
muscles of the hip.

→ T 43

Muscles of the thigh and the hip

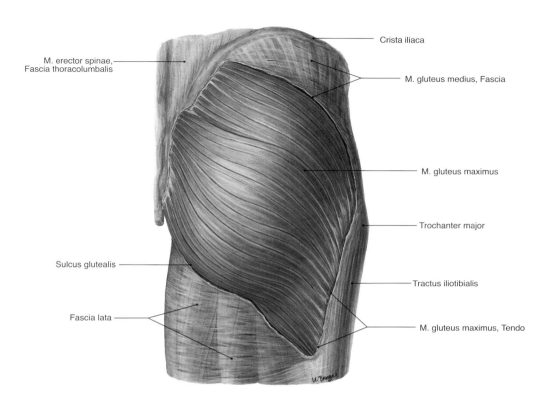

Crista iliaca

M. erector spinae,
Fascia thoracolumbalis

M. gluteus medius, Fascia

M. gluteus maximus

Trochanter major

Sulcus glutealis

Tractus iliotibialis

Fascia lata

M. gluteus maximus, Tendo

Fig. 1338   Muscles of the thigh and the hip.

$\rightarrow$ T 43

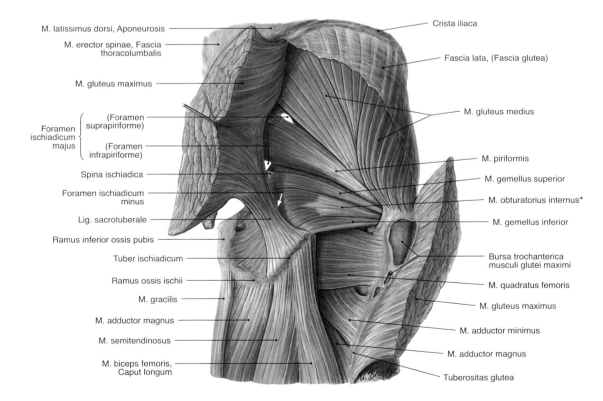

M. latissimus dorsi, Aponeurosis

Crista iliaca

M. erector spinae, Fascia
thoracolumbalis

Fascia lata, (Fascia glutea)

M. gluteus maximus

M. gluteus medius

Foramen
ischiadicum
majus
(Foramen
suprapiriforme)

(Foramen
infrapiriforme)

M. piriformis

M. gemellus superior

Spina ischiadica

M. obturatorius internus*

Foramen ischiadicum
minus

Lig. sacrotuberale

M. gemellus inferior

Ramus inferior ossis pubis

Bursa trochanterica
musculi glutei maximi

Tuber ischiadicum

M. quadratus femoris

Ramus ossis ischii

M. gluteus maximus

M. gracilis

M. adductor magnus

M. adductor minimus

M. semitendinosus

M. adductor magnus

M. biceps femoris,
Caput longum

Tuberositas glutea

Fig. 1339   Muscles of the thigh and the hip;
the gluteus maximus muscle has been sectioned;
dorsal view.

* The part of the obturator internus muscle between the curved edge
of the lesser sciatic notch and the insertion in the trochanteric fossa
frequently consists of tendinous bands.

$\rightarrow$ T 43, T 45, T 46

Muscles of the thigh and the hip

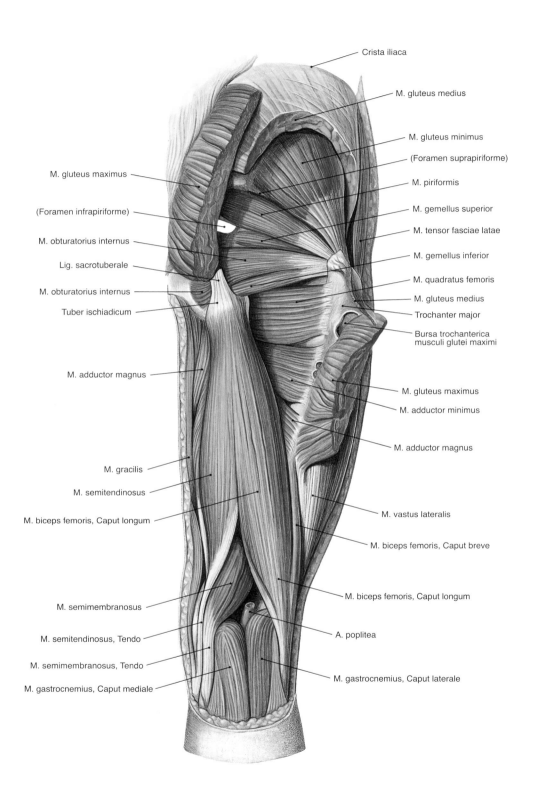

Crista iliaca

M. gluteus medius

M. gluteus minimus

(Foramen suprapiriforme)

M. gluteus maximus

M. piriformis

(Foramen infrapiriforme)

M. gemellus superior

M. obturatorius internus

M. tensor fasciae latae

Lig. sacrotuberale

M. gemellus inferior

M. obturatorius internus

M. quadratus femoris

Tuber ischiadicum

M. gluteus medius

Trochanter major

Bursa trochanterica musculi glutei maximi

M. adductor magnus

M. gluteus maximus

M. adductor minimus

M. adductor magnus

M. gracilis

M. semitendinosus

M. vastus lateralis

M. biceps femoris, Caput longum

M. biceps femoris, Caput breve

M. biceps femoris, Caput longum

M. semimembranosus

A. poplitea

M. semitendinosus, Tendo

M. semimembranosus, Tendo

M. gastrocnemius, Caput laterale

M. gastrocnemius, Caput mediale

→ T 43, T 45, T 46

Fig. 1340   Muscles of the thigh and the hip;
the gluteus maximus and medius muscles have
been partially removed;
dorsal view.

Muscles of the thigh and the hip

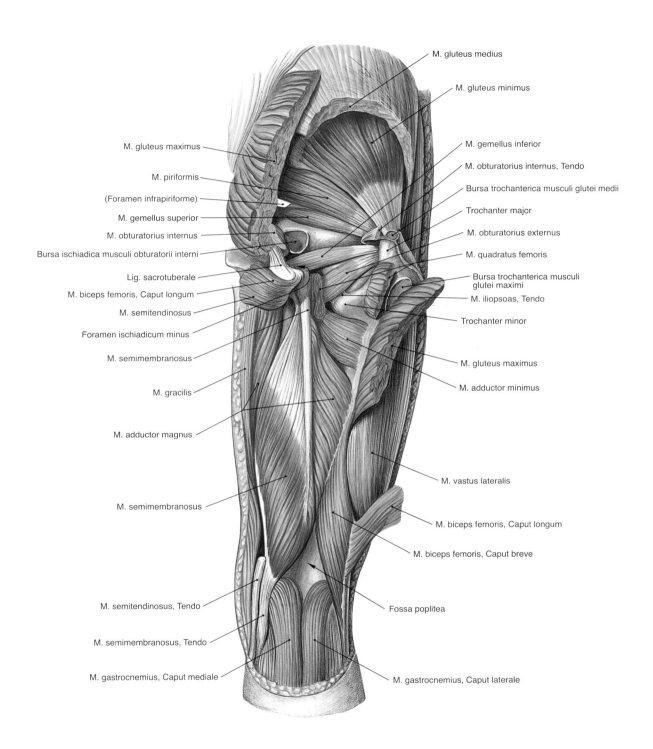

M. gluteus medius

M. gluteus minimus

M. gluteus maximus

M. piriformis

(Foramen infrapiriforme)

M. gemellus superior

M. obturatorius internus

Bursa ischiadica musculi obturatorii interni

Lig. sacrotuberale

M. biceps femoris, Caput longum

M. semitendinosus

Foramen ischiadicum minus

M. semimembranosus

M. gracilis

M. adductor magnus

M. semimembranosus

M. semitendinosus, Tendo

M. semimembranosus, Tendo

M. gastrocnemius, Caput mediale

M. gemellus inferior

M. obturatorius internus, Tendo

Bursa trochanterica musculi glutei medii

Trochanter major

M. obturatorius externus

M. quadratus femoris

Bursa trochanterica musculi glutei maximi

M. iliopsoas, Tendo

Trochanter minor

M. gluteus maximus

M. adductor minimus

M. vastus lateralis

M. biceps femoris, Caput longum

M. biceps femoris, Caput breve

Fossa poplitea

M. gastrocnemius, Caput laterale

Fig. 1341 Muscles of the thigh and the hip; deep layer after almost complete removal of the superficial gluteal and the ischiocrural muscles; dorsal view.

→ T 43, T 45, T 46

Muscles of the thigh and the hip

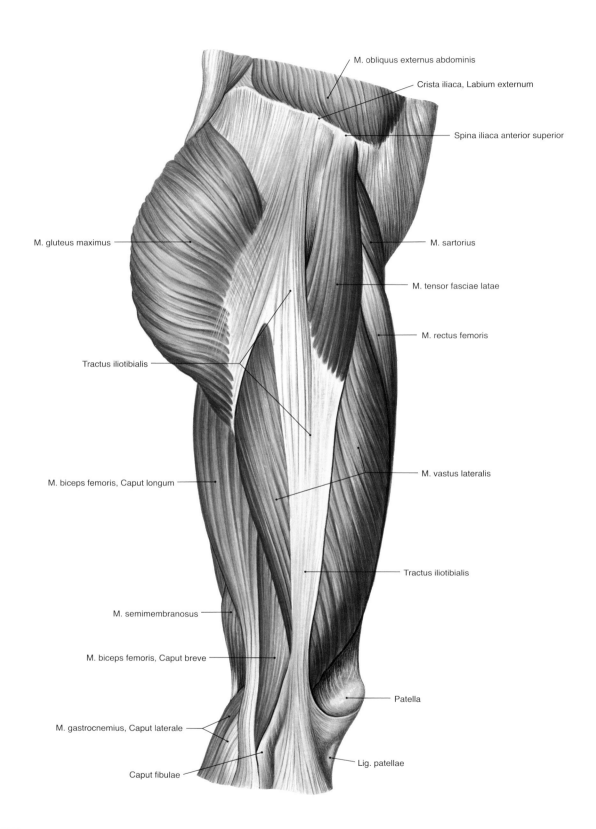

M. obliquus externus abdominis

Crista iliaca, Labium externum

Spina iliaca anterior superior

M. gluteus maximus

M. sartorius

M. tensor fasciae latae

M. rectus femoris

Tractus iliotibialis

M. biceps femoris, Caput longum

M. vastus lateralis

Tractus iliotibialis

M. semimembranosus

M. biceps femoris, Caput breve

Patella

M. gastrocnemius, Caput laterale

Caput fibulae

Lig. patellae

→ T 43, T 44, T 46

Fig. 1342 Muscles of the thigh and the hip;
after removal of the fascia lata except for the iliotibial tract.

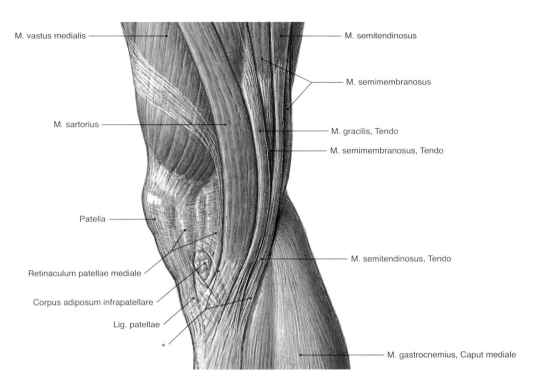

M. vastus medialis

M. semitendinosus

M. semimembranosus

M. sartorius

M. gracilis, Tendo

M. semimembranosus, Tendo

Patella

M. semitendinosus, Tendo

Retinaculum patellae mediale

Corpus adiposum infrapatellare

Lig. patellae

*

M. gastrocnemius, Caput mediale

Fig. 1343 Muscles in the region of the knee joint;
medial view.

* Common insertion just below the medial condyle of the tibia
(formerly known as superficial pes anserinus, Pes anserinus superficialis)

→ T 44–T 46, T 49

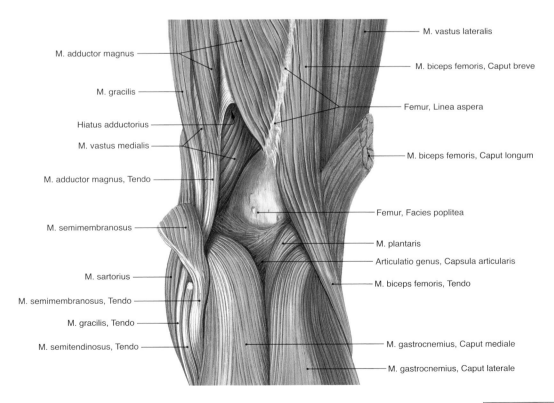

M. vastus lateralis

M. adductor magnus

M. biceps femoris, Caput breve

M. gracilis

Femur, Linea aspera

Hiatus adductorius

M. vastus medialis

M. biceps femoris, Caput longum

M. adductor magnus, Tendo

Femur, Facies poplitea

M. semimembranosus

M. plantaris

Articulatio genus, Capsula articularis

M. sartorius

M. biceps femoris, Tendo

M. semimembranosus, Tendo

M. gracilis, Tendo

M. semitendinosus, Tendo

M. gastrocnemius, Caput mediale

M. gastrocnemius, Caput laterale

Fig. 1344 Muscles in the region of the knee joint;
after almost complete removal of the ischiocrural muscles;
dorsal view.

→ T 44–T 46, T 49

Origins and insertions of the muscles of the thigh and the ventral part of the leg

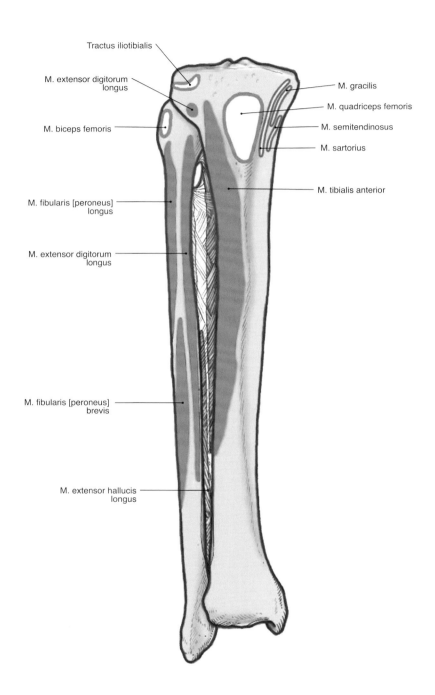

Tractus iliotibialis

M. extensor digitorum longus

M. biceps femoris

M. fibularis [peroneus] longus

M. extensor digitorum longus

M. fibularis [peroneus] brevis

M. extensor hallucis longus

M. gracilis

M. quadriceps femoris

M. semitendinosus

M. sartorius

M. tibialis anterior

→ T 44–T 47

Fig. 1345 Origins and insertions of the muscles at the bones of the leg; ventral view.

Origins and insertions of the muscles of the thigh and the dorsal part of the leg

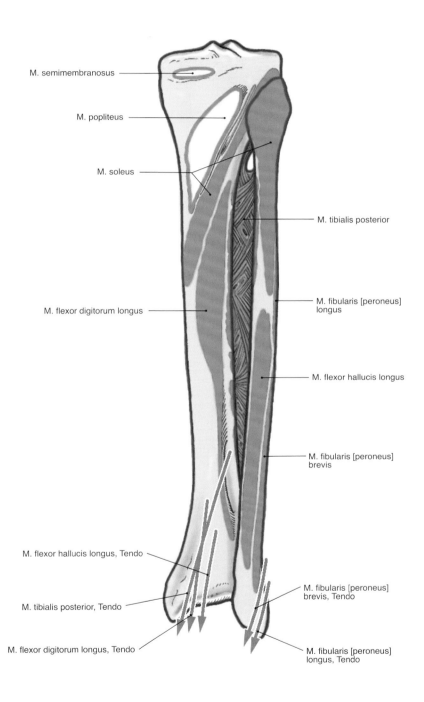

M. semimembranosus

M. popliteus

M. soleus

M. tibialis posterior

M. flexor digitorum longus

M. fibularis [peroneus] longus

M. flexor hallucis longus

M. fibularis [peroneus] brevis

M. flexor hallucis longus, Tendo

M. tibialis posterior, Tendo

M. fibularis [peroneus] brevis, Tendo

M. flexor digitorum longus, Tendo

M. fibularis [peroneus] longus, Tendo

Fig. 1346 Origins and insertions of the muscles at the bones of the leg; dorsal view.

→ T 46, T 48–T 50

Muscles of the leg

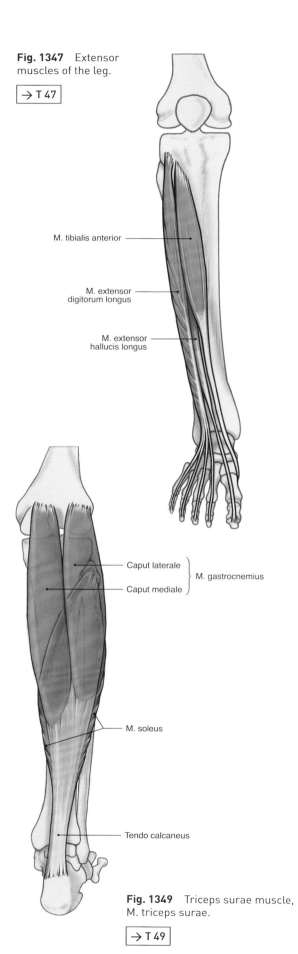

Fig. 1347 Extensor muscles of the leg.

→ T 47

M. tibialis anterior

M. extensor digitorum longus

M. extensor hallucis longus

Caput laterale ⎫
                    ⎬ M. gastrocnemius
Caput mediale ⎭

M. soleus

Tendo calcaneus

Fig. 1349 Triceps surae muscle, M. triceps surae.

→ T 49

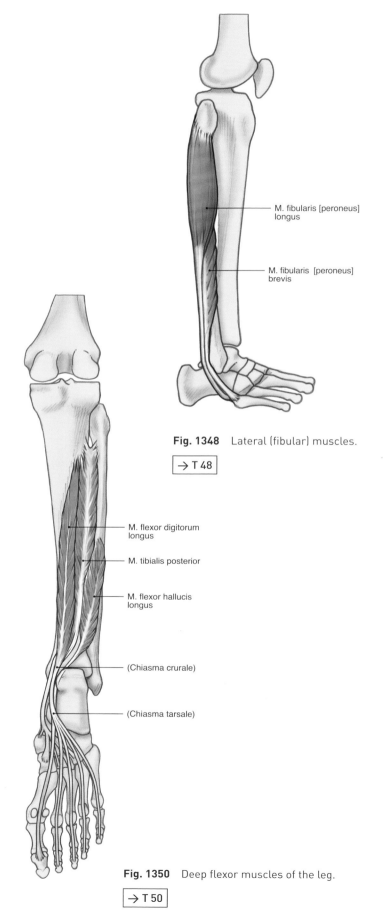

M. fibularis [peroneus] longus

M. fibularis [peroneus] brevis

Fig. 1348 Lateral (fibular) muscles.

→ T 48

M. flexor digitorum longus

M. tibialis posterior

M. flexor hallucis longus

(Chiasma crurale)

(Chiasma tarsale)

Fig. 1350 Deep flexor muscles of the leg.

→ T 50

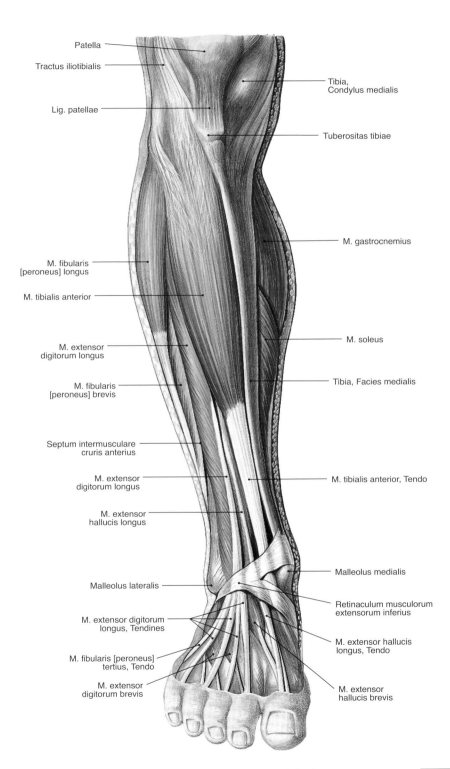

Patella

Tractus iliotibialis

Lig. patellae

Tibia, Condylus medialis

Tuberositas tibiae

M. gastrocnemius

M. fibularis [peroneus] longus

M. tibialis anterior

M. soleus

M. extensor digitorum longus

Tibia, Facies medialis

M. fibularis [peroneus] brevis

Septum intermusculare cruris anterius

M. extensor digitorum longus

M. tibialis anterior, Tendo

M. extensor hallucis longus

Malleolus medialis

Malleolus lateralis

Retinaculum musculorum extensorum inferius

M. extensor digitorum longus, Tendines

M. extensor hallucis longus, Tendo

M. fibularis [peroneus] tertius, Tendo

M. extensor digitorum brevis

M. extensor hallucis brevis

Fig. 1351   Muscles of the leg and the foot.

→ T 47, T 48

Muscles of the leg

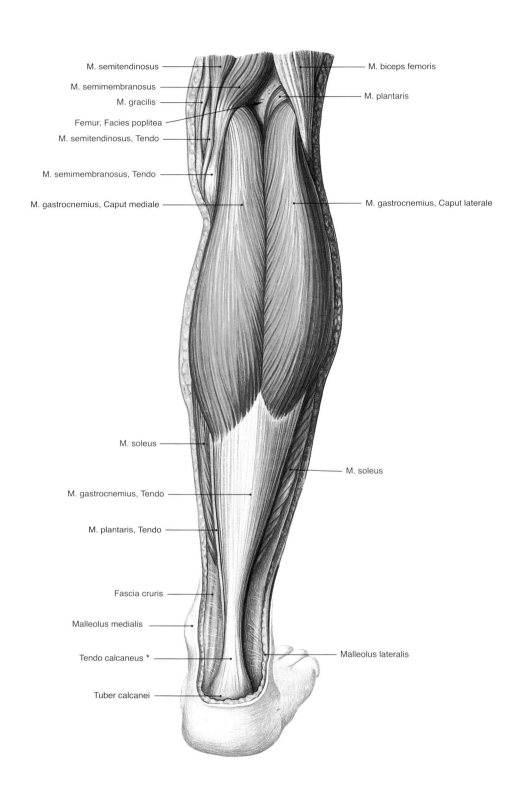

M. semitendinosus

M. semimembranosus

M. gracilis

Femur, Facies poplitea

M. semitendinosus, Tendo

M. semimembranosus, Tendo

M. gastrocnemius, Caput mediale

M. soleus

M. gastrocnemius, Tendo

M. plantaris, Tendo

Fascia cruris

Malleolus medialis

Tendo calcaneus *

Tuber calcanei

M. biceps femoris

M. plantaris

M. gastrocnemius, Caput laterale

M. soleus

Malleolus lateralis

→ T 49

Fig. 1352 Muscles of the leg;
superficial layer.
* Also: Achilles tendon

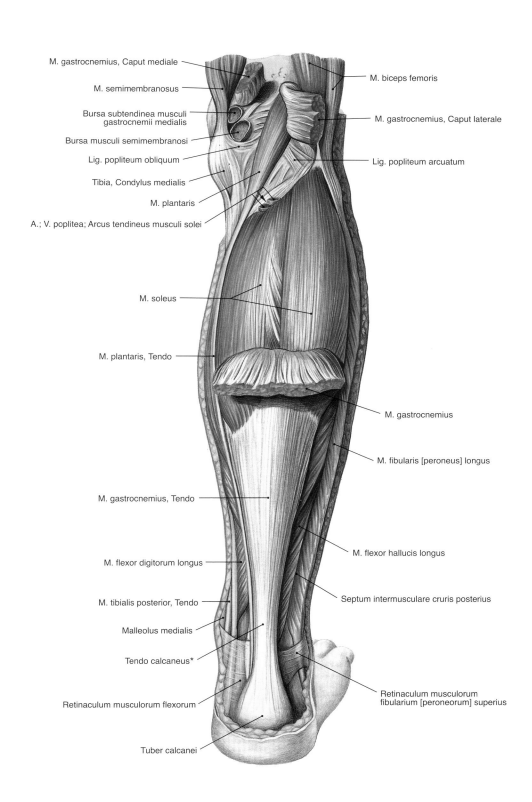

M. gastrocnemius, Caput mediale

M. semimembranosus

Bursa subtendinea musculi gastrocnemii medialis

Bursa musculi semimembranosi

Lig. popliteum obliquum

Tibia, Condylus medialis

M. plantaris

A.; V. poplitea; Arcus tendineus musculi solei

M. soleus

M. plantaris, Tendo

M. gastrocnemius, Tendo

M. flexor digitorum longus

M. tibialis posterior, Tendo

Malleolus medialis

Tendo calcaneus*

Retinaculum musculorum flexorum

Tuber calcanei

M. biceps femoris

M. gastrocnemius, Caput laterale

Lig. popliteum arcuatum

M. gastrocnemius

M. fibularis [peroneus] longus

M. flexor hallucis longus

Septum intermusculare cruris posterius

Retinaculum musculorum fibularium [peroneorum] superius

Fig. 1353 Muscles of the leg; superficial layer after partial removal of the gastrocnemius muscle.
* Also: Achilles tendon

 → T 49

Muscles of the leg

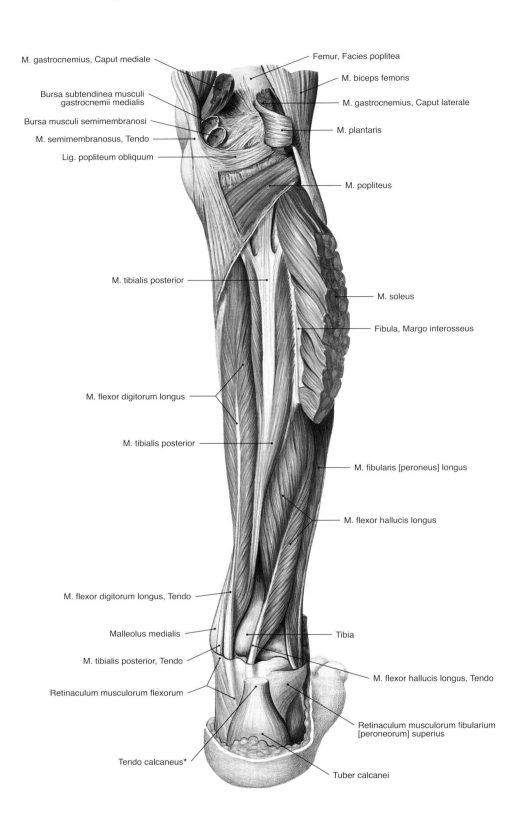

M. gastrocnemius, Caput mediale

Bursa subtendinea musculi gastrocnemii medialis

Bursa musculi semimembranosi

M. semimembranosus, Tendo

Lig. popliteum obliquum

M. tibialis posterior

M. flexor digitorum longus

M. tibialis posterior

M. flexor digitorum longus, Tendo

Malleolus medialis

M. tibialis posterior, Tendo

Retinaculum musculorum flexorum

Tendo calcaneus*

Femur, Facies poplitea

M. biceps femoris

M. gastrocnemius, Caput laterale

M. plantaris

M. popliteus

M. soleus

Fibula, Margo interosseus

M. fibularis [peroneus] longus

M. flexor hallucis longus

Tibia

M. flexor hallucis longus, Tendo

Retinaculum musculorum fibularium [peroneorum] superius

Tuber calcanei

→ T 50

Fig. 1354 Muscles of the leg; deep layer.
* Also: Achilles tendon

Muscles of the leg

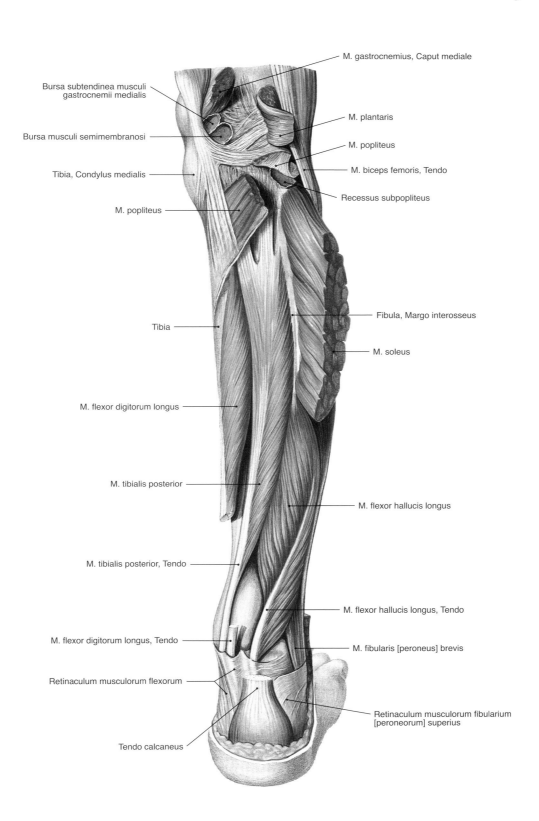

M. gastrocnemius, Caput mediale

Bursa subtendinea musculi
gastrocnemii medialis

M. plantaris

Bursa musculi semimembranosi

M. popliteus

M. biceps femoris, Tendo

Tibia, Condylus medialis

Recessus subpopliteus

M. popliteus

Tibia

Fibula, Margo interosseus

M. soleus

M. flexor digitorum longus

M. tibialis posterior

M. flexor hallucis longus

M. tibialis posterior, Tendo

M. flexor hallucis longus, Tendo

M. flexor digitorum longus, Tendo

M. fibularis [peroneus] brevis

Retinaculum musculorum flexorum

Retinaculum musculorum fibularium
[peroneorum] superius

Tendo calcaneus

Fig. 1355   Muscles of the leg;
deepest layer.

→ T 50

Muscles of the leg

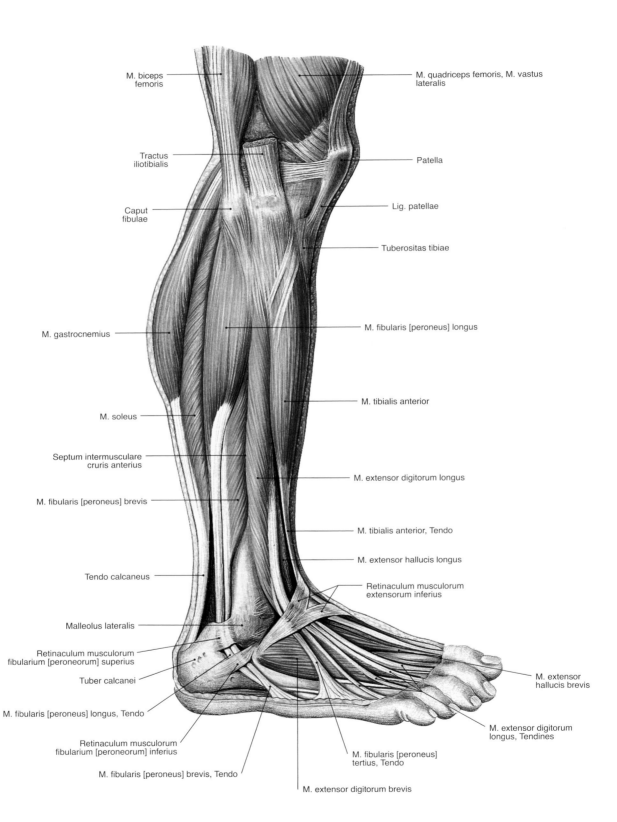

M. biceps femoris

M. quadriceps femoris, M. vastus lateralis

Tractus iliotibialis

Patella

Caput fibulae

Lig. patellae

Tuberositas tibiae

M. gastrocnemius

M. fibularis [peroneus] longus

M. tibialis anterior

M. soleus

Septum intermusculare cruris anterius

M. extensor digitorum longus

M. fibularis [peroneus] brevis

M. tibialis anterior, Tendo

M. extensor hallucis longus

Tendo calcaneus

Retinaculum musculorum extensorum inferius

Malleolus lateralis

Retinaculum musculorum fibularium [peroneorum] superius

Tuber calcanei

M. extensor hallucis brevis

M. fibularis [peroneus] longus, Tendo

M. extensor digitorum longus, Tendines

Retinaculum musculorum fibularium [peroneorum] inferius

M. fibularis [peroneus] brevis, Tendo

M. fibularis [peroneus] tertius, Tendo

M. extensor digitorum brevis

→ T 47 – T 49, T 51

Fig. 1356 Muscles of the leg and the foot.

Origins and insertions of the muscles of the the foot and the leg

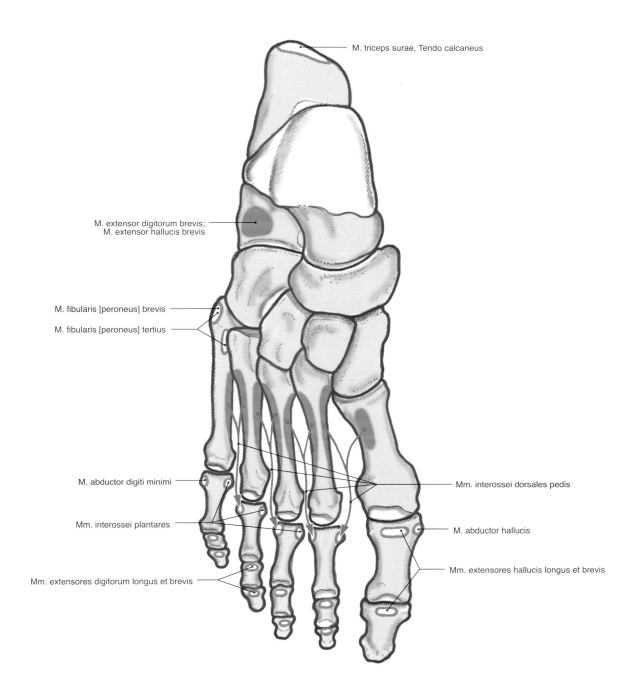

M. triceps surae, Tendo calcaneus

M. extensor digitorum brevis;
M. extensor hallucis brevis

M. fibularis [peroneus] brevis

M. fibularis [peroneus] tertius

M. abductor digiti minimi

Mm. interossei plantares

Mm. extensores digitorum longus et brevis

Mm. interossei dorsales pedis

M. abductor hallucis

Mm. extensores hallucis longus et brevis

Fig. 1357 Origins and insertions of the muscles
at the bones of the foot;
dorsal view.

→ T 47, T 48, T 51,
T 53, T 54

Tendon sheaths of the foot

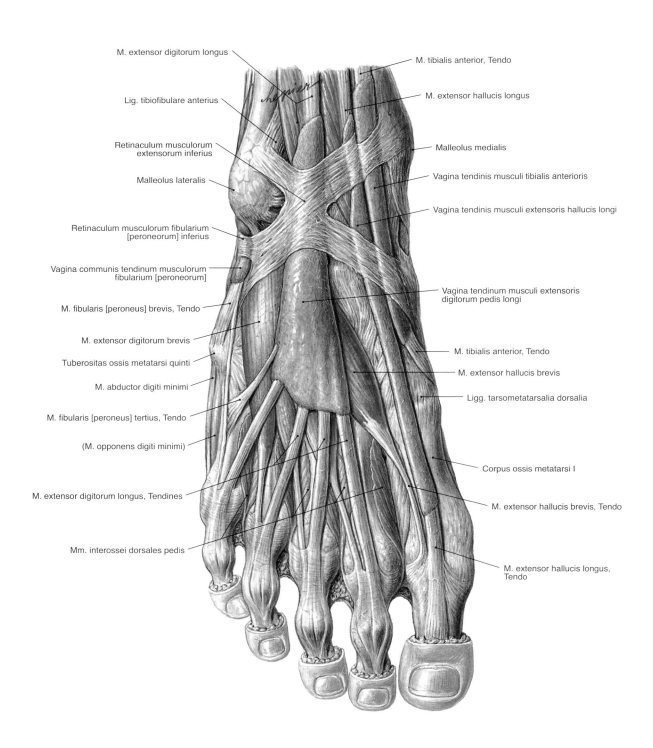

M. extensor digitorum longus

M. tibialis anterior, Tendo

Lig. tibiofibulare anterius

M. extensor hallucis longus

Retinaculum musculorum extensorum inferius

Malleolus medialis

Malleolus lateralis

Vagina tendinis musculi tibialis anterioris

Vagina tendinis musculi extensoris hallucis longi

Retinaculum musculorum fibularium [peroneorum] inferius

Vagina communis tendinum musculorum fibularium [peroneorum]

Vagina tendinum musculi extensoris digitorum pedis longi

M. fibularis [peroneus] brevis, Tendo

M. extensor digitorum brevis

Tuberositas ossis metatarsi quinti

M. tibialis anterior, Tendo

M. abductor digiti minimi

M. extensor hallucis brevis

M. fibularis [peroneus] tertius, Tendo

Ligg. tarsometatarsalia dorsalia

(M. opponens digiti minimi)

Corpus ossis metatarsi I

M. extensor digitorum longus, Tendines

M. extensor hallucis brevis, Tendo

Mm. interossei dorsales pedis

M. extensor hallucis longus, Tendo

Fig. 1358 Tendon sheaths, Vaginae tendinum, of the foot.

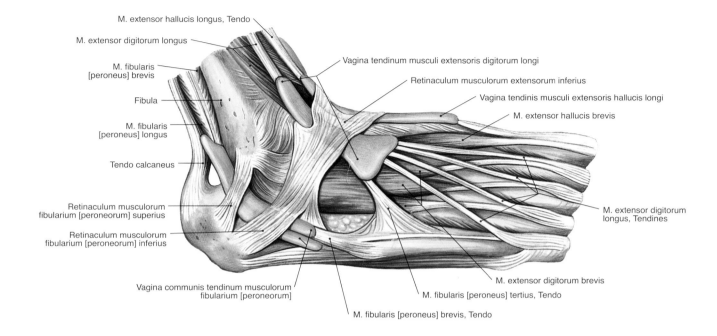

M. extensor hallucis longus, Tendo

M. extensor digitorum longus

M. fibularis [peroneus] brevis

Fibula

M. fibularis [peroneus] longus

Tendo calcaneus

Retinaculum musculorum fibularium [peroneorum] superius

Retinaculum musculorum fibularium [peroneorum] inferius

Vagina communis tendinum musculorum fibularium [peroneorum]

Vagina tendinum musculi extensoris digitorum longi

Retinaculum musculorum extensorum inferius

Vagina tendinis musculi extensoris hallucis longi

M. extensor hallucis brevis

M. extensor digitorum longus, Tendines

M. extensor digitorum brevis

M. fibularis [peroneus] tertius, Tendo

M. fibularis [peroneus] brevis, Tendo

Fig. 1359 Tendon sheaths, Vaginae tendinum, of the foot.

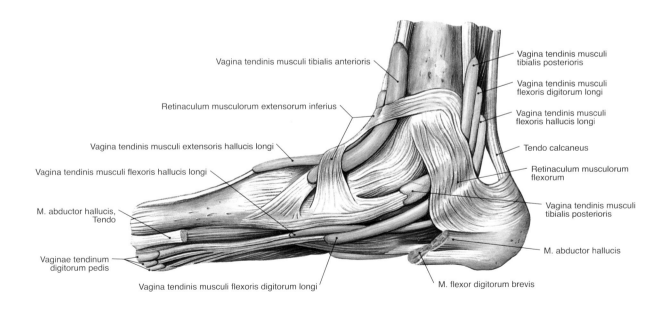

Vagina tendinis musculi tibialis anterioris

Retinaculum musculorum extensorum inferius

Vagina tendinis musculi extensoris hallucis longi

Vagina tendinis musculi flexoris hallucis longi

M. abductor hallucis, Tendo

Vaginae tendinum digitorum pedis

Vagina tendinis musculi flexoris digitorum longi

Vagina tendinis musculi tibialis posterioris

Vagina tendinis musculi flexoris digitorum longi

Vagina tendinis musculi flexoris hallucis longi

Tendo calcaneus

Retinaculum musculorum flexorum

Vagina tendinis musculi tibialis posterioris

M. abductor hallucis

M. flexor digitorum brevis

Fig. 1360 Tendon sheaths, Vaginae tendinum, of the foot.

Muscles of the foot

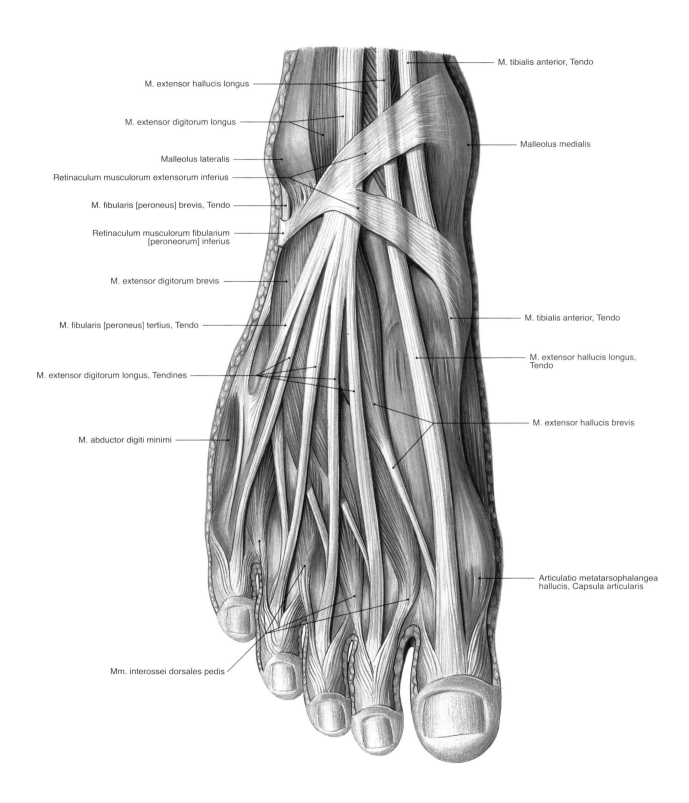

M. tibialis anterior, Tendo

M. extensor hallucis longus

M. extensor digitorum longus

Malleolus medialis

Malleolus lateralis

Retinaculum musculorum extensorum inferius

M. fibularis [peroneus] brevis, Tendo

Retinaculum musculorum fibularium [peroneorum] inferius

M. extensor digitorum brevis

M. fibularis [peroneus] tertius, Tendo

M. tibialis anterior, Tendo

M. extensor digitorum longus, Tendines

M. extensor hallucis longus, Tendo

M. abductor digiti minimi

M. extensor hallucis brevis

Articulatio metatarsophalangea hallucis, Capsula articularis

Mm. interossei dorsales pedis

→ T 47, T 51, T 53

Fig. 1361 Muscles of the foot; after removal of the tendon sheaths.

Muscles of the foot

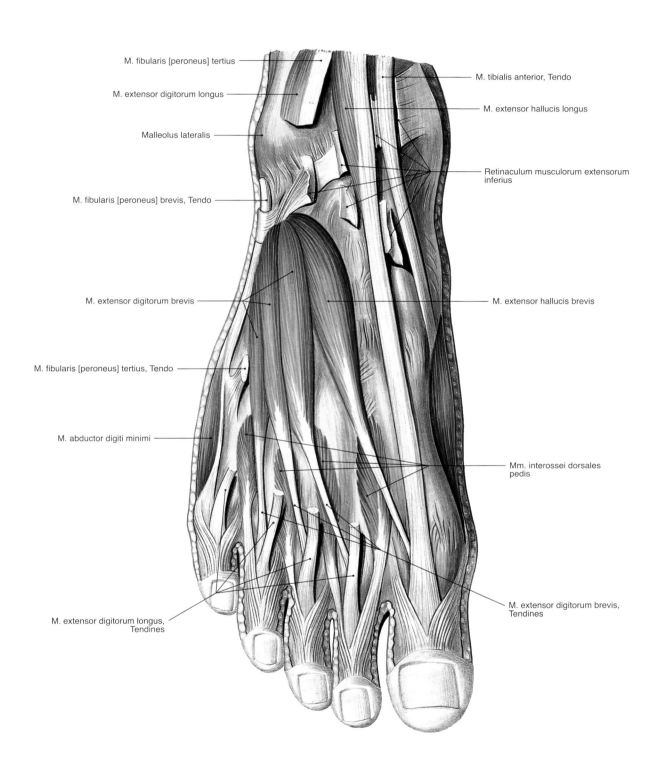

M. fibularis [peroneus] tertius

M. extensor digitorum longus

Malleolus lateralis

M. fibularis [peroneus] brevis, Tendo

M. extensor digitorum brevis

M. fibularis [peroneus] tertius, Tendo

M. abductor digiti minimi

M. extensor digitorum longus, Tendines

M. tibialis anterior, Tendo

M. extensor hallucis longus

Retinaculum musculorum extensorum inferius

M. extensor hallucis brevis

Mm. interossei dorsales pedis

M. extensor digitorum brevis, Tendines

Fig. 1362   Muscles of the foot; after section of the inferior extensor retinaculum.

→ T 47, T 51, T 53

Muscles of the foot

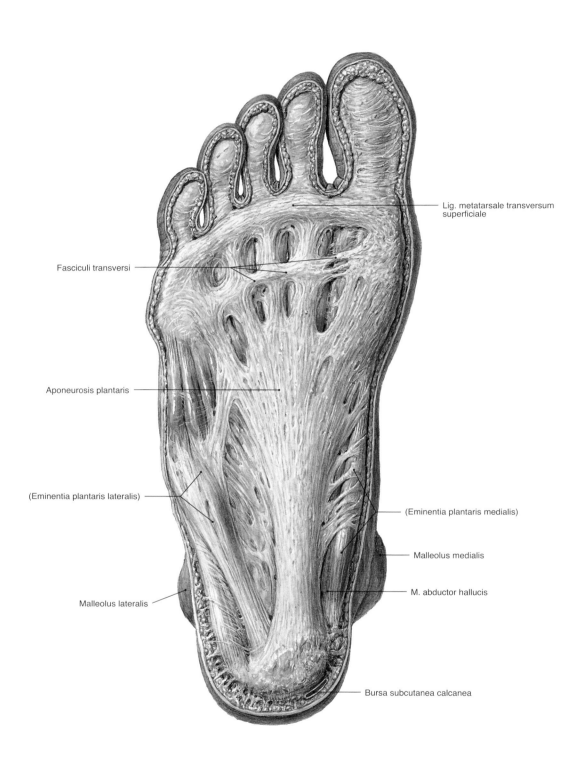

Lig. metatarsale transversum superficiale

Fasciculi transversi

Aponeurosis plantaris

(Eminentia plantaris lateralis)

(Eminentia plantaris medialis)

Malleolus medialis

M. abductor hallucis

Malleolus lateralis

Bursa subcutanea calcanea

Fig. 1363 Muscles of the foot;
plantar aponeurosis, Aponeurosis plantaris.

Origins and insertions of the muscles of the foot and the leg

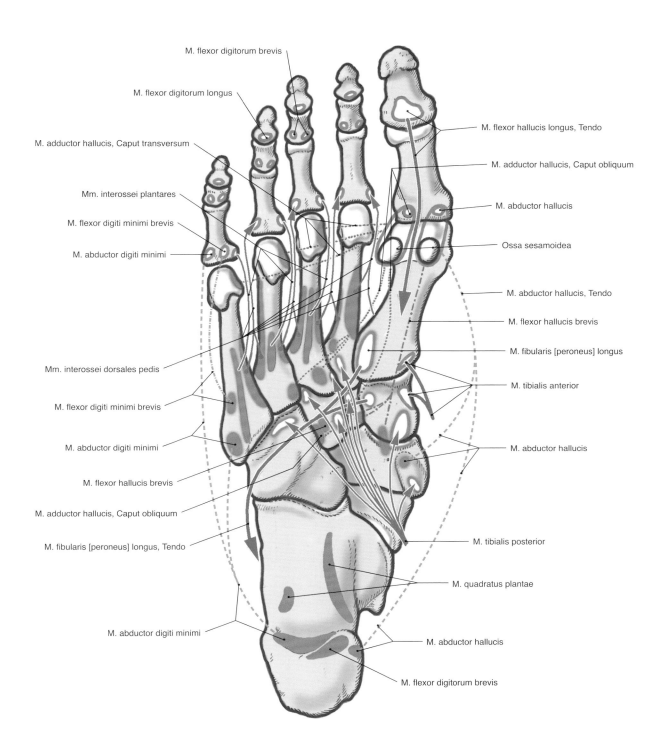

M. flexor digitorum brevis

M. flexor digitorum longus

M. adductor hallucis, Caput transversum

Mm. interossei plantares

M. flexor digiti minimi brevis

M. abductor digiti minimi

Mm. interossei dorsales pedis

M. flexor digiti minimi brevis

M. abductor digiti minimi

M. flexor hallucis brevis

M. adductor hallucis, Caput obliquum

M. fibularis [peroneus] longus, Tendo

M. abductor digiti minimi

M. flexor hallucis longus, Tendo

M. adductor hallucis, Caput obliquum

M. abductor hallucis

Ossa sesamoidea

M. abductor hallucis, Tendo

M. flexor hallucis brevis

M. fibularis [peroneus] longus

M. tibialis anterior

M. abductor hallucis

M. tibialis posterior

M. quadratus plantae

M. abductor hallucis

M. flexor digitorum brevis

Fig. 1364 Origins and insertions of the muscles at the bones of the foot; plantar view.

→ T 47, T 48, T 50, T 52–T 54

Muscles of the foot

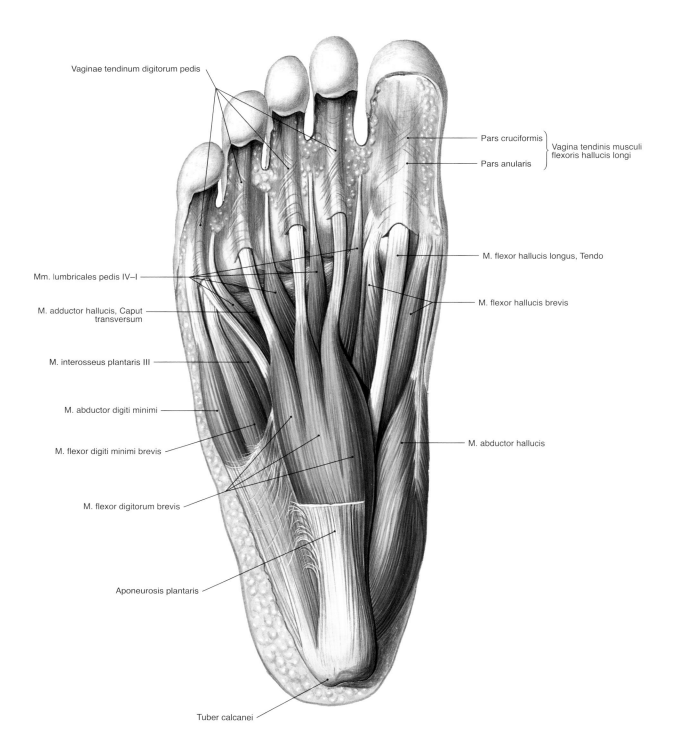

Vaginae tendinum digitorum pedis

Pars cruciformis ⎫ Vagina tendinis musculi
                    ⎬ flexoris hallucis longi
Pars anularis   ⎭

M. flexor hallucis longus, Tendo

Mm. lumbricales pedis IV–I

M. adductor hallucis, Caput transversum

M. flexor hallucis brevis

M. interosseus plantaris III

M. abductor digiti minimi

M. flexor digiti minimi brevis

M. abductor hallucis

M. flexor digitorum brevis

Aponeurosis plantaris

Tuber calcanei

→ T 52 – T 54

Fig. 1365 Muscles of the foot;
the plantar aponeurosis has been removed.

Muscles of the foot

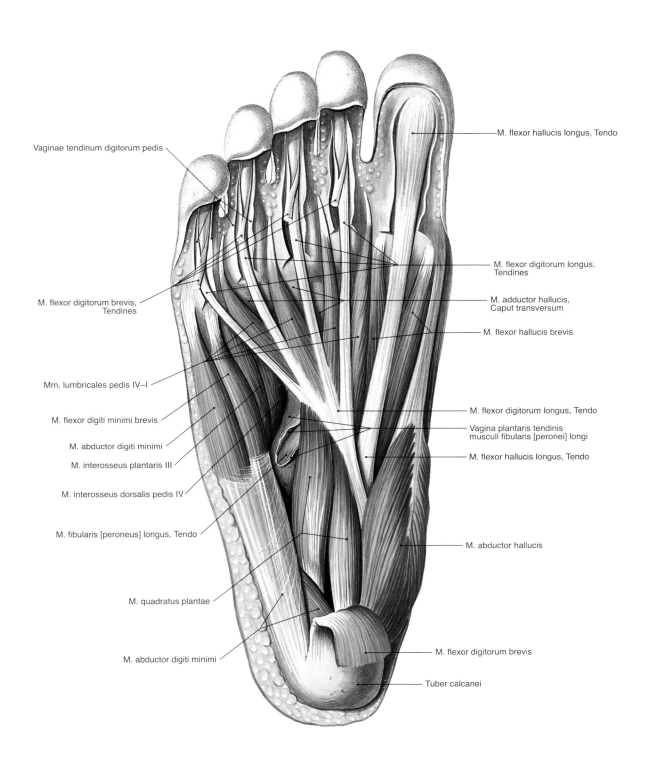

Vaginae tendinum digitorum pedis

M. flexor digitorum brevis, Tendines

Mm. lumbricales pedis IV–I

M. flexor digiti minimi brevis

M. abductor digiti minimi

M. interosseus plantaris III

M. interosseus dorsalis pedis IV

M. fibularis [peroneus] longus, Tendo

M. quadratus plantae

M. abductor digiti minimi

M. flexor hallucis longus, Tendo

M. flexor digitorum longus, Tendines

M. adductor hallucis, Caput transversum

M. flexor hallucis brevis

M. flexor digitorum longus, Tendo

Vagina plantaris tendinis musculi fibularis [peronei] longi

M. flexor hallucis longus, Tendo

M. abductor hallucis

M. flexor digitorum brevis

Tuber calcanei

Fig. 1366   Muscles of the foot;
middle layer after almost complete removal of the
flexor digitorum brevis muscle.

→ T 50, T 52 – T 54

Muscles of the foot

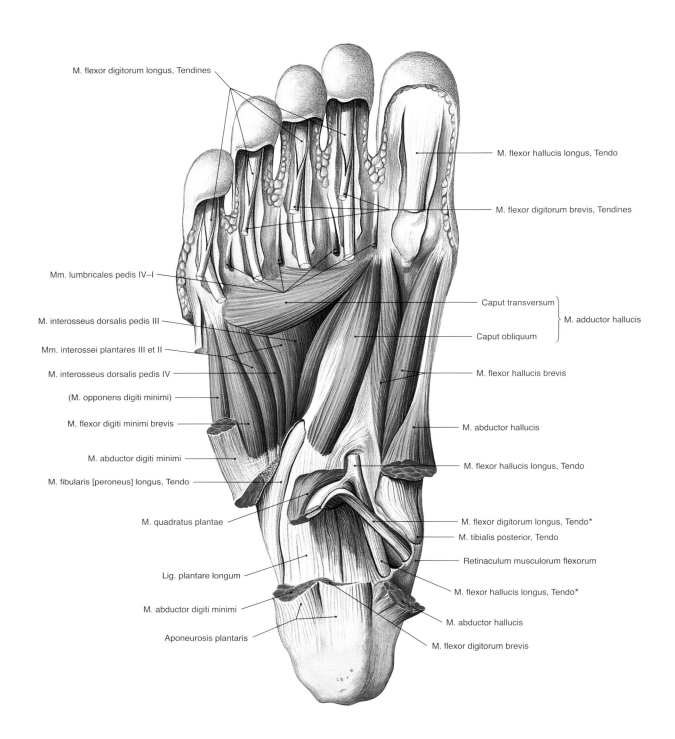

M. flexor digitorum longus, Tendines

M. flexor hallucis longus, Tendo

M. flexor digitorum brevis, Tendines

Mm. lumbricales pedis IV–I

M. interosseus dorsalis pedis III

Mm. interossei plantares III et II

M. interosseus dorsalis pedis IV

(M. opponens digiti minimi)

M. flexor digiti minimi brevis

M. abductor digiti minimi

M. fibularis [peroneus] longus, Tendo

M. quadratus plantae

Lig. plantare longum

M. abductor digiti minimi

Aponeurosis plantaris

Caput transversum

Caput obliquum

M. adductor hallucis

M. flexor hallucis brevis

M. abductor hallucis

M. flexor hallucis longus, Tendo

M. flexor digitorum longus, Tendo*

M. tibialis posterior, Tendo

Retinaculum musculorum flexorum

M. flexor hallucis longus, Tendo*

M. abductor hallucis

M. flexor digitorum brevis

→ T 50, T 52 – T 54

Fig. 1367 Muscles of the foot;
deep layer.

* The site where the tendon of the flexor digitorum longus muscle crosses the tendon of the flexor hallucis longus muscle is commonly referred to as plantar chiasm, Chiasma plantare.

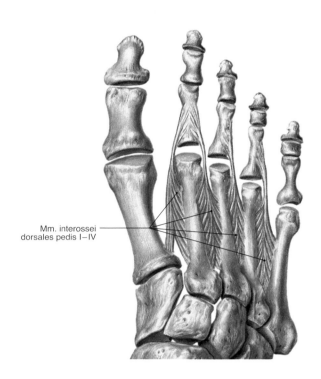

Mm. interossei
dorsales pedis I–IV

Fig. 1368   Dorsal interossei muscles, Mm. interossei dorsales pedis;
dorsal view.   → T 53

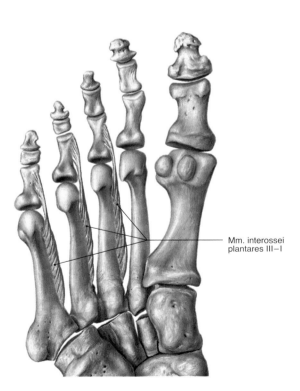

Mm. interossei
plantares III–I

Fig. 1369   Plantar interossei muscles, Mm. interossei plantares;
plantar view.   → T 53

Lumbosacral plexus

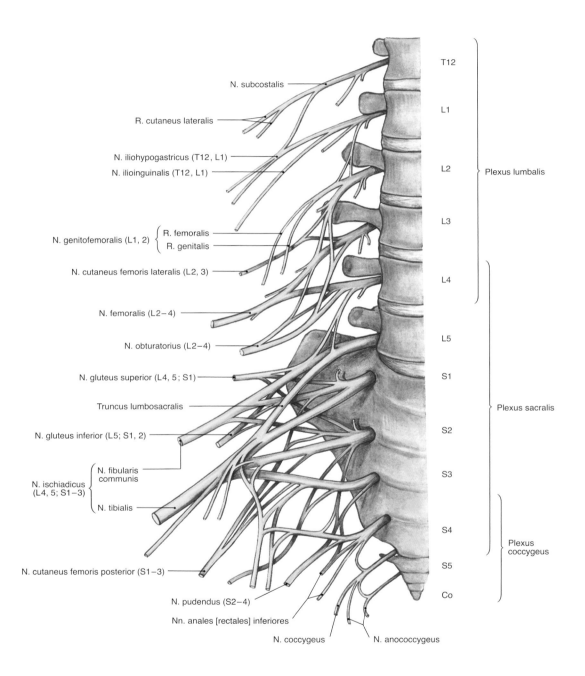

N. subcostalis

R. cutaneus lateralis

N. iliohypogastricus (T12, L1)

N. ilioinguinalis (T12, L1)

N. genitofemoralis (L1, 2) { R. femoralis
R. genitalis

N. cutaneus femoris lateralis (L2, 3)

N. femoralis (L2–4)

N. obturatorius (L2–4)

N. gluteus superior (L4, 5; S1)

Truncus lumbosacralis

N. gluteus inferior (L5; S1, 2)

N. ischiadicus (L4, 5; S1–3) { N. fibularis communis
N. tibialis

N. cutaneus femoris posterior (S1–3)

N. pudendus (S2–4)

Nn. anales [rectales] inferiores

N. coccygeus

N. anococcygeus

T12

L1

L2

L3

L4

L5

S1

S2

S3

S4

S5

Co

Plexus lumbalis

Plexus sacralis

Plexus coccygeus

→ 863

Fig. 1370 Lumbosacral and coccygeal plexus, Plexus lumbosacralis (Plexus lumbalis et sacralis) et coccygeus; segmental organisation of nerves.

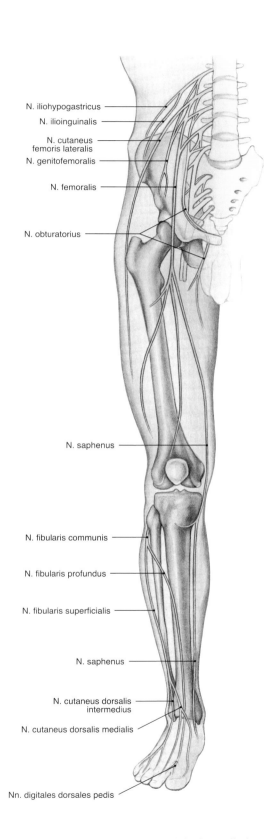

N. iliohypogastricus

N. ilioinguinalis

N. cutaneus
femoris lateralis

N. genitofemoralis

N. femoralis

N. obturatorius

N. saphenus

N. fibularis communis

N. fibularis profundus

N. fibularis superficialis

N. saphenus

N. cutaneus dorsalis
intermedius

N. cutaneus dorsalis medialis

Nn. digitales dorsales pedis

Fig. 1371 Nerves of the lower limb;
overview.

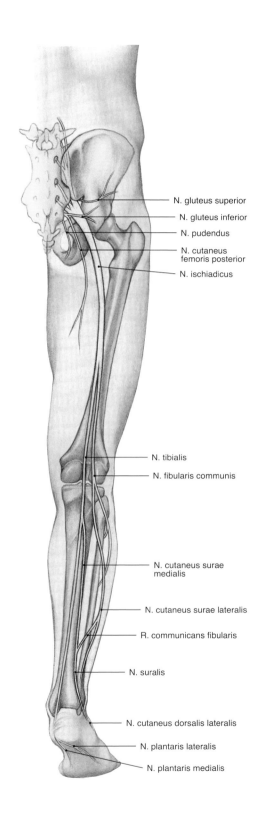

N. gluteus superior

N. gluteus inferior

N. pudendus

N. cutaneus
femoris posterior

N. ischiadicus

N. tibialis

N. fibularis communis

N. cutaneus surae
medialis

N. cutaneus surae lateralis

R. communicans fibularis

N. suralis

N. cutaneus dorsalis lateralis

N. plantaris lateralis

N. plantaris medialis

Fig. 1372 Nerves of the lower limb;
overview.

Cutaneous innervation

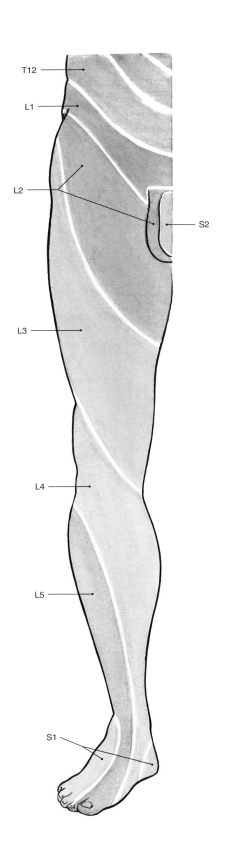

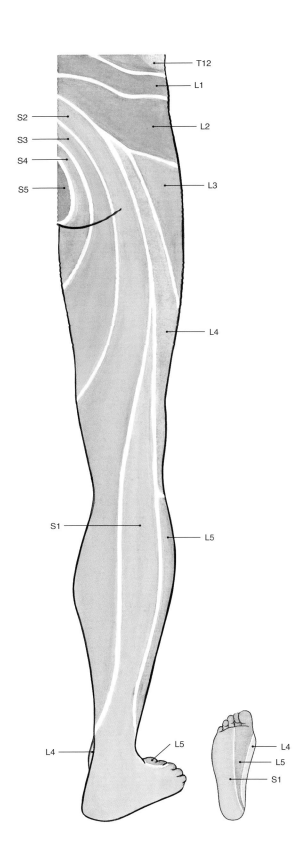

Fig. 1373 Segmental cutaneous innervation (dermatomes) of the lower limb.

Fig. 1374 Segmental cutaneous innervation (dermatomes) of the lower limb.

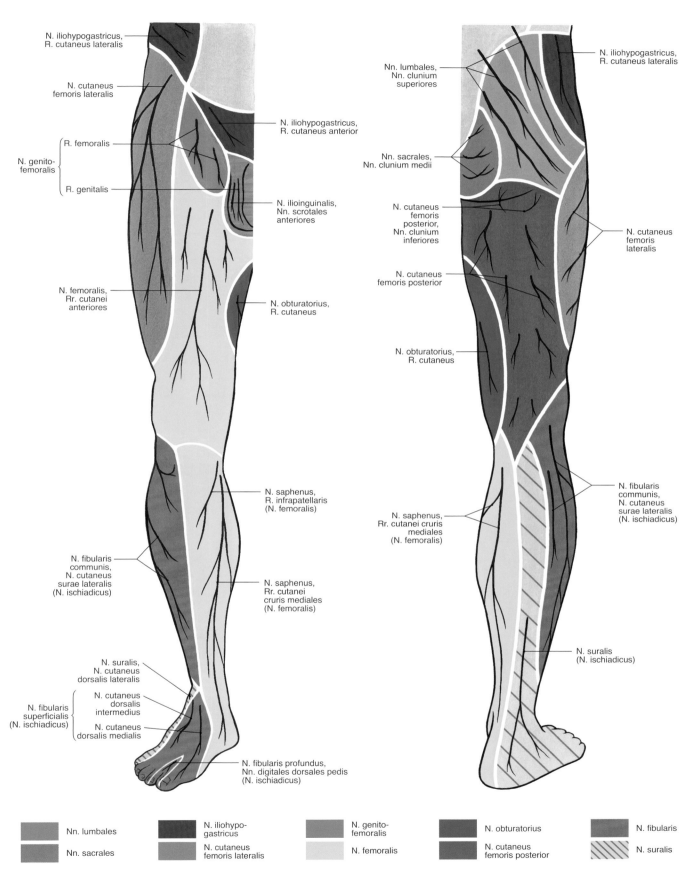

N. iliohypogastricus,
R. cutaneus lateralis

N. cutaneus
femoris lateralis

N. genito-
femoris
{ R. femoralis

R. genitalis }

N. femoralis,
Rr. cutanei
anteriores

N. fibularis
communis,
N. cutaneus
surae lateralis
(N. ischiadicus)

N. suralis,
N. cutaneus
dorsalis lateralis

N. fibularis
superficialis
(N. ischiadicus)
{ N. cutaneus
dorsalis
intermedius

N. cutaneus
dorsalis medialis }

N. iliohypogastricus,
R. cutaneus anterior

N. ilioinguinalis,
Nn. scrotales
anteriores

N. obturatorius,
R. cutaneus

N. saphenus,
R. infrapatellaris
(N. femoralis)

N. saphenus,
Rr. cutanei
cruris mediales
(N. femoralis)

N. fibularis profundus,
Nn. digitales dorsales pedis
(N. ischiadicus)

Nn. lumbales,
Nn. clunium
superiores

Nn. sacrales,
Nn. clunium medii

N. cutaneus
femoris
posterior,
Nn. clunium
inferiores

N. cutaneus
femoris posterior

N. obturatorius,
R. cutaneus

N. saphenus,
Rr. cutanei cruris
mediales
(N. femoralis)

N. iliohypogastricus,
R. cutaneus lateralis

N. cutaneus
femoris
lateralis

N. fibularis
communis,
N. cutaneus
surae lateralis
(N. ischiadicus)

N. suralis
(N. ischiadicus)

| | Nn. lumbales | | N. iliohypo-gastricus | | N. genito-femoralis | | N. obturatorius | | N. fibularis |
| | Nn. sacrales | | N. cutaneus femoris lateralis | | N. femoralis | | N. cutaneus femoris posterior | | N. suralis |

Fig. 1375 Cutaneous nerves of the lower limb.

Fig. 1376 Cutaneous nerves of the lower limb.

Femoral and obturator nerve

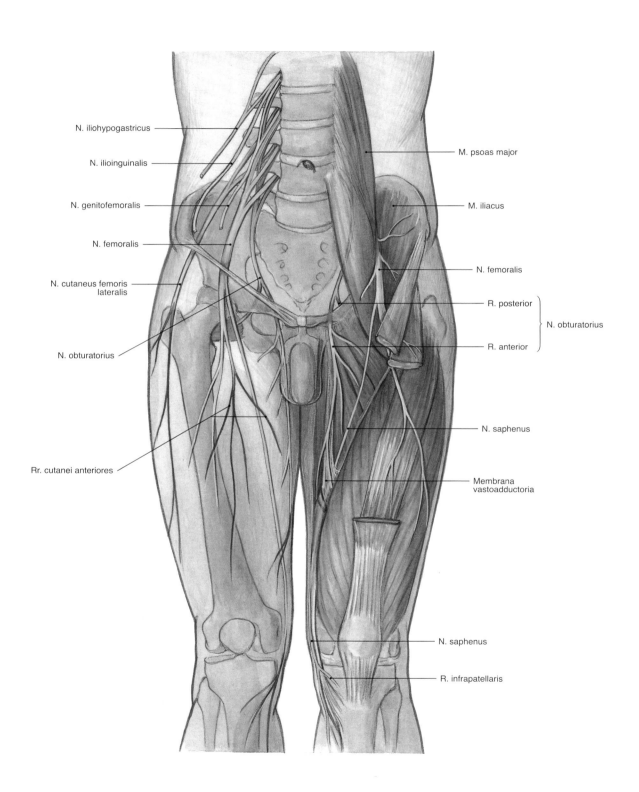

N. iliohypogastricus

N. ilioinguinalis

N. genitofemoralis

N. femoralis

N. cutaneus femoris lateralis

N. obturatorius

Rr. cutanei anteriores

M. psoas major

M. iliacus

N. femoralis

R. posterior ⎫
⎬ N. obturatorius
R. anterior ⎭

N. saphenus

Membrana vastoadductoria

N. saphenus

R. infrapatellaris

Fig. 1377 Femoral and obturator nerve, Nn. femoralis et obturatorius; overview; cutaneous innervation illustrated with purple.

Gluteal nerves and sciatic nerve

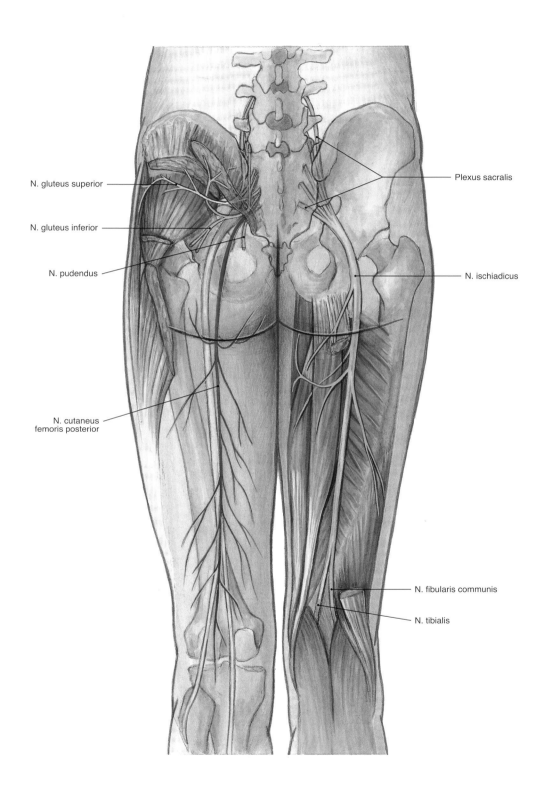

N. gluteus superior

N. gluteus inferior

N. pudendus

N. cutaneus femoris posterior

Plexus sacralis

N. ischiadicus

N. fibularis communis

N. tibialis

Fig. 1378   Gluteal nerves, Nn. glutei, and sciatic nerve, N. ischiadicus; overview;
cutaneous innervation illustrated with purple.

Tibial and fibular nerve

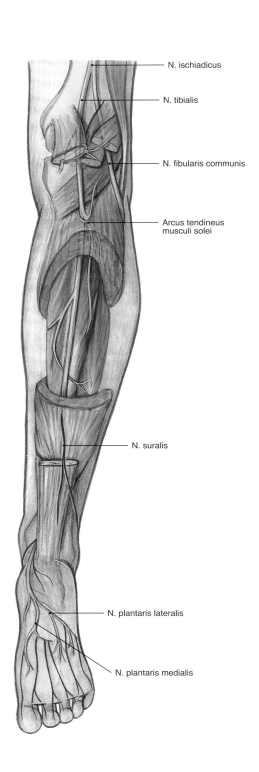

N. ischiadicus

N. tibialis

N. fibularis communis

Arcus tendineus
musculi solei

N. suralis

N. plantaris lateralis

N. plantaris medialis

Fig. 1379 Tibial nerve, N. tibialis;
overview;
cutaneous innervation illustrated with purple.

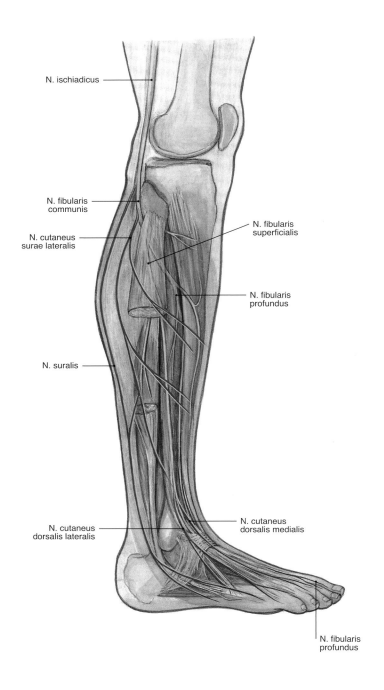

N. ischiadicus

N. fibularis
communis

N. cutaneus
surae lateralis

N. fibularis
superficialis

N. fibularis
profundus

N. suralis

N. cutaneus
dorsalis lateralis

N. cutaneus
dorsalis medialis

N. fibularis
profundus

Fig. 1380 Fibular nerve, N. fibularis;
overview;
cutaneous innervation illustrated with purple.

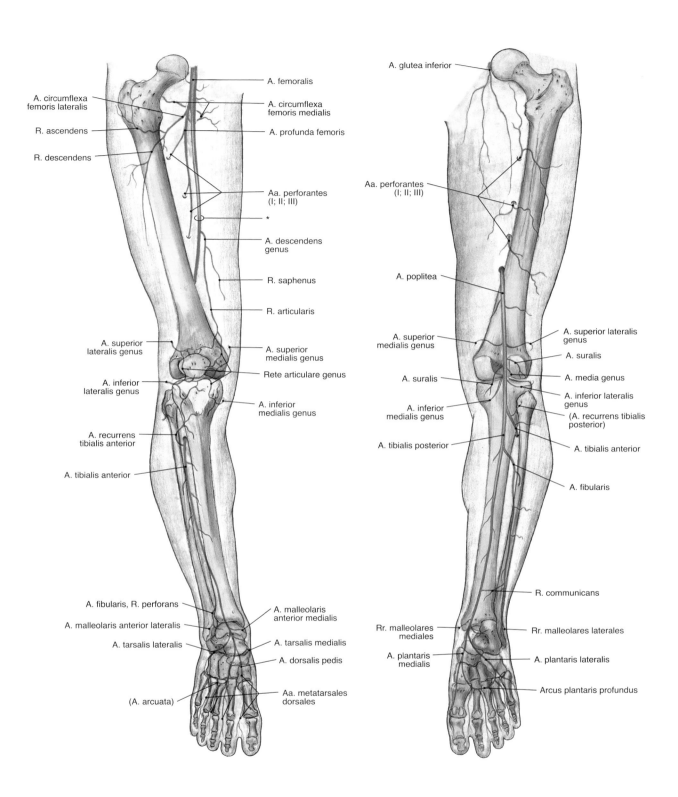

A. circumflexa
femoris lateralis

A. femoralis

R. ascendens

A. circumflexa
femoris medialis

R. descendens

A. profunda femoris

Aa. perforantes
(I; II; III)

*

A. descendens
genus

R. saphenus

R. articularis

A. superior
lateralis genus

A. superior
medialis genus

A. inferior
lateralis genus

Rete articulare genus

A. recurrens
tibialis anterior

A. inferior
medialis genus

A. tibialis anterior

A. fibularis, R. perforans

A. malleolaris
anterior medialis

A. malleolaris anterior lateralis

A. tarsalis lateralis

A. tarsalis medialis

A. dorsalis pedis

(A. arcuata)

Aa. metatarsales
dorsales

A. glutea inferior

Aa. perforantes
(I; II; III)

A. poplitea

A. superior
medialis genus

A. suralis

A. inferior
medialis genus

A. tibialis posterior

A. superior lateralis
genus

A. suralis

A. media genus

A. inferior lateralis
genus
(A. recurrens tibialis
posterior)

A. tibialis anterior

A. fibularis

R. communicans

Rr. malleolares
mediales

Rr. malleolares laterales

A. plantaris
medialis

A. plantaris lateralis

Arcus plantaris profundus

Fig. 1381   Arteries of the lower limb;
overview;
ventral view.
The segment of the femoral artery between the point where
the deep artery of thigh branches off and the point of entry
into the adductor canal (*) is known clinically as superficial
femoral artery.

Fig. 1382   Arteries of the lower limb;
overview;
dorsal view.

Veins and lymphatics of the lower limb

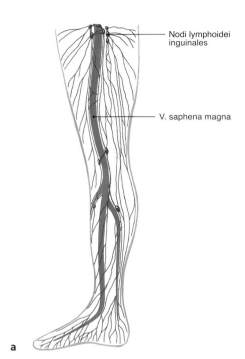

Nodi lymphoidei inguinales

V. saphena magna

a

Fig. 1383 a, b Veins and lymphatics of the lower limb; overview.

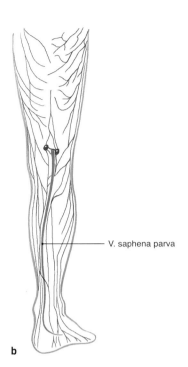

V. saphena parva

b

a Medial view
b Dorsal view

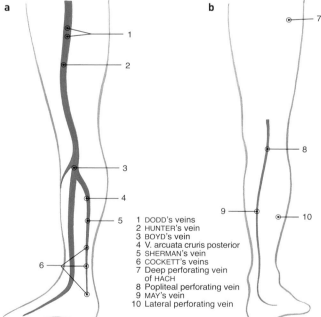

a

1
2
3
4
5
6

b

7
8
9
10

1 DODD's veins
2 HUNTER's vein
3 BOYD's vein
4 V. arcuata cruris posterior
5 SHERMAN's vein
6 COCKETT's veins
7 Deep perforating vein of HACH
8 Popliteal perforating vein
9 MAY's vein
10 Lateral perforating vein

Fig. 1384 a, b Perforating veins, Vv. perforantes; overview (according to HACH, 1986).
a Medial view
b Dorsal view

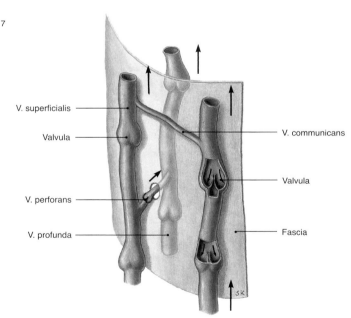

V. superficialis

Valvula

V. perforans

V. profunda

V. communicans

Valvula

Fascia

SK

Fig. 1385 Veins of the lower limb; principle of organisation.
Disturbances of the venous flow of the lower limb, especially varicosis, are a common cause of vascular disorders.
If one of the venous systems is entirely occluded, the perforating veins may be of crucial importance to maintain the venous drainage.

Vessels and nerves of the thigh

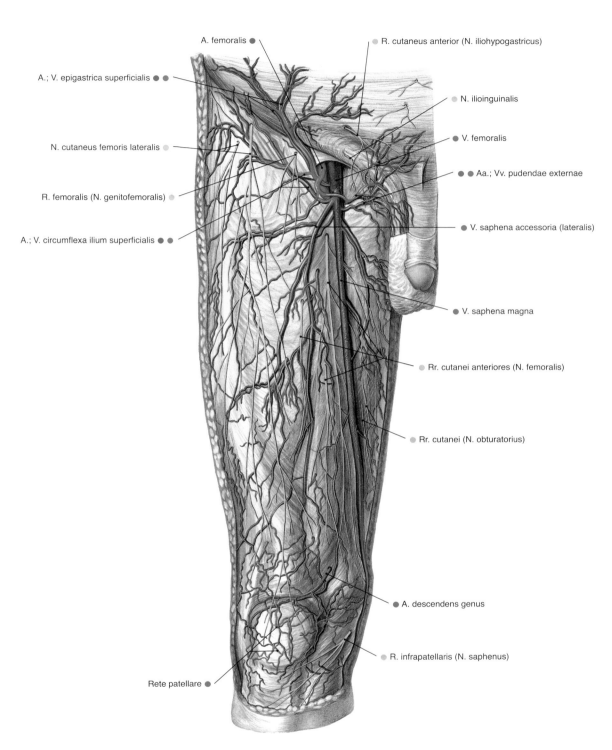

A. femoralis ●

R. cutaneus anterior (N. iliohypogastricus) ●

A.; V. epigastrica superficialis ● ●

● N. ilioinguinalis

N. cutaneus femoris lateralis ●

● V. femoralis

R. femoralis (N. genitofemoralis) ●

● ● Aa.; Vv. pudendae externae

A.; V. circumflexa ilium superficialis ● ●

● V. saphena accessoria (lateralis)

● V. saphena magna

● Rr. cutanei anteriores (N. femoralis)

● Rr. cutanei (N. obturatorius)

● A. descendens genus

● R. infrapatellaris (N. saphenus)

Rete patellare ●

860
1391
1403

Fig. 1386 Epifascial vessels and nerves of the inguinal region, Regio inguinalis, the anterior region of thigh, Regio femoris anterior, and the anterior region of knee, Regio genus anterior.

Lymphatics of the inguinal region

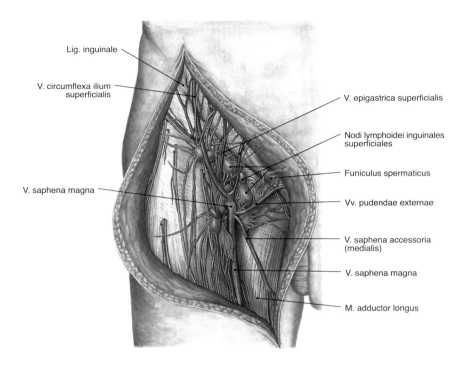

Lig. inguinale

V. circumflexa ilium superficialis

V. saphena magna

V. epigastrica superficialis

Nodi lymphoidei inguinales superficiales

Funiculus spermaticus

Vv. pudendae externae

V. saphena accessoria (medialis)

V. saphena magna

M. adductor longus

Fig. 1387   Superficial lymphatics, lymph nodes and major veins of the inguinal region, Regio inguinalis.

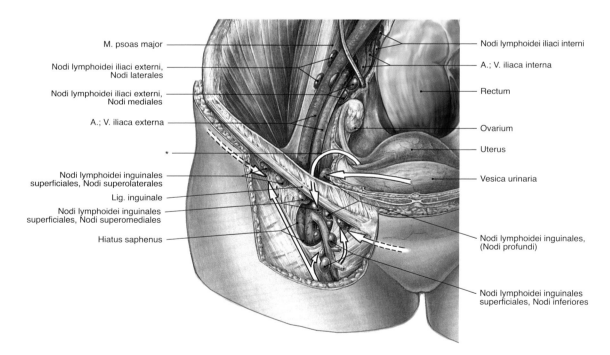

M. psoas major

Nodi lymphoidei iliaci externi, Nodi laterales

Nodi lymphoidei iliaci externi, Nodi mediales

A.; V. iliaca externa

*

Nodi lymphoidei inguinales superficiales, Nodi superolaterales

Lig. inguinale

Nodi lymphoidei inguinales superficiales, Nodi superomediales

Hiatus saphenus

Nodi lymphoidei iliaci interni

A.; V. iliaca interna

Rectum

Ovarium

Uterus

Vesica urinaria

Nodi lymphoidei inguinales, (Nodi profundi)

Nodi lymphoidei inguinales superficiales, Nodi inferiores

Fig. 1388   Draining areas of the lymph nodes in the inguinal region, Regio inguinalis, of the female; overview.
The arrows indicate possible directions of the flow of lymph.

* In some rare cases, the medial parts of the uterine tube and the fundus of the uterus may be drained by superficial lymph nodes in the inguinal region via the round ligament of uterus.

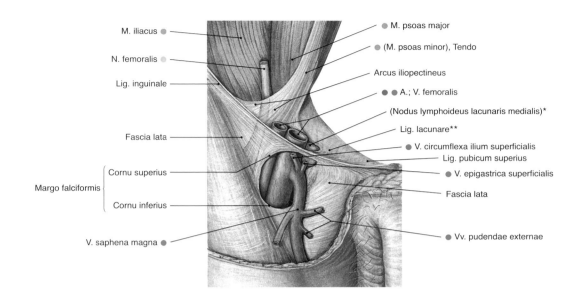

M. iliacus

M. psoas major

N. femoralis

(M. psoas minor), Tendo

Lig. inguinale

Arcus iliopectineus

A.; V. femoralis

(Nodus lymphoideus lacunaris medialis)*

Fascia lata

Lig. lacunare**

V. circumflexa ilium superficialis

Lig. pubicum superius

Cornu superius

V. epigastrica superficialis

Margo falciformis

Fascia lata

Cornu inferius

V. saphena magna

Vv. pudendae externae

Fig. 1389   Saphenous opening, Hiatus saphenus,
and vascular space, Lacuna vasorum;
after removal of the anterior abdominal wall and the
contents of the abdomen, as well as dissection of the
iliac fascia and the femoral septum [CLOQUET].
* Also: ROSENMÜLLER's node
** Also: GIMBERNAT's ligament

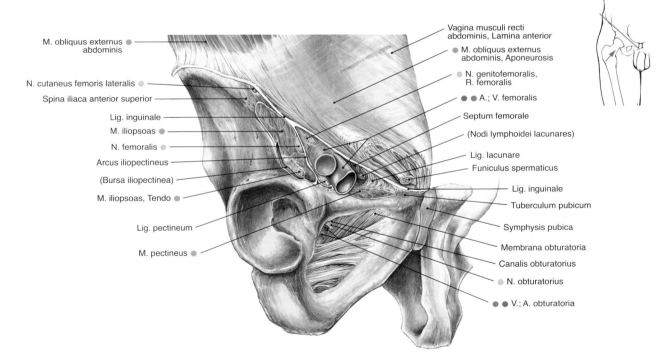

M. obliquus externus
abdominis

Vagina musculi recti
abdominis, Lamina anterior

M. obliquus externus
abdominis, Aponeurosis

N. cutaneus femoris lateralis

N. genitofemoralis,
R. femoralis

Spina iliaca anterior superior

A.; V. femoralis

Lig. inguinale

Septum femorale

M. iliopsoas

(Nodi lymphoidei lacunares)

N. femoralis

Arcus iliopectineus

Lig. lacunare

(Bursa iliopectinea)

Funiculus spermaticus

M. iliopsoas, Tendo

Lig. inguinale

Tuberculum pubicum

Lig. pectineum

Symphysis pubica

M. pectineus

Membrana obturatoria

Canalis obturatorius

N. obturatorius

V.; A. obturatoria

Fig. 1390   Muscular and vascular space,
Lacunae musculorum et vasorum;
oblique section at the level of the inguinal ligament.

Vessels and nerves of the thigh

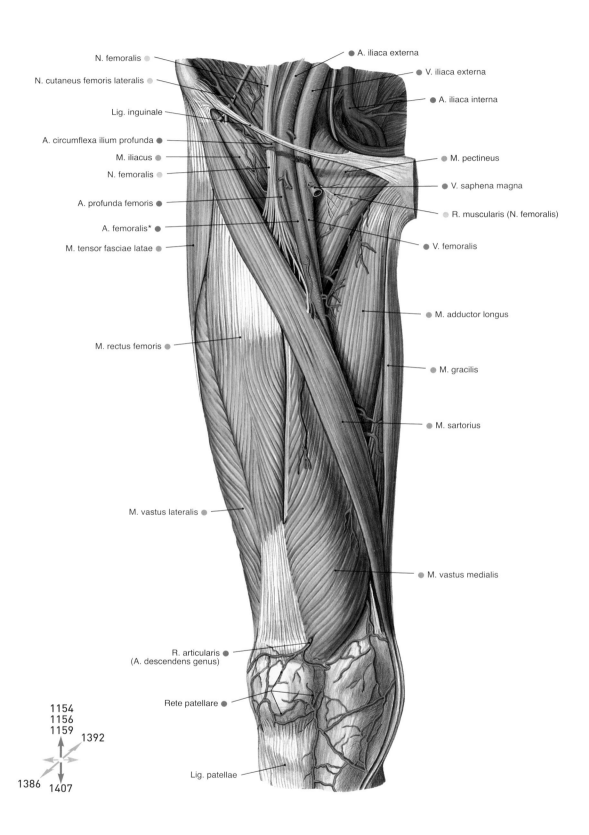

N. femoralis

N. cutaneus femoris lateralis

Lig. inguinale

A. circumflexa ilium profunda

M. iliacus

N. femoralis

A. profunda femoris

A. femoralis*

M. tensor fasciae latae

M. rectus femoris

M. vastus lateralis

R. articularis
(A. descendens genus)

Rete patellare

Lig. patellae

A. iliaca externa

V. iliaca externa

A. iliaca interna

M. pectineus

V. saphena magna

R. muscularis (N. femoralis)

V. femoralis

M. adductor longus

M. gracilis

M. sartorius

M. vastus medialis

1154
1156
1159   1392

1386 1407

Fig. 1391   Vessels and nerves of the anterior region of thigh,
Regio femoris anterior;
after removal of the fascia lata except for the iliotibial tract.

* Clinically the femoral artery is commonly referred to as superficial
femoral artery to distinguish it from the deep artery of thigh.

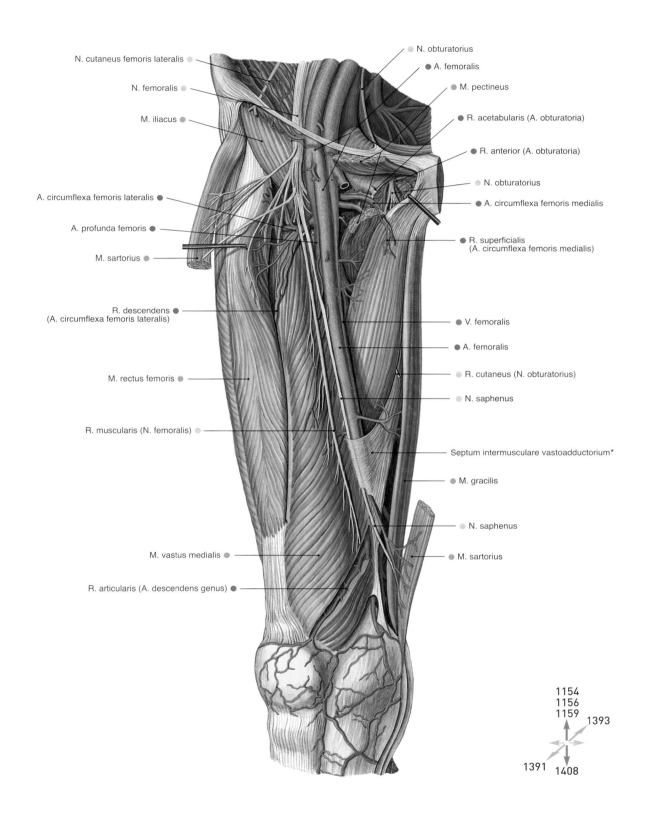

N. cutaneus femoris lateralis

N. femoralis

M. iliacus

A. circumflexa femoris lateralis

A. profunda femoris

M. sartorius

R. descendens
(A. circumflexa femoris lateralis)

M. rectus femoris

R. muscularis (N. femoralis)

M. vastus medialis

R. articularis (A. descendens genus)

N. obturatorius

A. femoralis

M. pectineus

R. acetabularis (A. obturatoria)

R. anterior (A. obturatoria)

N. obturatorius

A. circumflexa femoris medialis

R. superficialis
(A. circumflexa femoris medialis)

V. femoralis

A. femoralis

R. cutaneus (N. obturatorius)

N. saphenus

Septum intermusculare vastoadductorium*

M. gracilis

N. saphenus

M. sartorius

1154
1156
1159   1393

1391 1408

Fig. 1392   Vessels and nerves of the anterior region of thigh,
Regio femoris anterior;
after partial removal of the sartorius muscle and dissection of
the pectineus muscle.

* The entrance into the adductor canal is formed by the vastus medialis
and adductor longus muscles as well as by the anteromedial
intermuscular septum spanning between them.

Vessels and nerves of the thigh

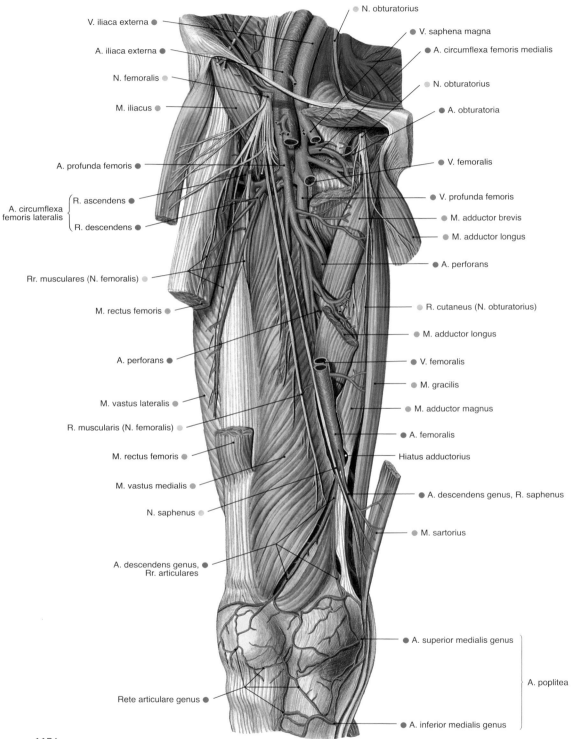

- V. iliaca externa ●
- A. iliaca externa ●
- N. femoralis ●
- M. iliacus ●
- A. profunda femoris ●
- A. circumflexa femoris lateralis { R. ascendens ● / R. descendens ● }
- Rr. musculares (N. femoralis) ●
- M. rectus femoris ●
- A. perforans ●
- M. vastus lateralis ●
- R. muscularis (N. femoralis) ●
- M. rectus femoris ●
- M. vastus medialis ●
- N. saphenus ●
- A. descendens genus, ● Rr. articulares
- Rete articulare genus ●

- ● N. obturatorius
- ● V. saphena magna
- ● A. circumflexa femoris medialis
- ● N. obturatorius
- ● A. obturatoria
- ● V. femoralis
- ● V. profunda femoris
- ● M. adductor brevis
- ● M. adductor longus
- ● A. perforans
- ● R. cutaneus (N. obturatorius)
- ● M. adductor longus
- ● V. femoralis
- ● M. gracilis
- ● M. adductor magnus
- ● A. femoralis
- Hiatus adductorius
- ● A. descendens genus, R. saphenus
- ● M. sartorius
- ● A. superior medialis genus
- ● A. inferior medialis genus
- A. poplitea

1154
1156
1159

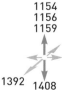

1392 1408

Fig. 1393 Vessels and nerves of the anterior region of thigh, Regio femoris anterior; deep layer after partial removal of the sartorius and rectus femoris muscles, the pectineus and adductor longus muscles have been dissected; the adductor canal is almost entirely opened.

Arteries of the pelvis and the hip

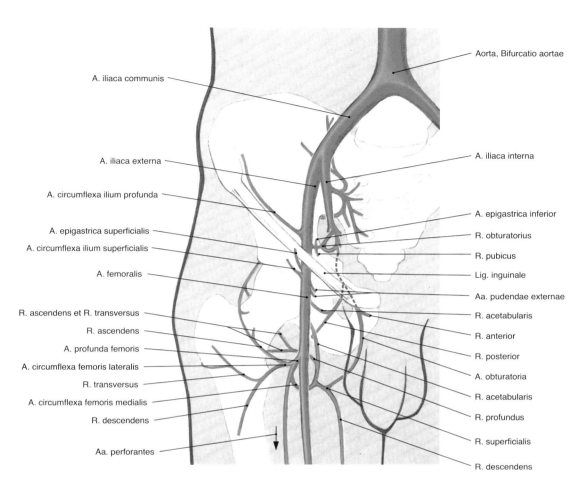

A. iliaca communis
A. iliaca externa
A. circumflexa ilium profunda
A. epigastrica superficialis
A. circumflexa ilium superficialis
A. femoralis
R. ascendens et R. transversus
R. ascendens
A. profunda femoris
A. circumflexa femoris lateralis
R. transversus
A. circumflexa femoris medialis
R. descendens
Aa. perforantes

Aorta, Bifurcatio aortae
A. iliaca interna
A. epigastrica inferior
R. obturatorius
R. pubicus
Lig. inguinale
Aa. pudendae externae
R. acetabularis
R. anterior
R. posterior
A. obturatoria
R. acetabularis
R. profundus
R. superficialis
R. descendens

Fig. 1394 Arteries of the hip and the thigh;
overview.

The branching pattern of these arteries varies considerably.
This type of origin and arborisation of the deep artery of thigh
occurs in approximately 58% of cases.

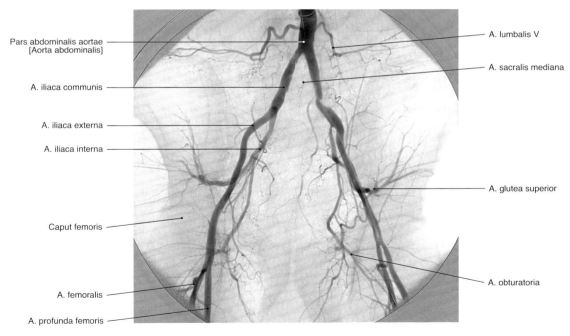

Pars abdominalis aortae
[Aorta abdominalis]
A. iliaca communis
A. iliaca externa
A. iliaca interna
Caput femoris
A. femoralis
A. profunda femoris

A. lumbalis V
A. sacralis mediana
A. glutea superior
A. obturatoria

Fig. 1395 Arteries of the pelvis and the thigh;
digital subtraction angiography (DSA).

Veins and nerves of the thigh

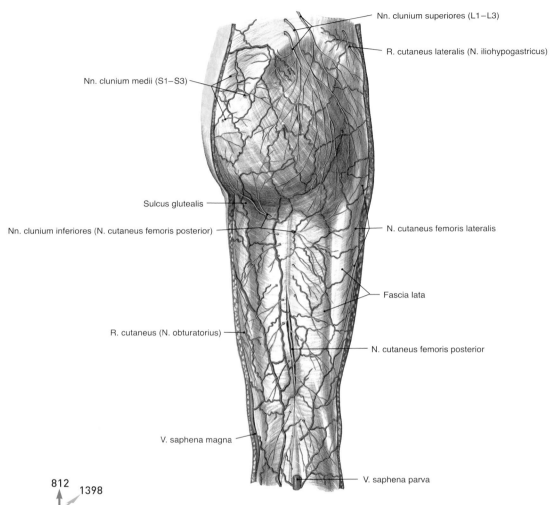

Nn. clunium superiores (L1−L3)

R. cutaneus lateralis (N. iliohypogastricus)

Nn. clunium medii (S1−S3)

Sulcus glutealis

Nn. clunium inferiores (N. cutaneus femoris posterior)

N. cutaneus femoris lateralis

Fascia lata

R. cutaneus (N. obturatorius)

N. cutaneus femoris posterior

V. saphena magna

V. saphena parva

812 1398

1404

Fig. 1396 Epifascial veins and nerves of the posterior region of thigh, Regio femoris posterior, the gluteal region, Regio glutealis, and the popliteal fossa, Fossa poplitea.

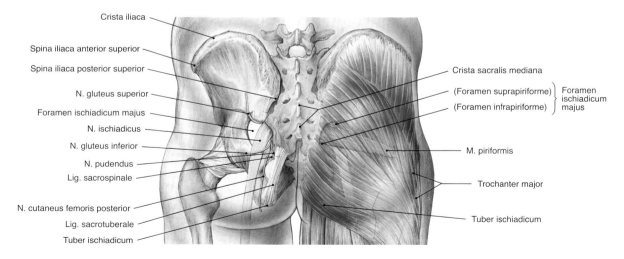

Crista iliaca

Spina iliaca anterior superior

Spina iliaca posterior superior

N. gluteus superior

Foramen ischiadicum majus

N. ischiadicus

N. gluteus inferior

N. pudendus

Lig. sacrospinale

N. cutaneus femoris posterior

Lig. sacrotuberale

Tuber ischiadicum

Crista sacralis mediana

(Foramen suprapiriforme) Foramen
ischiadicum
(Foramen infrapiriforme) majus

M. piriformis

Trochanter major

Tuber ischiadicum

Fig. 1397 Skeleton contour and sciatic nerve, N. ischiadicus, projected onto the surface of the gluteal region, Regio glutealis.

Vessels and nerves of the thigh

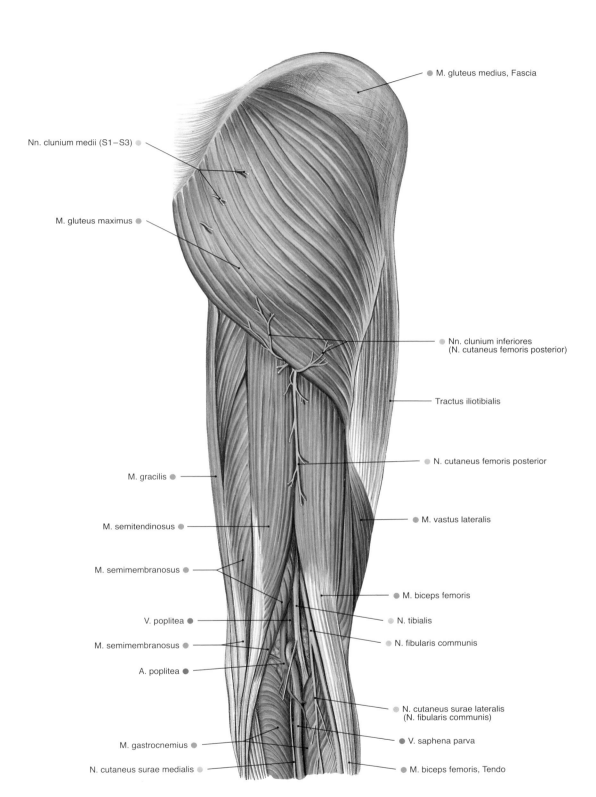

● M. gluteus medius, Fascia

Nn. clunium medii (S1–S3) ●

M. gluteus maximus ●

● Nn. clunium inferiores
(N. cutaneus femoris posterior)

Tractus iliotibialis

● N. cutaneus femoris posterior

M. gracilis ●

● M. vastus lateralis

M. semitendinosus ●

M. semimembranosus ●

● M. biceps femoris

V. poplitea ●

● N. tibialis

M. semimembranosus ●

● N. fibularis communis

A. poplitea ●

● N. cutaneus surae lateralis
(N. fibularis communis)

● V. saphena parva

M. gastrocnemius ●

N. cutaneus surae medialis ●

● M. biceps femoris, Tendo

Fig. 1398   Vessels and nerves of the gluteal region,
Regio glutealis, the posterior region of thigh, Regio femoris
posterior, and the popliteal fossa, Fossa poplitea.

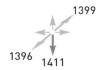

1399

1396 1411

Vessels and nerves of the thigh

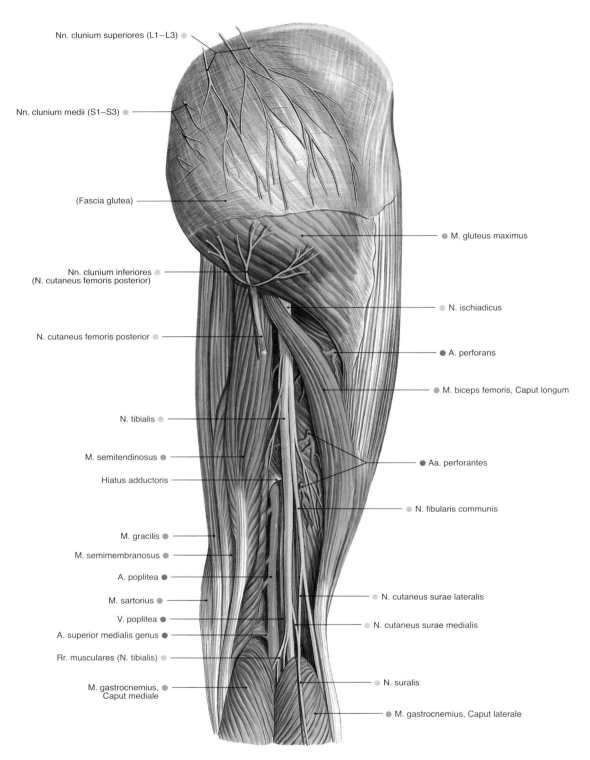

Nn. clunium superiores (L1–L3) ●

Nn. clunium medii (S1–S3) ●

(Fascia glutea)

Nn. clunium inferiores ●
(N. cutaneus femoris posterior)

N. cutaneus femoris posterior ●

N. tibialis ●

M. semitendinosus ●

Hiatus adductoris

M. gracilis ●

M. semimembranosus ●

A. poplitea ●

M. sartorius ●

V. poplitea ●

A. superior medialis genus ●

Rr. musculares (N. tibialis) ●

M. gastrocnemius, ●
Caput mediale

● M. gluteus maximus

● N. ischiadicus

● A. perforans

● M. biceps femoris, Caput longum

● Aa. perforantes

● N. fibularis communis

● N. cutaneus surae lateralis

● N. cutaneus surae medialis

● N. suralis

● M. gastrocnemius, Caput laterale

1400

1398

Fig. 1399   Vessels and nerves of the gluteal region, Regio glutealis,
the posterior region of thigh, Regio femoris posterior,
and the popliteal fossa, Fossa poplitea;
the long head of the biceps femoris muscle has been retracted
laterally.
In this specimen, the medial and lateral sural cutaneous nerves branch
off quite far proximally.

Vessels and nerves of the thigh

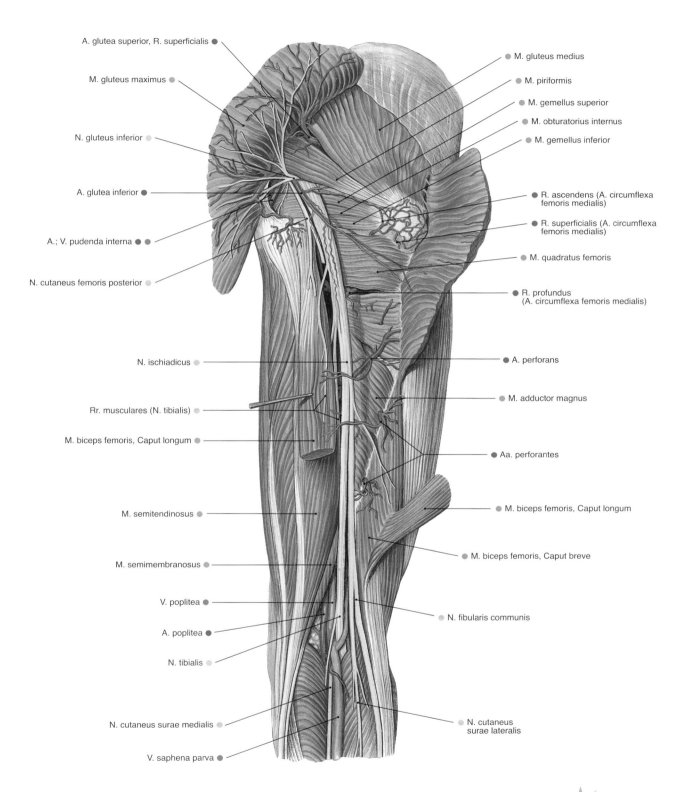

A. glutea superior, R. superficialis ●

M. gluteus maximus ●

N. gluteus inferior ●

A. glutea inferior ●

A.; V. pudenda interna ● ●

N. cutaneus femoris posterior ●

N. ischiadicus ●

Rr. musculares (N. tibialis) ●

M. biceps femoris, Caput longum ●

M. semitendinosus ●

M. semimembranosus ●

V. poplitea ●

A. poplitea ●

N. tibialis ●

N. cutaneus surae medialis ●

V. saphena parva ●

● M. gluteus medius

● M. piriformis

● M. gemellus superior

● M. obturatorius internus

● M. gemellus inferior

● R. ascendens (A. circumflexa femoris medialis)

● R. superficialis (A. circumflexa femoris medialis)

● M. quadratus femoris

● R. profundus (A. circumflexa femoris medialis)

● A. perforans

● M. adductor magnus

● Aa. perforantes

● M. biceps femoris, Caput longum

● M. biceps femoris, Caput breve

● N. fibularis communis

● N. cutaneus surae lateralis

Fig. 1400 Vessels and nerves of the gluteal region, Regio glutealis, the posterior region of thigh, Regio femoris posterior, and the popliteal fossa, Fossa poplitea; after dissection of the gluteus maximus muscle and the long head of the biceps femoris muscle.

1399

1411
1413
1414

Vessels and nerves of the gluteal region

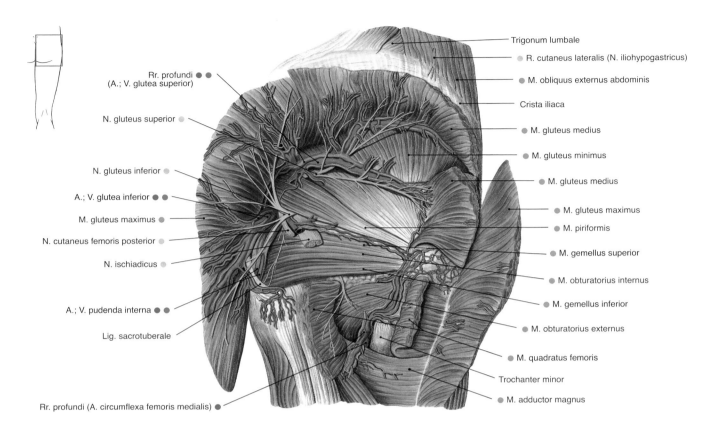

Rr. profundi ● ●
(A.; V. glutea superior)

N. gluteus superior ●

N. gluteus inferior ●

A.; V. glutea inferior ● ●

M. gluteus maximus ●

N. cutaneus femoris posterior ●

N. ischiadicus ●

A.; V. pudenda interna ● ●

Lig. sacrotuberale

Rr. profundi (A. circumflexa femoris medialis) ●

Trigonum lumbale

● R. cutaneus lateralis (N. iliohypogastricus)

● M. obliquus externus abdominis

Crista iliaca

● M. gluteus medius

● M. gluteus minimus

● M. gluteus medius

● M. gluteus maximus

● M. piriformis

● M. gemellus superior

● M. obturatorius internus

● M. gemellus inferior

● M. obturatorius externus

● M. quadratus femoris

Trochanter minor

● M. adductor magnus

Fig. 1401   Vessels and nerves of the gluteal region, Regio glutealis;
after dissection and partial removal of the gluteus maximus and medius muscles;
the sciatic nerve has been removed after its passage through the infrapiriform foramen.

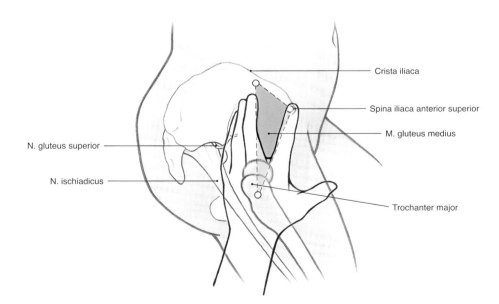

Crista iliaca

Spina iliaca anterior superior

M. gluteus medius

N. gluteus superior

N. ischiadicus

Trochanter major

Fig. 1402   Ventrogluteal injection (according to v. HOCHSTETTER).
In order to avoid the superior gluteal nerve and, in particular,
the superior gluteal artery the injection is made into the
triangular field formed by the two spread fingers and the iliac
crest. The index finger – or when using the right hand, the
middle finger – is placed on the anterior superior iliac spine
and the palm of the hand on the greater trochanter. Since the
injected material should be deposited within the belly of the
gluteus medius muscle as far away as possible from any vessel,
the needle should not cross the lines of the triangle. However,
some risk remains for the nerve branch that runs from the
superior gluteal nerve to the tensor fasciae latae muscle.

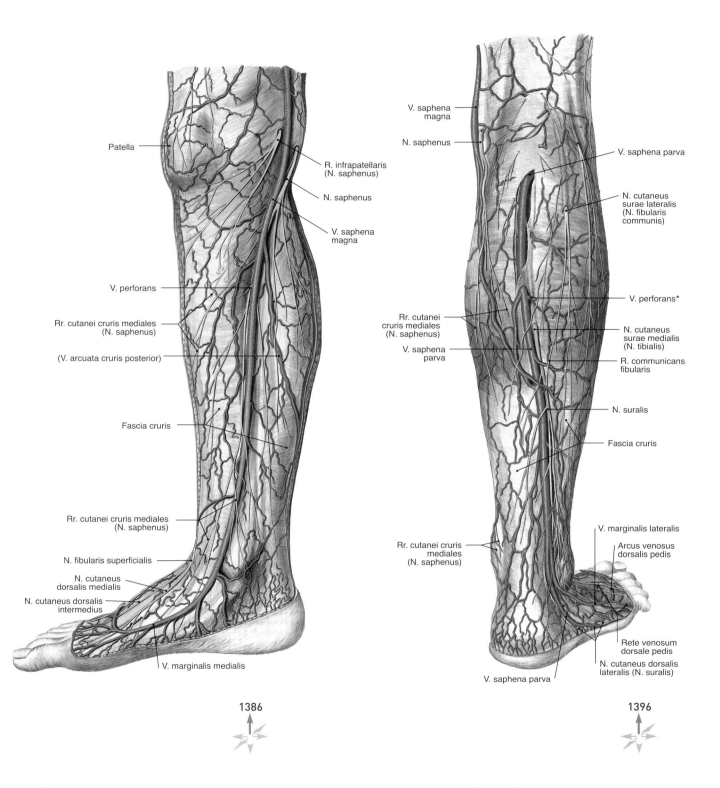

Patella

R. infrapatellaris
(N. saphenus)

N. saphenus

V. saphena
magna

V. perforans

Rr. cutanei cruris mediales
(N. saphenus)

(V. arcuata cruris posterior)

Fascia cruris

Rr. cutanei cruris mediales
(N. saphenus)

N. fibularis superficialis

N. cutaneus
dorsalis medialis

N. cutaneus dorsalis
intermedius

V. marginalis medialis

1386

V. saphena
magna

N. saphenus

V. saphena parva

N. cutaneus
surae lateralis
(N. fibularis
communis)

V. perforans*

Rr. cutanei
cruris mediales
(N. saphenus)

N. cutaneus
surae medialis
(N. tibialis)

V. saphena
parva

R. communicans
fibularis

N. suralis

Fascia cruris

V. marginalis lateralis

Arcus venosus
dorsalis pedis

Rr. cutanei cruris
mediales
(N. saphenus)

Rete venosum
dorsale pedis

N. cutaneus dorsalis
lateralis (N. suralis)

V. saphena parva

1396

Fig. 1403 Epifascial veins and nerves of the leg
and the foot, Regiones cruris et pedis.

Fig. 1404 Epifascial veins and nerves of the leg
and the foot, Regiones cruris et pedis;
the deep fascia of leg has been dissected
proximally.

* Clinical term: MAY's vein

Vessels and nerves of the leg

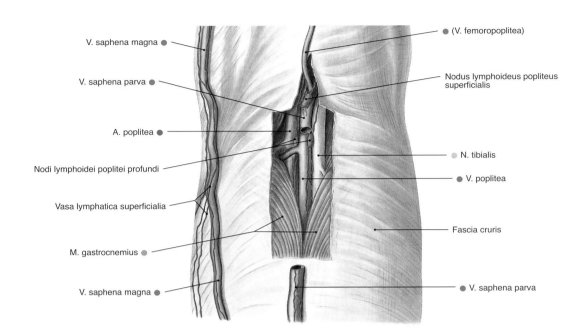

V. saphena magna ●

V. saphena parva ●

A. poplitea ●

Nodi lymphoidei poplitei profundi

Vasa lymphatica superficialia

M. gastrocnemius ●

V. saphena magna ●

● (V. femoropoplitea)

Nodus lymphoideus popliteus superficialis

● N. tibialis

● V. poplitea

Fascia cruris

● V. saphena parva

Fig. 1405   Vessels and nerves of the popliteal fossa, Fossa poplitea;
after dissection of the deep fascia of leg and partial removal of the small saphenous vein.

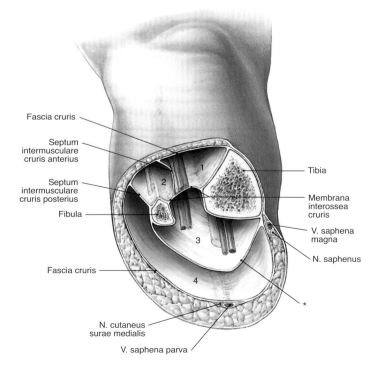

Fascia cruris

Septum intermusculare cruris anterius

Septum intermusculare cruris posterius

Fibula

Fascia cruris

N. cutaneus surae medialis

V. saphena parva

Tibia

Membrana interossea cruris

V. saphena magna

N. saphenus

*

1 Compartimentum cruris anterius:
A.; V. tibialis anterior
N. fibularis profundus
M. tibialis anterior
M. extensor digitorum longus
M. extensor hallucis longus
M. fibularis [peroneus] tertius

2 Compartimentum cruris laterale:
N. fibularis superficialis
M. fibularis [peroneus] longus
M. fibularis [peroneus] brevis

3 Compartimentum cruris posterius, Pars profunda:
A.; V. tibialis posterior
A.; V. fibularis
N. tibialis
M. flexor digitorum longus
M. tibialis posterior
M. flexor hallucis longus

4 Compartimentum cruris posterius, Pars super-ficialis:
M. triceps surae
M. plantaris

Fig. 1406   Osteofibrous tubes of the leg;
cross-section superior to the middle of the leg.
These osteofibrous tubes together with their contents are clinically known as compartments.
* Deep part of the deep fascia of leg

→ 1425

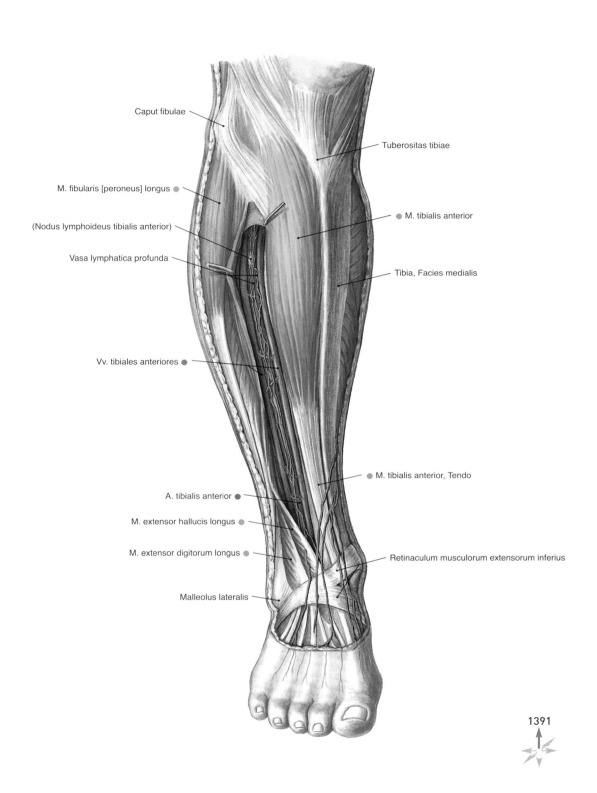

Caput fibulae

Tuberositas tibiae

M. fibularis [peroneus] longus ●

● M. tibialis anterior

(Nodus lymphoideus tibialis anterior)

Vasa lymphatica profunda

Tibia, Facies medialis

Vv. tibiales anteriores ●

● M. tibialis anterior, Tendo

A. tibialis anterior ●

M. extensor hallucis longus ●

M. extensor digitorum longus ●

Retinaculum musculorum extensorum inferius

Malleolus lateralis

1391

Abb. 1407 Vessels of the anterior region of leg, Regio cruris anterior; the extensor muscles spread by retractors.

The superficial lymphatics regularly follow the major epifascial veins and converge along the great saphenous vein to the medial side of the leg. The deep lymphatics are found within the connective tissue sheaths of the deep arteries and veins of the leg.

Arteries and nerves of the leg

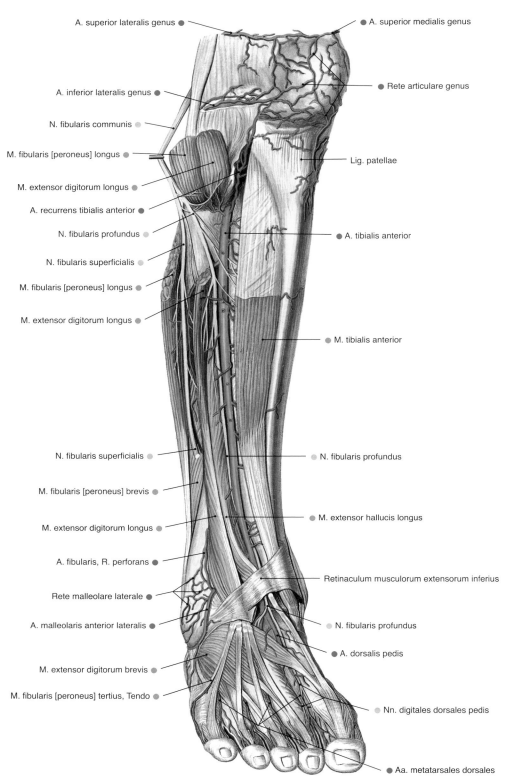

A. superior lateralis genus ●

● A. superior medialis genus

A. inferior lateralis genus ●

● Rete articulare genus

N. fibularis communis ●

M. fibularis [peroneus] longus ●

M. extensor digitorum longus ●

Lig. patellae

A. recurrens tibialis anterior ●

N. fibularis profundus ●

N. fibularis superficialis ●

● A. tibialis anterior

M. fibularis [peroneus] longus ●

M. extensor digitorum longus ●

● M. tibialis anterior

N. fibularis superficialis ●

● N. fibularis profundus

M. fibularis [peroneus] brevis ●

M. extensor digitorum longus ●

● M. extensor hallucis longus

A. fibularis, R. perforans ●

Retinaculum musculorum extensorum inferius

Rete malleolare laterale ●

A. malleolaris anterior lateralis ●

● N. fibularis profundus

● A. dorsalis pedis

M. extensor digitorum brevis ●

M. fibularis [peroneus] tertius, Tendo ●

● Nn. digitales dorsales pedis

● Aa. metatarsales dorsales

1391
1392
1416

1407

Fig. 1408 Arteries and nerves of the anterior region of leg,
Regio cruris anterior, and the dorsum of foot, Dorsum pedis;
after removal of the deep fascia of leg and dissection of the extensor
digitorum longus and fibularis [peroneus] longus muscles.

Arteries and nerves of the popliteal fossa

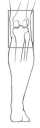

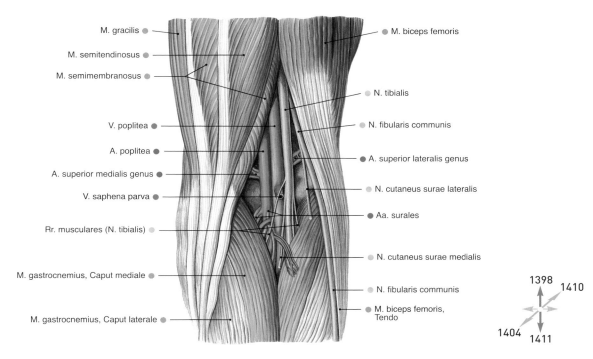

M. gracilis

M. semitendinosus

M. semimembranosus

V. poplitea

A. poplitea

A. superior medialis genus

V. saphena parva

Rr. musculares (N. tibialis)

M. gastrocnemius, Caput mediale

M. gastrocnemius, Caput laterale

M. biceps femoris

N. tibialis

N. fibularis communis

A. superior lateralis genus

N. cutaneus surae lateralis

Aa. surales

N. cutaneus surae medialis

N. fibularis communis

M. biceps femoris, Tendo

1398   1410
1404   1411

Fig. 1409 Vessels and nerves of the popliteal fossa, Fossa poplitea; after removal of the fascia lata and the deep fascia of leg.

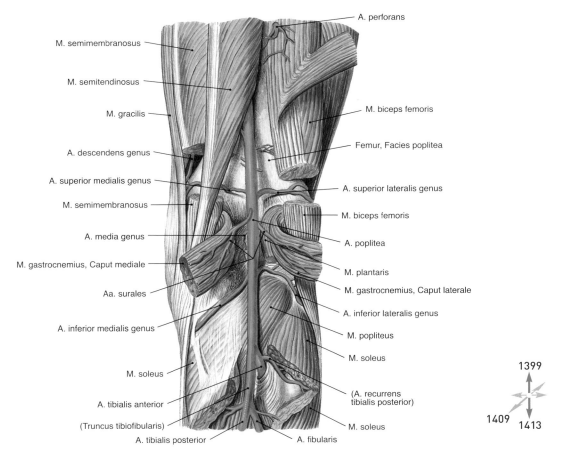

M. semimembranosus

M. semitendinosus

M. gracilis

A. descendens genus

A. superior medialis genus

M. semimembranosus

A. media genus

M. gastrocnemius, Caput mediale

Aa. surales

A. inferior medialis genus

M. soleus

A. tibialis anterior

(Truncus tibiofibularis)

A. tibialis posterior

A. perforans

M. biceps femoris

Femur, Facies poplitea

A. superior lateralis genus

M. biceps femoris

A. poplitea

M. plantaris

M. gastrocnemius, Caput laterale

A. inferior lateralis genus

M. popliteus

M. soleus

(A. recurrens tibialis posterior)

M. soleus

A. fibularis

1399

1409   1413

Fig. 1410 Arteries of the popliteal fossa, Fossa poplitea; demonstration of the arterial supply after partial removal of the covering muscles. This branching pattern is found in about 90% of the cases.

Vessels and nerves of the popliteal fossa and the leg

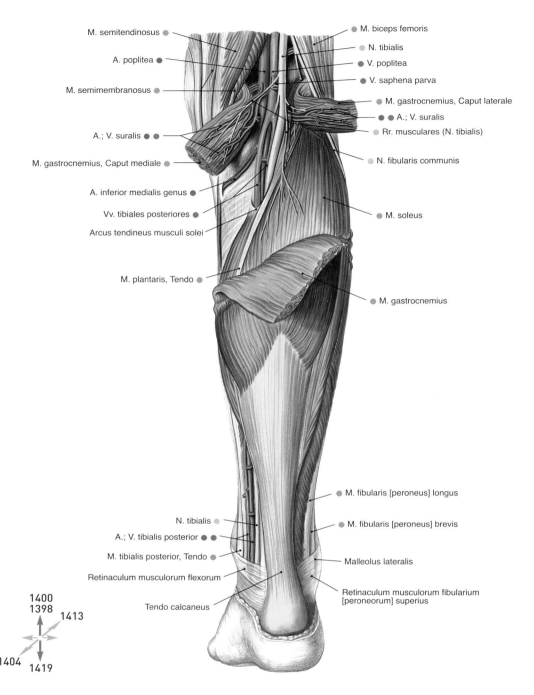

M. semitendinosus ●
A. poplitea ●
M. semimembranosus ●
A.; V. suralis ● ●
M. gastrocnemius, Caput mediale ●
A. inferior medialis genus ●
Vv. tibiales posteriores ●
Arcus tendineus musculi solei
M. plantaris, Tendo ●

● M. biceps femoris
● N. tibialis
● V. poplitea
● V. saphena parva
● M. gastrocnemius, Caput laterale
● ● A.; V. suralis
● Rr. musculares (N. tibialis)
● N. fibularis communis
● M. soleus
● M. gastrocnemius

N. tibialis ●
A.; V. tibialis posterior ● ●
M. tibialis posterior, Tendo ●
Retinaculum musculorum flexorum
Tendo calcaneus

● M. fibularis [peroneus] longus
● M. fibularis [peroneus] brevis
Malleolus lateralis
Retinaculum musculorum fibularium [peroneorum] superius

1400
1398
1413
1404　1419

Fig. 1411 Vessels and nerves of the popliteal fossa, Fossa poplitea, and the posterior region of leg, Regio cruris posterior; after removal of the deep fascia of leg and dissection of the gastrocnemius muscle.

Fig. 1412 a–d Variations in the branching pattern of the popliteal artery, A. poplitea.
a Common trunk of the anterior and posterior tibial artery, Aa. tibiales anterior et posterior, along with the fibular artery, A. fibularis
b The popliteal artery, A. poplitea, branches off proximally to the superior border of the popliteal muscle, M. popliteus.
c Posterior tibial and fibular artery, Aa. tibialis posterior et fibularis, originate from a common proximal trunk.
d The anterior tibial artery, A. tibialis anterior, passes ventrally to the popliteal muscle, M. popliteus.

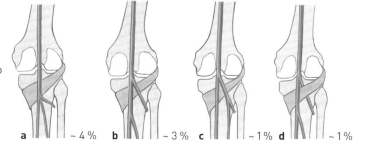

a ~ 4 %　**b** ~ 3 %　**c** ~ 1 %　**d** ~ 1 %

Vessels and nerves of the popliteal fossa and the leg

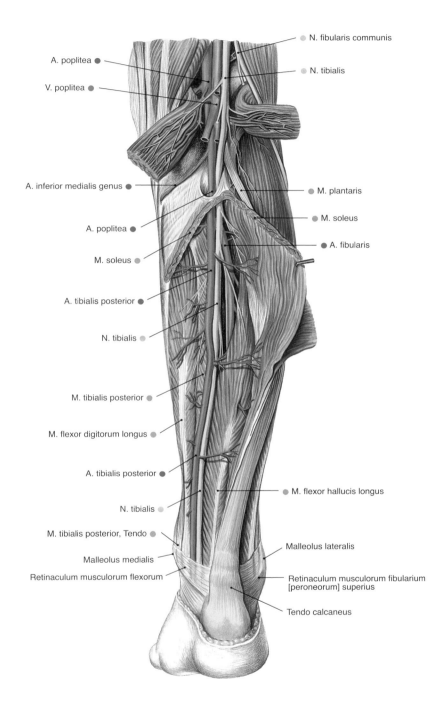

A. poplitea ●

V. poplitea ●

A. inferior medialis genus ●

A. poplitea ●

M. soleus ●

A. tibialis posterior ●

N. tibialis ○

M. tibialis posterior ●

M. flexor digitorum longus ●

A. tibialis posterior ●

N. tibialis ○

M. tibialis posterior, Tendo ●

Malleolus medialis

Retinaculum musculorum flexorum

● N. fibularis communis

● N. tibialis

● M. plantaris

● M. soleus

● A. fibularis

● M. flexor hallucis longus

Malleolus lateralis

Retinaculum musculorum fibularium
[peroneorum] superius

Tendo calcaneus

1398
1400
1414
1411
1420

Fig. 1413 Vessels and nerves of the popliteal fossa, Fossa poplitea, and the posterior region of leg, Regio cruris posterior; deep layer.

Arteries and nerves of the leg

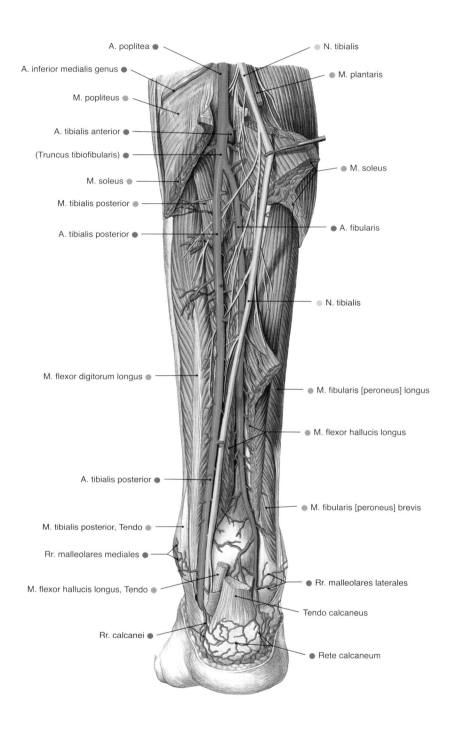

A. poplitea ●
A. inferior medialis genus ●
M. popliteus ●
A. tibialis anterior ●
(Truncus tibiofibularis) ●
M. soleus ●
M. tibialis posterior ●
A. tibialis posterior ●
M. flexor digitorum longus ●
A. tibialis posterior ●
M. tibialis posterior, Tendo ●
Rr. malleolares mediales ●
M. flexor hallucis longus, Tendo ●
Rr. calcanei ●

● N. tibialis
● M. plantaris
● M. soleus
● A. fibularis
● N. tibialis
● M. fibularis [peroneus] longus
● M. flexor hallucis longus
● M. fibularis [peroneus] brevis
● Rr. malleolares laterales
Tendo calcaneus
● Rete calcaneum

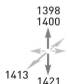

1398
1400

1413 1421

Fig. 1414 Arteries and nerves of the popliteal fossa, Fossa poplitea, and the posterior region of leg, Regio cruris posterior; deepest layer.

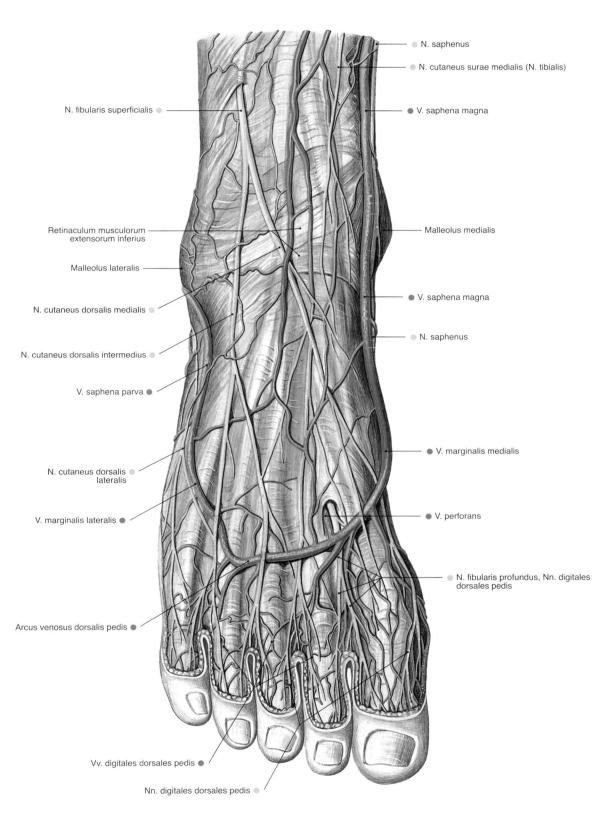

N. saphenus

N. cutaneus surae medialis (N. tibialis)

N. fibularis superficialis

V. saphena magna

Retinaculum musculorum extensorum inferius

Malleolus medialis

Malleolus lateralis

N. cutaneus dorsalis medialis

V. saphena magna

N. saphenus

N. cutaneus dorsalis intermedius

V. saphena parva

V. marginalis medialis

N. cutaneus dorsalis lateralis

V. marginalis lateralis

V. perforans

N. fibularis profundus, Nn. digitales dorsales pedis

Arcus venosus dorsalis pedis

Vv. digitales dorsales pedis

Nn. digitales dorsales pedis

1403

1416

Fig. 1415 Epifascial veins and nerves of the dorsum of foot, Dorsum pedis.

Arteries and nerves of the foot

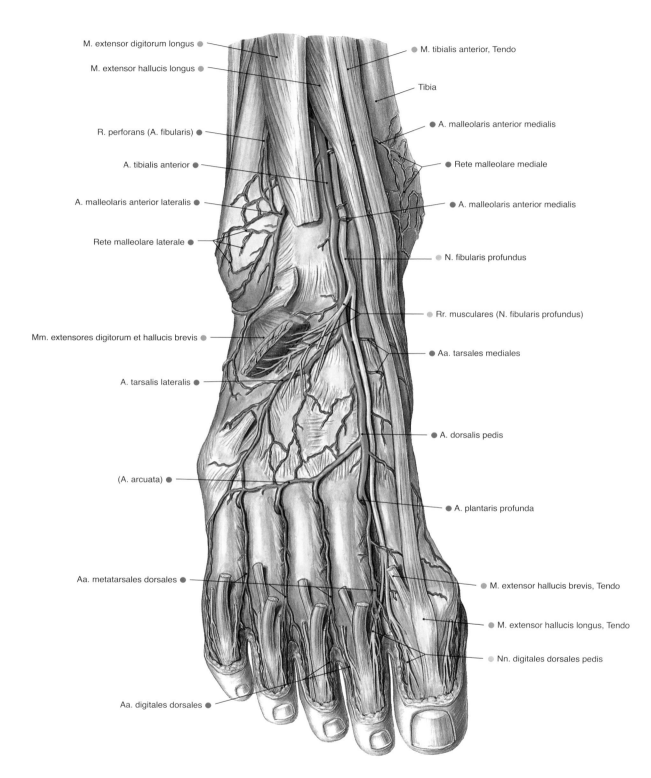

M. extensor digitorum longus ●

M. extensor hallucis longus ●

R. perforans (A. fibularis) ●

A. tibialis anterior ●

A. malleolaris anterior lateralis ●

Rete malleolare laterale ●

Mm. extensores digitorum et hallucis brevis ●

A. tarsalis lateralis ●

(A. arcuata) ●

Aa. metatarsales dorsales ●

Aa. digitales dorsales ●

● M. tibialis anterior, Tendo

Tibia

● A. malleolaris anterior medialis

● Rete malleolare mediale

● A. malleolaris anterior medialis

● N. fibularis profundus

● Rr. musculares (N. fibularis profundus)

● Aa. tarsales mediales

● A. dorsalis pedis

● A. plantaris profunda

● M. extensor hallucis brevis, Tendo

● M. extensor hallucis longus, Tendo

● Nn. digitales dorsales pedis

1408

1415

Fig. 1416 Arteries and nerves of the dorsum of foot, Dorsum pedis.

Arteries of the foot

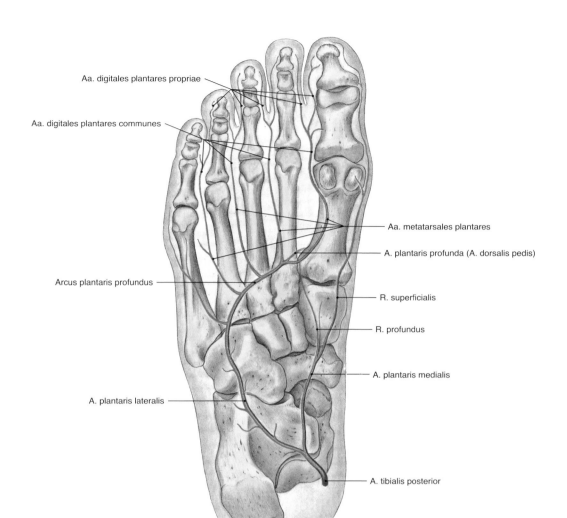

Aa. digitales plantares propriae

Aa. digitales plantares communes

Aa. metatarsales plantares

A. plantaris profunda (A. dorsalis pedis)

Arcus plantaris profundus

R. superficialis

R. profundus

A. plantaris medialis

A. plantaris lateralis

A. tibialis posterior

Fig. 1417   Arteries of the sole of foot, Planta; overview.

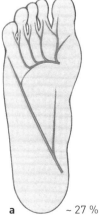
a   ~ 27 %

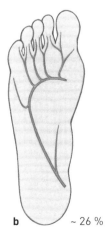
b   ~ 26 %

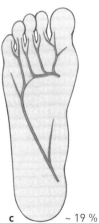
c   ~ 19 %

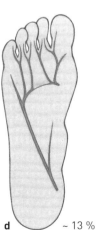
d   ~ 13 %

Fig. 1418 a–d   Variations in the arterial supply of the sole of foot, Planta.
a   Dorsalis pedis artery, A. dorsalis pedis, as major supply for the deep plantar arch, Arcus plantaris profundus
b   Posterior tibial artery, A. tibialis posterior, as major supply for the deep plantar arch, Arcus plantaris profundus
c   The fifth toe and lateral parts of the fourth toe are supplied by the posterior tibial artery, A. tibialis posterior, whereas the

remaining medially located toes receive their arterial supply through the dorsalis pedis artery, A. dorsalis pedis.
d   The fifth and fourth toe as well as lateral parts of the third toe are supplied by the posterior tibial artery, A. tibialis posterior, whereas all remaining medially located toes receive their arterial supply through the dorsalis pedis artery, A. dorsalis pedis.

Arteries and nerves of the foot

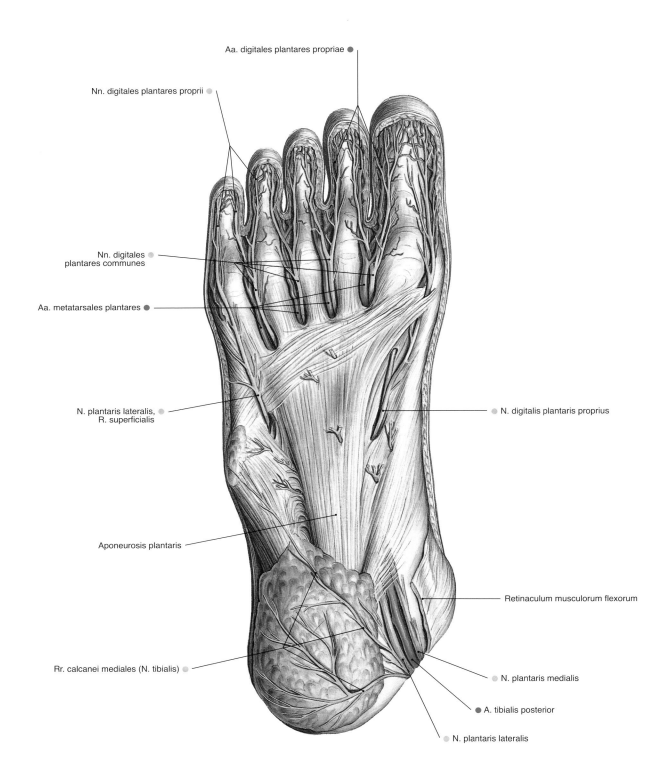

Aa. digitales plantares propriae ●

Nn. digitales plantares proprii ●

Nn. digitales plantares communes ●

Aa. metatarsales plantares ●

N. plantaris lateralis, R. superficialis ●

● N. digitalis plantaris proprius

Aponeurosis plantaris

Retinaculum musculorum flexorum

Rr. calcanei mediales (N. tibialis) ●

● N. plantaris medialis

● A. tibialis posterior

● N. plantaris lateralis

1411
1420

Fig. 1419   Arteries and nerves of the sole of foot, Planta.

Arteries and nerves of the foot

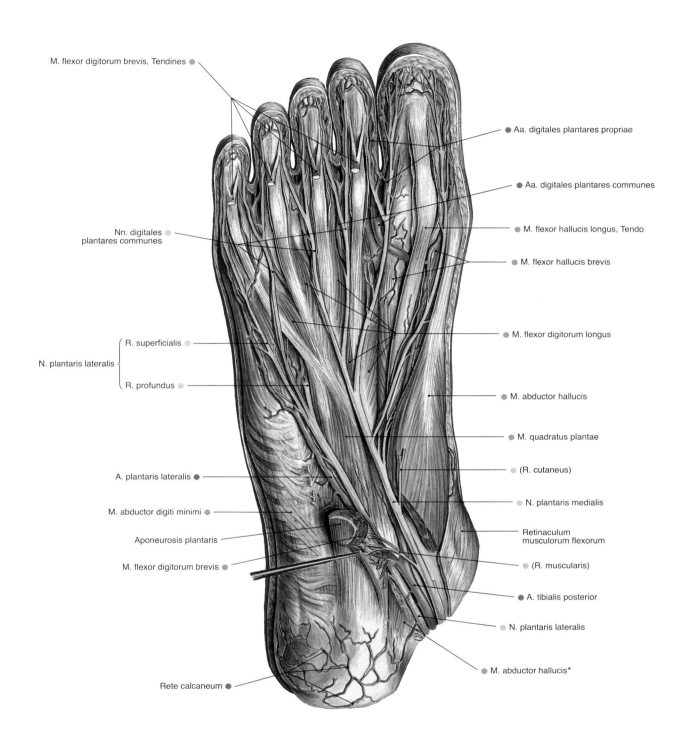

M. flexor digitorum brevis, Tendines ●

● Aa. digitales plantares propriae

● Aa. digitales plantares communes

Nn. digitales ●
plantares communes

● M. flexor hallucis longus, Tendo

● M. flexor hallucis brevis

R. superficialis ●

N. plantaris lateralis

R. profundus ●

● M. flexor digitorum longus

● M. abductor hallucis

● M. quadratus plantae

○ (R. cutaneus)

A. plantaris lateralis ●

○ N. plantaris medialis

M. abductor digiti minimi ●

Retinaculum
musculorum flexorum

Aponeurosis plantaris

○ (R. muscularis)

M. flexor digitorum brevis ●

● A. tibialis posterior

○ N. plantaris lateralis

● M. abductor hallucis*

Rete calcaneum ●

Fig. 1420 Arteries and nerves of the sole of foot, Planta;
deep layer.
* The distal extension of the medial retromalleolar space
beneath the abductor hallucis muscle is also known as tarsal
tunnel.

Arteries of the foot

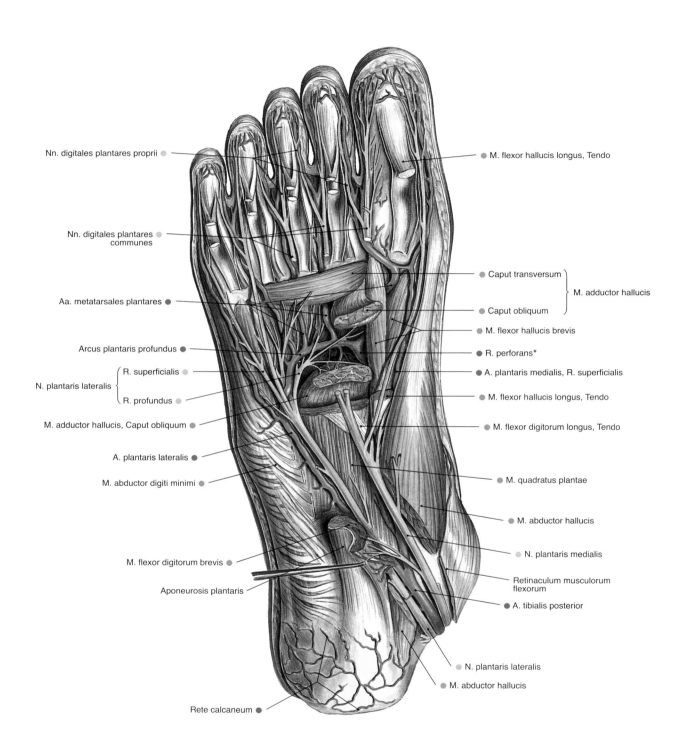

Nn. digitales plantares proprii ●

Nn. digitales plantares ●
communes

Aa. metatarsales plantares ●

Arcus plantaris profundus ●

N. plantaris lateralis { R. superficialis ●
                        R. profundus ●

M. adductor hallucis, Caput obliquum ●

A. plantaris lateralis ●

M. abductor digiti minimi ●

M. flexor digitorum brevis ●

Aponeurosis plantaris

Rete calcaneum ●

● M. flexor hallucis longus, Tendo

● Caput transversum }
                     } M. adductor hallucis
● Caput obliquum }

● M. flexor hallucis brevis

● R. perforans*

● A. plantaris medialis, R. superficialis

● M. flexor hallucis longus, Tendo

● M. flexor digitorum longus, Tendo

● M. quadratus plantae

● M. abductor hallucis

● N. plantaris medialis

Retinaculum musculorum
flexorum

● A. tibialis posterior

● N. plantaris lateralis

● M. abductor hallucis

1414

1420

Fig. 1421   Arteries and nerves of the sole of foot, Planta;
deepest layer.
* Anastomosis with the dorsalis pedis artery

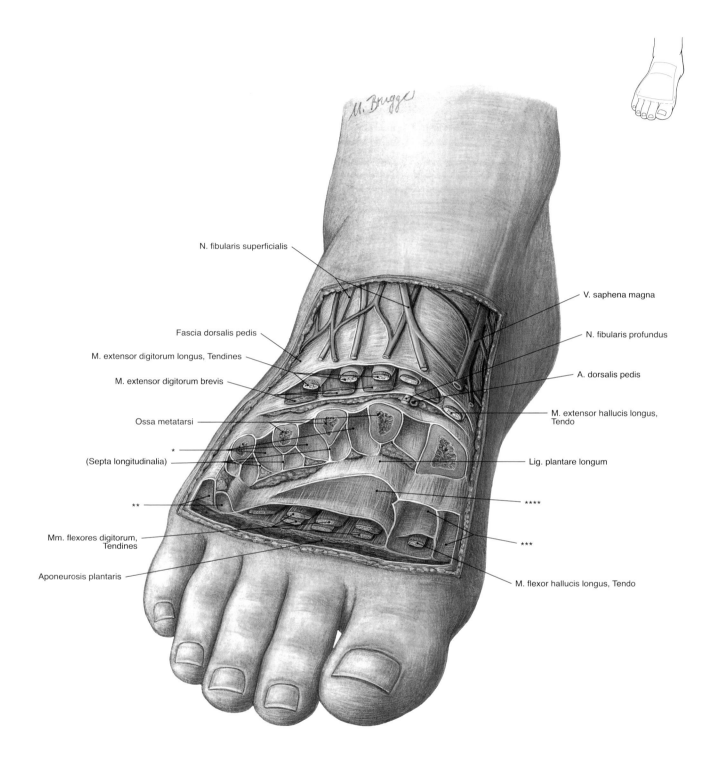

N. fibularis superficialis

V. saphena magna

Fascia dorsalis pedis

N. fibularis profundus

M. extensor digitorum longus, Tendines

M. extensor digitorum brevis

A. dorsalis pedis

M. extensor hallucis longus, Tendo

Ossa metatarsi

*

(Septa longitudinalia)

Lig. plantare longum

****

**

***

Mm. flexores digitorum, Tendines

Aponeurosis plantaris

M. flexor hallucis longus, Tendo

Fig. 1422 Compartments of the foot;
stepwise section.
*   Space of the interossei muscles
**   Lateral compartment
***   Medial compartment
**** Intermediate compartment

Thigh, oblique section

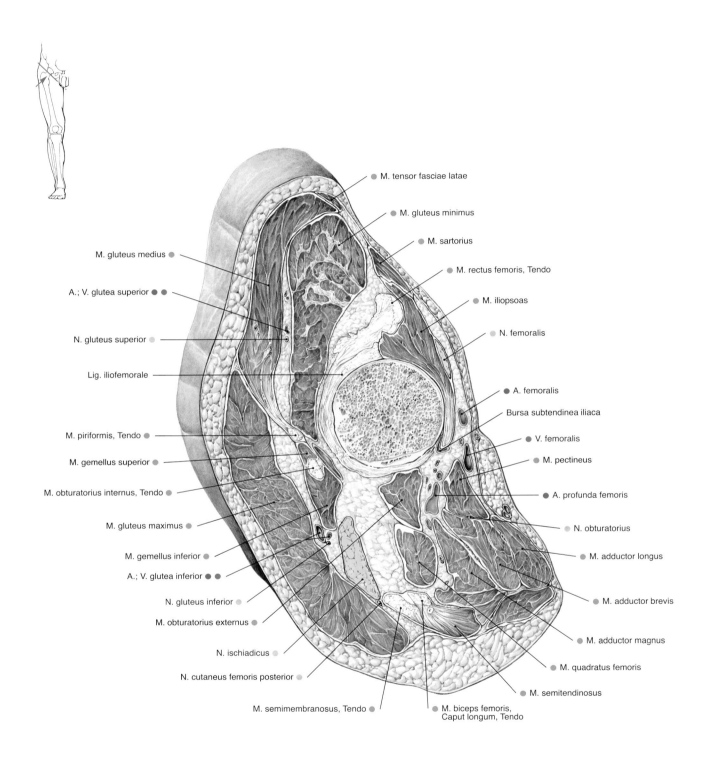

M. tensor fasciae latae

M. gluteus minimus

M. sartorius

M. rectus femoris, Tendo

M. iliopsoas

N. femoralis

A. femoralis

Bursa subtendinea iliaca

V. femoralis

M. pectineus

A. profunda femoris

N. obturatorius

M. adductor longus

M. adductor brevis

M. adductor magnus

M. quadratus femoris

M. semitendinosus

M. biceps femoris, Caput longum, Tendo

M. semimembranosus, Tendo

N. cutaneus femoris posterior

N. ischiadicus

M. obturatorius externus

N. gluteus inferior

A.; V. glutea inferior

M. gemellus inferior

M. gluteus maximus

M. obturatorius internus, Tendo

M. gemellus superior

M. piriformis, Tendo

Lig. iliofemorale

N. gluteus superior

A.; V. glutea superior

M. gluteus medius

Fig. 1423 Thigh, Femur; oblique section through the hip joint.

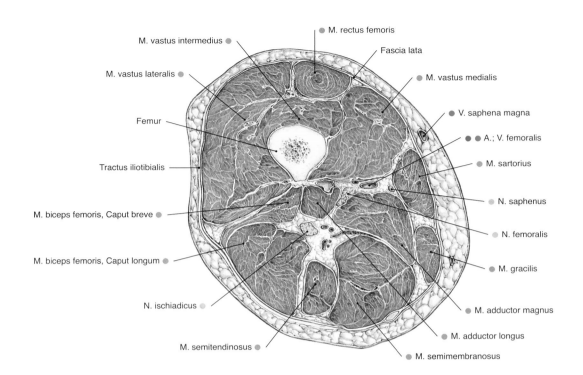

M. vastus intermedius ●
M. vastus lateralis ●
Femur
Tractus iliotibialis
M. biceps femoris, Caput breve ●
M. biceps femoris, Caput longum ●
N. ischiadicus ●
M. semitendinosus ●

● M. rectus femoris
Fascia lata
● M. vastus medialis
● V. saphena magna
● ● A.; V. femoralis
● M. sartorius
● N. saphenus
● N. femoralis
● M. gracilis
● M. adductor magnus
● M. adductor longus
● M. semimembranosus

Fig. 1424 Thigh, Femur;
cross-section through the middle of the thigh.

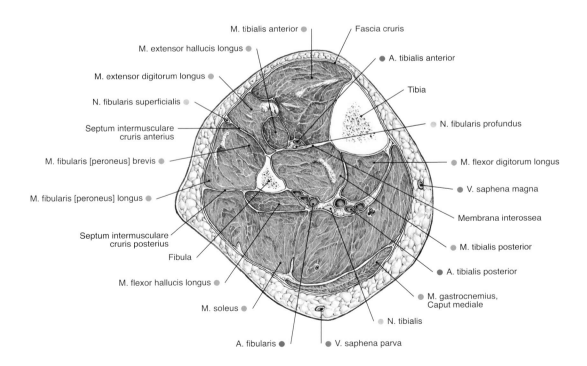

M. tibialis anterior ●
M. extensor hallucis longus ●
M. extensor digitorum longus ●
N. fibularis superficialis ●
Septum intermusculare
cruris anterius
M. fibularis [peroneus] brevis ●
M. fibularis [peroneus] longus ●
Septum intermusculare
cruris posterius
Fibula
M. flexor hallucis longus ●
M. soleus ●
A. fibularis ●

Fascia cruris
● A. tibialis anterior
Tibia
● N. fibularis profundus
● M. flexor digitorum longus
● V. saphena magna
Membrana interossea
● M. tibialis posterior
● A. tibialis posterior
● M. gastrocnemius,
Caput mediale
● N. tibialis
● V. saphena parva

Fig. 1425 Leg, Crus;
cross-section through the middle of the leg.

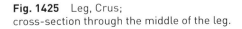

→ 1406

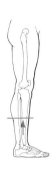

Leg and foot, sections

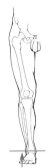

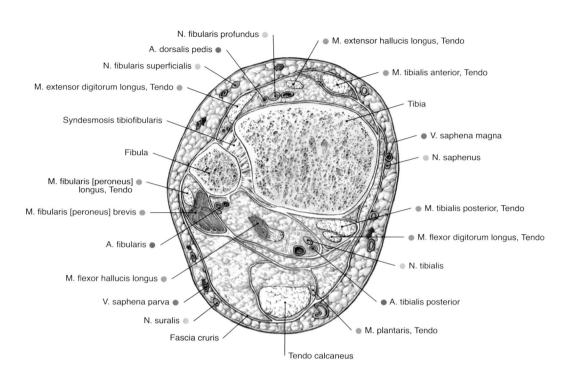

N. fibularis profundus

A. dorsalis pedis

N. fibularis superficialis

M. extensor digitorum longus, Tendo

Syndesmosis tibiofibularis

Fibula

M. fibularis [peroneus] longus, Tendo

M. fibularis [peroneus] brevis

A. fibularis

M. flexor hallucis longus

V. saphena parva

N. suralis

Fascia cruris

Tendo calcaneus

M. extensor hallucis longus, Tendo

M. tibialis anterior, Tendo

Tibia

V. saphena magna

N. saphenus

M. tibialis posterior, Tendo

M. flexor digitorum longus, Tendo

N. tibialis

A. tibialis posterior

M. plantaris, Tendo

Fig. 1426 Leg, Crus;
cross-section just above the ankle joint.

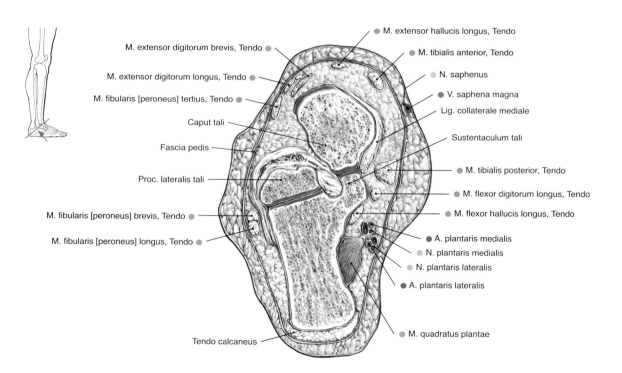

M. extensor digitorum brevis, Tendo

M. extensor digitorum longus, Tendo

M. fibularis [peroneus] tertius, Tendo

Caput tali

Fascia pedis

Proc. lateralis tali

M. fibularis [peroneus] brevis, Tendo

M. fibularis [peroneus] longus, Tendo

Tendo calcaneus

M. extensor hallucis longus, Tendo

M. tibialis anterior, Tendo

N. saphenus

V. saphena magna

Lig. collaterale mediale

Sustentaculum tali

M. tibialis posterior, Tendo

M. flexor digitorum longus, Tendo

M. flexor hallucis longus, Tendo

A. plantaris medialis

N. plantaris medialis

N. plantaris lateralis

A. plantaris lateralis

M. quadratus plantae

Fig. 1427 Foot, Pes;
oblique section through the calcaneus and the head of the talus.

Foot, sagittal sections

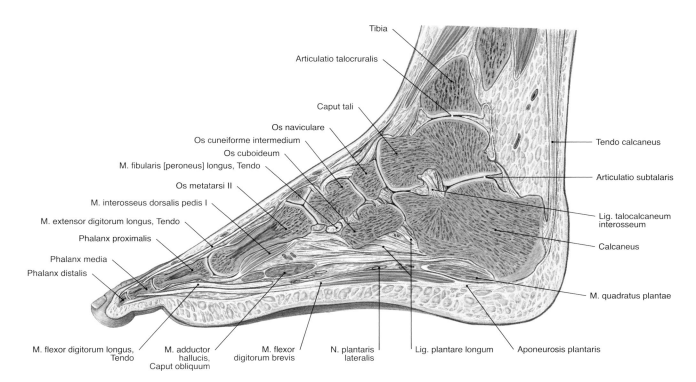

Tibia

Articulatio talocruralis

Caput tali

Os naviculare

Os cuneiforme intermedium

Os cuboideum

M. fibularis [peroneus] longus, Tendo

Os metatarsi II

M. interosseus dorsalis pedis I

M. extensor digitorum longus, Tendo

Phalanx proximalis

Phalanx media

Phalanx distalis

Tendo calcaneus

Articulatio subtalaris

Lig. talocalcaneum interosseum

Calcaneus

M. quadratus plantae

M. flexor digitorum longus, Tendo

M. adductor hallucis, Caput obliquum

M. flexor digitorum brevis

N. plantaris lateralis

Lig. plantare longum

Aponeurosis plantaris

Fig. 1428   Foot, Pes;
sagittal section through the second toe.

→ 1315, 1316

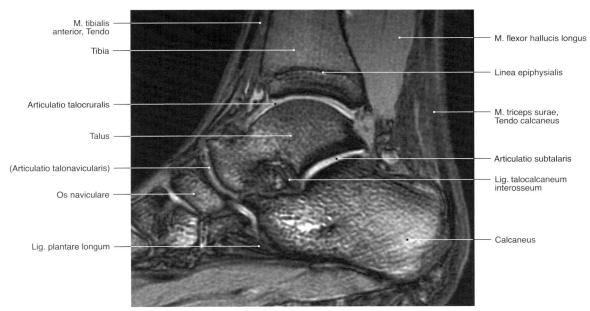

M. tibialis anterior, Tendo

Tibia

Articulatio talocruralis

Talus

(Articulatio talonavicularis)

Os naviculare

Lig. plantare longum

M. flexor hallucis longus

Linea epiphysialis

M. triceps surae, Tendo calcaneus

Articulatio subtalaris

Lig. talocalcaneum interosseum

Calcaneus

Fig. 1429   Foot, Pes;
magnetic resonance tomography image (MRI); sagittal section.

→ 1317, 1318

Foot, cross-section and pedograms

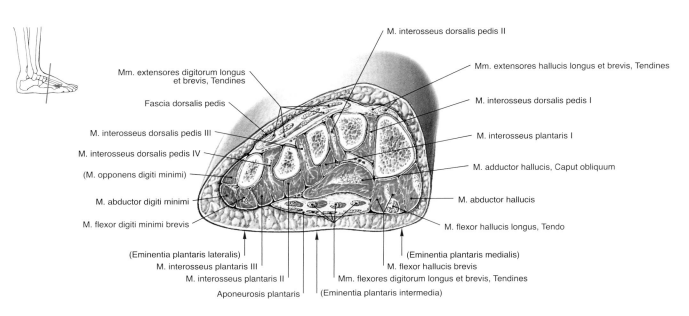

Fig. 1430 Osteofibrous tubes of the foot; frontal section through the metatarsus.

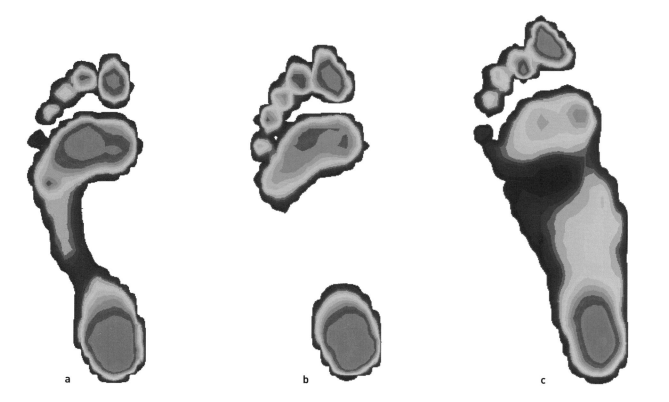

Fig. 1431 a–c Foot prints, pedograms.
a Normal foot
b Pes cavus
c Flat foot

Index

The numbers refer to the page numbers.
The numbers with „T" refer to the numbers of the tables in the separate booklet enclosed in Volume 1.

Nervus(-i)
- obturatorius 68, 71, 220–221, 225, 229, 231, 236–237, 256–257, 261, 317, 344–345, 348–349, 353, 355, 357–358, 360, 380, T40, T45
- occipitalis major 37–40
- – minor 36–38
- – tertius 37, 40
- pectoralis lateralis 60, T26
- – medialis 60, T26
- perineales 234, 240–241, 260–261, T40
- phrenicus 63, 89, 110–113, 115, 118, 120–121, 124–127, T21
- – course 118
- plantaris lateralis 304, 345, 350, 376–378, 382–383, T40, T52–T54
- – medialis 304, 345, 350, 376–378, 382, T40, T52–T53
- pudendus 214, 222–223, 225, 234, 236, 240–241, 257, 260–261, 344–345, 349, 360, T22, T40
- radialis 36–37
- rectales inferiores s. Nervus(-i) anales inferiores
- sacrales 223, 225–226, 243, 349, T22
- saphenus 345, 348–349, 353, 357–358, 365–366, 373, 381–382, T40
- scrotales anteriores T40
- – posteriores 222, 240, T40
- spinales 36, 41, 43, 45, 251
- spinalis 24, 29
- spinalis(-es) 24, 35, 40–41
- splanchnici lumbales 214
- – pelvici s. Radix parasympathica
- splanchnicus major 63, 112–113, 115–117, 120–121, 220–221, 245, 249
- – minor 63, 115, 117, 121, 245, 249
- subcostalis 68, 73, 115–117, 217, 220–221, 344
- suboccipitalis 37, 39–40, T20
- subscapulares 37, T26
- supraclaviculares 66
- – laterales 36–37
- suprascapularis 123
- suralis 345, 349–350, 362, 365, 382, T40
- thoracici 37, 60, 66, 70, 112–113, 115–117, 120–121, 220, 249, T15, T19–T20
- thoracicus longus 122, 124–126, T17
- thoracodorsalis 122, T18
- tibialis 284, 344–345, 349–350, 361–363, 365–366, 369–373, 376, 381–382, T40, T49–T50, T52–T53
- vaginalis 223
- vagus [X] 83, 88–89, 111–113, 115, 117–118, 120–121, 123–127, 220
Node of ROSENMÜLLER 355
Nodulus(-i)
- lymphoideus(-i) aggregati 137, 139
- – solitarii 130, 136–137, 139, 150, 210
- valvulae semilunaris 79
Nodus(-i)
- atrioventricularis 82–83
- lymphoideus(-i) aortici laterales 229
- – axillaris(-es) 65, 122, 124
- – – apicalis 124

Nodus(-i) lymphoideus(-i)
- – brachiales 65
- – bronchopulmonales 125–127
- – cervicales anteriores 65
- – – profundi 65
- – – laterales 120
- – – profundi inferiores 120
- – deltopectorales 65
- – gastrici 131, 218
- – gastroomentales 131, 249
- – hepatici 131
- – ileocolici 243
- – iliaci communes 218, 229
- – – externi 218, 229, 236, 354
- – – – laterales 229, 354
- – – mediales 229, 354
- – – interni 218, 229, 354
- – infraclaviculares 65
- – inguinales 352
- – – profundi 218, 354
- – – superficiales 218–219, 354
- – – – inferiores 218, 354
- – – – superolaterales 218, 354
- – – – superomediales 218, 256, 354
- – juxtaoesophageales 107, 127
- – lacunaris(-es) 355
- – – medialis 355
- – ligamenti arteriosi 88
- – lumbales dextri 218
- – – intermedii 218
- – mediastinales anteriores 88, 111, 113
- – – posteriores 107, 245
- – obturatorii 229
- – pancreaticus 250
- – paramammarii 65
- – pararectales 122, 229
- – parasternales 65
- – paratracheales 88, 120, 124
- – parietales 218
- – phrenici inferiores 218
- – – superiores 88, 119
- – popliteus profundus 366
- – – superficialis 366
- – preaortici 229, 251
- – precavales 229
- – promontorii 218
- – pylorici 131
- – rectalis superior 229
- – retroaortici 229
- – retrocavales 243
- – splenici 245, 249
- – submammarii 65
- – supraclaviculares 65
- – thoracis 107, 120
- – tibialis anterior 367
- – tracheobronchiales 95, 98–99, 113, 122
- – – inferiores 88, 95, 107, 119, 127
- – – superiores 88, 107, 119
- sinuatrialis 82
Nucleus pulposus 24–25, 29

O

Oesophagoscopy 108, 133
Oesophagus 62–63, 67, 104–109, 112–113, 115–117, 119–121, 123–130, 132–133, 157, 180, 220, 242, 245
- constrictions 108–109
- diverticulum 109
- radiography 108

Olisthesis 9
Omentum
- majus 121, 131, 139–140, 149, 157–166, 172, 242–243, 245–247, 249, 252, 254
- minus 160–161, 166, 247, 249
Orchis s. Testis
Organum(-a)
- genitalia feminina externa 223, 233, 235, 241
- – interna 204, 209
- – masculina 222, 239
- – – externa 197, 238, 240
- – pelvis in the female 237
- – in the male 236
- – urogenitalia feminina, development 200
- – masculina, development 192
Orificium ductus pancreatici 150
Os(-sa)
- coccygis 2–4, 11, 207, 215, 230, 232–233, 242, 252, 256–257, 271, 273
- coxae 2, 16, 41, 263, 266–267
- – AP-radiograph 16
- – development 267
- cuboideum 295–296, 298–299, 303, 383
- cuneiforme(-ia) 299
- – intermedium 295–296, 298, 304, 383
- – laterale 295, 298
- – mediale 295–296, 298, 302
- digitorum (Pes) 263, 295–296
- hyoideum 12
- ilium 3, 15–16, 41, 71, 73, 230, 244, 258, 264, 272, 274, 280
- ischii 236, 256, 264, 274
- metatarsi 263, 295–296, 298–299, 303–304, 379, 383
- naviculare 295–296, 298–299, 303–305, 383
- occipitale 6, 12, 17–19
- pedis 295–296, 299
- – structure characteristics 299
- pubis 169, 215, 226, 234, 242, 244, 256–257, 264, 274, 279
- sacrum 2–5, 10–11, 15, 23, 26, 41, 215, 226, 230, 242–243, 252–254, 262, 264, 271–273, 317
- – sex differences 11
- sesamoidea (Pes) 295–296, 302, 339
- tarsi 263, 295–296, 298
- temporale 40
Ostium(-a)
- abdominale tubae uterinae 201, 204, 209
- appendicis vermiformis 139
- atrioventriculare dextrum 78
- – sinistrum 79, 126
- cardiacum 108, 121, 130, 166–167, 244–245, 247
- ileale 139
- pyloricum 135
- sinus coronarii 78, 82, 84
- ureteris 190–191, 195, 198, 205, 252–253, 260
- urethrae externum (Urethra feminina) 200, 231, 233, 235, 237, 241, 253, 261
- – – (Urethra masculina) 198–199, 252
- – internum (Urethra feminina) 205, 253
- – – (Urethra masculina) 190, 195, 198, 252, 260

Ostium(-a)
- uteri 201–202, 205, 207, 253
- uterinum tubae uterinae 201, 203
- vaginae 200, 233, 235, 237
- venae cavae inferioris 82
- – – superioris 82
Ovarium 140, 167, 200–202, 204, 209, 223, 228, 253, 354

P

Palatum osseum 12
Pancreas 121, 131, 134, 152–153, 157, 163–164, 172, 177, 242–243, 245, 249–250
- computed tomography 155
- low magnitude enlargement 153
- projection 134
- ultrasound image 154
Pancreatocyticus exocrinus 153
Panniculus adiposus 58, 72, 210, 232, 239
Papilla(-ae)
- duodeni major 135, 150, 152–153
- – minor 152–153
- ilealis 139
- mammaria 52, 64, 127
- renales 183–184, 186, 245
- of Vater s. Papilla(-ae) duodeni major
Paracystium 260–261
Paradidymis 192
Parametrium s. Ligamentum cardinale
Paraproctium s. Spatium pararectale
Parasympathetic nervous system 214, 222–223
Paries
- anterior (Gaster) 133, 160–161
- membranaceus (Trachea) 91, 99, 107, 119
- posterior (Gaster) 133, 155
Paroophoron 200
Pars
- abdominalis aortae 35, 62–63, 69, 104, 115, 117, 148, 154–155, 157, 168, 172, 174, 177–179, 185, 187–189, 212, 214, 216–218, 221, 225, 227, 229, 242, 245, 250–251, 359
- – – ultrasound image 178
- – autonomica 220
- – (M. pectoralis major) 52, 54, 56, 58, 60, T26
- – (Oesophagus) 62–63, 104, 106, 108–109, 117, 128, 130
- – (Ureter) 163, 216
- anterior (Facies diaphragmatica hepatis) 145
- – (Fornix vaginae) 202, 205
- anularis vaginae fibrosae 340
- ascendens aortae 75, 78–80, 84, 109, 114–115, 117, 119–121, 125–126, 255
- – (Duodenum) 134, 139–140, 152, 165, 167
- – (M. trapezius) 26, T17
- atlantica (A. vertebralis) 34, 40
- basalis (Aa. lobares inferiores dextrae) 98
- – (Aa. lobares inferiores sinistrae) 98–99
- basilaris (Os occipitale) 17–19